Sterilization, Disinfection and Infection Control

Sterilization, Disinfection and Infection Control

Joan F. Gardner AO MSc(Melb) DPhil(Oxon)
Formerly Senior Lecturer, Department of Microbiology and Immunology,
University of Melbourne

Margaret M. Peel BSc(Qld) DipBact(Lond) PhD(Lond) MAIMS FASM MASM(USA)
Principal Microbiologist, Microbiological Diagnostic Unit,
Department of Microbiology and Immunology, University of Melbourne

THIRD EDITION

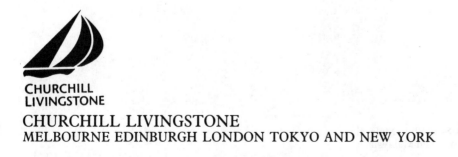

CHURCHILL LIVINGSTONE
MELBOURNE EDINBURGH LONDON TOKYO AND NEW YORK

Churchill Livingstone

An imprint of
Harcourt Brace & Company, Australia
30–52 Smidmore Street, Marrickville, NSW 2204

Harcourt Brace & Company
Orlando. Florida 32887

First edition 1986
Second edition 1991
  Reprinted 1992, 1996
Third edition 1998

First edition published under the title
Introduction to Sterilization and Disinfection

Second edition published under the title *Introduction to
Sterilization, Disinfection and Infection Control*

National Library of Australia Cataloguing-in-Publication Data:

Gardner, Joan F.
  Sterilization, disinfection and infection control.

  3rd ed.
  Includes index.
  ISBN 0443 05435 5.

1. Sterilization. 2. Disinfection and disinfectants.
I. Peel, Margaret M. II. Title.

614.48

Publishing editor: Gina Brandwood
Production editor: Sarah Connelley
Cover design: Maria Miranda

Typeset by Syarikat Seng Teik Sdn. Bhd., Malaysia
Printed by Addison Wesley Longman Malaysia

Contents

Preface to the third edition

The forever evolving microbial world continues to present new challenges. Examples include multidrug-resistant strains of *Mycobacterium tuberculosis*, the emergence of which coincided with a resurgence in tuberculosis, especially in those infected by the human immunodeficiency virus. Newly emerged, but already rapidly disseminated, are vancomycin-resistant enterococci, which pose therapeutic problems for the patients they infect. Of even more concern is the recent discovery in Japan of strains of *Staphylococcus aureus* with increased resistance to vancomycin. Fundamental to the control of these and other microorganisms and to the prevention of nosocomial infection is the understanding and implementation of the principles and practices of sterilization, disinfection and infection control.

The third edition of this book has been updated to take account of recommendations for the control and prevention of infections caused by emerging resistant microorganisms, among others. It also describes new developments in sterilization technology and progress in the understanding of microbial resistance to chemical disinfection. In addition, the importance of guidelines, recommendations and standards in implementing and maintaining quality in sterile supplies and services is emphasized. The updating of the book has been accomplished by substitution, with no increase in size; it remains a relatively slim and easily transportable volume.

The phasing out of chlorofluorocarbons because of damage to the ozone layer has resulted in the use of low-temperature sterilization processes based solely on pure ethylene oxide, instead of ethylene oxide/chlorofluorocarbon-12 mixtures. In addition, two different systems of gas plasma sterilization have been developed as alternatives for low-temperature, gaseous sterilization in hospitals. The use of vapour phase hydrogen peroxide for decontamination in the pharmaceutical and biotechnology industries is now also established. These advances in low-temperature sterilization technology are presented in Chapter 7. The powerful activity of the liquid chemical, peracetic acid, has been harnessed in a self-contained, sterilization system for use with instruments such as endoscopes. References to this system and its applications are given in Chapters 10, 11 and 14. Improvements in the design and efficiency of washer/disinfectors have resulted in their increased usage with a concomitant reduction in exposure to hazards associated with the cleaning of contaminated articles and equipment (Chapter 3).

Further investigations into the remarkable resistance of prions have cast doubt on the efficacy and reliability of currently recommended methods for their inactivation. Apparently, even more stringent processes are needed. Included in this group are the agents causing Creutzfeldt–Jacob disease in man and bovine spongiform encephalopathy ('mad cow disease'). The importance of biofilms in protecting microorganisms from the action of chemical disinfectants is being increasingly recognized. Biofilms form on the surfaces and along the walls of tubing in devices and equipment as diverse as cooling towers, respiratory therapy equipment, intravascular catheters and dental water units. In these sites, biofilms can act as a source of contamination and infection.

References are made to the latest versions of many guidelines, recommendations and standards throughout the new edition. A trend towards uniformity and international harmonization in this area is evidenced by the increasing availability of International (ISO) Standards. The infection control policy of 'Universal Precautions' has been superseded by the more inclusive 'Standard Precautions'. The second tier of this infection control system provides precautions and procedures which are specifically tailored to the prevention of nosocomial infections with different modes of transmission. Their application to the prevention of airborne transmission of tuberculosis and contact transmission of vancomycin-resistant enterococci is described in Chapter 13.

Represented in this third edition are the results of our access to a body of published literature not only from current contributors but also from past pioneers. We trust that the results of our efforts will serve to advise, guide, inform and support those who are involved in, or have responsibility for, the provision of sterile supplies and services or the application of infection control principles and practices in health care.

Melbourne 1997   J. F. Gardner
                                         M. M. Peel

Preface to the first edition

The presentation of sterilization and disinfection in this book has been tailored to the requirements of hospital staff who hold positions of responsibility in the supply and use of sterile equipment and pharmaceuticals and also in the broader field of infection control. A balance has been sought between principles and practice, the number of references cited in the text being reduced in order to avoid undue interruption for the reader. The book is also intended to provide background information for engineers whose duties include the maintenance and servicing of sterilizers and ancillary equipment, for manufacturers of such equipment and for companies that produce sterile medical devices or chemical disinfectants.

The proper use of chemical disinfectants and a sound knowledge of the conditions that determine whether the solutions fulfil their intended purpose of killing microorganisms are important to all who rely on the products for control of microbial contamination in situations ranging from hospitals, dental surgeries and other health services to community-based services such as podiatry and hair-dressing.

This new, enlarged book has been developed from a former publication (Rubbo S. D., Gardner J. F. 1965 A review of sterilization and disinfection. Lloyd-Luke, London). Like its predecessor, it is designed for use as a textbook in specialized courses for microbiologists and for post-basic education or training of hospital staff. It should also be suitable as a reference text for students reading for medical, dental or science degrees in universities and other tertiary education institutions.

Melbourne 1986

J. F. Gardner
M. M. Peel

Acknowledgements

The preparation of the third edition of this book has been assisted by consultation with several specialists in Australia and the United Kingdom, who have given generously of their expert advice. We record and acknowledge these contributions with gratitude.

Mrs Mary McCrorie (Infection Control Officer, Mercy Private Hospital, Melbourne) made available the proceedings of an international conference on the subject of sterile supply services, which also served to initiate us into the current status (in draft or final form) of several European and International Standards relating to sterilization. Mr Philip Robins (Sterile Supply Services Advisor, Health Department of Western Australia) provided valuable British technical publications relating to the validation and control of sterilization processes, the design and installation of sterile services departments and the special requirements for ethylene oxide sterilization. The staff of the Victorian branch of Standards Australia facilitated access to current American (ANSI/AAMI), Australian (AS), British (BS), European (EN) and International (ISO) Standards. Dr Ken R Davey (Department of Chemical Engineering, University of Adelaide) made contributions to Chapters 2 and 4 on basic principles of microbial inactivation.

From the United Kingdom, Miss Sheila Scott (Consultant in Healthcare Facility Planning) informed us of current developments concerning sterile services departments in Britain and Dr David Coates (Consultant in Sterilization and Disinfection) provided updated general information on chemical disinfectants and sterilants. Mr John R Babb and Emeritus Professor G A J Ayliffe of the Hospital Infection Research Laboratory, Birmingham, supplied recent publications on chemical disinfection and infection control, with particular reference to endoscopes (Chapter 14). Dr David M Taylor (BBRC and MRC Neuropathogenesis Unit, Institute for Animal Health, Edinburgh) continues to advise us on developments relating to the extraordinary resistance of prions to agents of sterilization and disinfection.

In the field of commercial expertise, Mr George West (General Manager, Steritech, Victoria) and Mr Frank Scalzo (Senior Applications Specialist, Millipore) assisted by providing information on recent developments in radiation sterilization (Chapter 8) and microbial filtration (Chapter 9) respectively. Mr Patrick McMahon (Marketing Manager, Advanced Sterilization Products) and Ms Merrilyn Little (Professional Services Manager, 3M Australia) kept us informed about new technological developments in the field of gas sterilization (Chapter 7).

About the authors

Joan F. Gardner graduated in Science (BSc, MSc) from the University of Melbourne. After a period as a research assistant in the Biochemistry Department, she travelled to England to work at the Dunn School of Pathology for four years, gaining the degree of DPhil (Oxon) during that time for investigations into anti-microbial chemotherapeutic agents. Her interest in the sterilization of medical equipment also commenced in the United Kingdom, where major advances in that area were being made in the early 1960s.

On her return from Oxford, Joan was appointed as a lecturer, subsequently a senior lecturer, in the Microbiology Department at the University of Melbourne. Sterilization, disinfection and other aspects of infection control comprised a major part of her research and teaching for the next 30 years until her retirement. She was also a member of various committees of Standards Australia that were responsible for preparing and updating standards for sterilizers and related hospital equipment.

In addition to her duties at the university, Joan became a founding, and later an Honorary Life Member, of the Sterilization and Disinfection Society (Vic.) in 1970 (now incorporated into the Sterilizing Research Advisory Council of Australia). She was an initial course organizer and continuing lecturer in the advanced training courses for staff in hospital sterilizing departments and infection control nurses, which commenced in 1971. In recognition of these hospital-associated activities, she received an Order of Australia award (AO) in 1992 for service to medicine in the field of sterilization, disinfection and infection control.

Margaret M. Peel holds a Diploma in Medical Laboratory Science and is a graduate in Science (Microbiology) from the University of Queensland. She was awarded the Academic Postgraduate Diploma in Bacteriology (with a mark of Distinction) and a PhD from the Faculty of Medicine at the London School of Hygiene and Tropical Medicine of the University of London. Her current position is that of Principal Microbiologist at the Microbiological Diagnostic Unit, a public health laboratory within the Department of Microbiology and Immunology in the Faculty of Medicine, Dentistry and Health Sciences at the University of Melbourne. Margaret is a fellow of the Australian Society for Microbiology, a member of the Australian Institute of Medical Scientists and a member of the American Society for Microbiology.

Margaret's interests in infection and contamination control range from the identification of infectious agents through prevention of infection and contamination to methods for the destruction of microorganisms. She is author or co-author of about 50 publications in national and international journals of microbiology and medicine.

Margaret is a member of the Standing Committee on Biosafety of the Australian Society for Microbiology and the Standing Committee on Infection Control and Legionella Monitoring Group of the Victorian Department of Human Services. She has contributed to the writing of guidelines, codes of practice and standards on biosafety, infection control and related issues through participation on committees, working parties and task forces of Standards Australia, national and state government bodies and professional scientific societies. Margaret belongs to the Australian Contamination Control Society; and, in 1994, was awarded Honorary Life Membership of the Sterilizing Research Advisory Council of Australia.

1. Sterilization, disinfection and the microbial target

The principles and practice of methods used for killing, removing or excluding microorganisms to assist in the prevention of infectious disease constitute the subject of this book. Their applications in hospitals, health clinics and microbiological laboratories will be described in detail and, when appropriate, reference will be made to the commercial production of sterile pharmaceuticals and processed foods.

In this chapter, the difference between sterilization and disinfection is explained and other relevant terms defined. This is followed by a summary of the essential prerequisites for sterilization and disinfection. A brief description of microorganisms is provided for readers who might not be familiar with their nature, activities and distribution.

STERILIZATION

The term 'sterile' refers to the inability of living organisms to reproduce. Sterility of microorganisms is synonymous with death because their activities are usually undetectable in the absence of multiplication. Articles that are free of living organisms are also termed sterile; as the presence of a single microorganism renders an article unsterile, terms such as 'almost sterile' or 'partially sterile' should not be used.

Sterilization is a process that kills or removes all types of microorganisms, including resistant bacterial spores. However, for reasons that will be explained in Chapter 2, it is impossible to guarantee that every microorganism exposed to a particular treatment has been killed or that every article has been sterilized. It is therefore realistic to define sterilization as a process that provides an

1

acceptably low probability (e.g. one chance in a million) that any microorganism will survive the treatment.

It is important to know when sterilization, which may involve severe treatment of equipment and materials, is required. It is essential for articles that enter the blood or tissues, such as surgical instruments, syringes, needles and solutions for injection or intravenous infusion. Diagnostic instruments that come in contact with delicate mucous membranes, such as those lining the urinary tract or peritoneal cavity, should also be used in a sterile condition. Sterile culture media, containers and laboratory apparatus are essential for microbiological research and investigation, including the diagnosis of infectious disease. It is also necessary to ensure that discarded cultures are sterilized before cleaning or disposal of the containers. Infectious medical waste should be sterilized before disposal, or incinerated.

Microorganisms that are sterile or dead cannot cause infectious disease but Gram-negative bacteria or their liberated cell wall constituents can cause serious febrile (pyrogenic) reactions if they are introduced into the blood or tissues in large numbers. Sterile solutions intended for parenteral use must therefore be pyrogen-free.

DISINFECTION

A disinfection process is intended to kill or remove pathogenic (disease-producing) microorganisms but cannot usually kill bacterial spores. Spores are killed by a sterilization process. Terminal disinfection of used equipment which may be contaminated with harmful microorganisms is commonly referred to as 'decontamination'. Antisepsis is not synonymous with disinfection; this term should be reserved for the prevention of infection by topical application of antimicrobial agents to injured tissue.

Disinfection is adequate for the preparation of many articles intended for use in patient care. These include bedpans, urinals, clinical thermometers and, if necessary, eating and drinking utensils. Floors, walls, tables, trolleys and work benches require disinfection as well as cleaning if contamination with blood, tissues, exudates or microbial cultures has occurred. Disinfection by chemical agents is the only method applicable to the skin of hands, operation sites and injection sites for killing transient contaminants or reducing the resident microbial flora to a low level.

Disinfection by pasteurization, boiling or chemical agents does not make surgical instruments safe to use. Disinfection should not be used as a substitute for sterilization; when this is unavoidable because a costly instrument, in short supply, is heat-sensitive and insufficient time is available for the slower process of gas sterilization a broad spectrum disinfectant, such as glutaraldehyde, should be chosen.

Definitions

Activation	Initiation of a chemical or biological process (e.g. germination of bacterial spores).
Airborne infection	Infection caused by inhaling airborne dust particles or droplet nuclei carrying microbial contaminants.
Antimicrobial	Adjective describing an agent or action that kills or inhibits the growth of microorganisms.
Antisepsis	Prevention of infection by topical application of biocidal or biostatic agents to injured tissues.
Antiseptic	A chemical agent used for antisepsis.
Asepsis	Prevention of microbial contamination of living tissues or sterile materials by excluding, removing or killing microorganisms.
Autoclave	A vessel fitted with a self-sealing door; not descriptive of modern pressure steam sterilizers but continued usage (as noun or verb) is convenient.
Bactericide	A chemical or physical agent that rapidly kills vegetative (non-sporing) bacteria.
Bacteriostat (Bacteristat)	An agent that prevents multiplication of bacteria.
Biocide	A physical or chemical agent that kills some or all types of microorganisms (often used in the inexact sense).
Biological safety cabinet	A completely or partly enclosed work station with laminar air flow through high-efficiency filters for personnel and product protection against infection and contamination.
Buffered solution	An aqueous solution containing chemicals which maintain a specified pH value.
Commensals	Non-pathogenic microorganisms that are living and reproducing as human or animal parasites.
Contact infection	Infection transmitted by direct personal contact or indirectly by contaminated droplets or fomites (inanimate objects).
Contamination	Introduction of microorganisms to sterile articles, materials or tissues.

Contamination level (Bioburden)	The number, or density, of microorganisms on a particular object or surface, or in a specified volume of liquid or air.
Culture medium	A nutrient solution or agar gel for isolating and identifying microorganisms.
Decontamination	Disinfection of used articles to make them safe to handle.
Detergent-sanitizer	A cleaning solution containing an antibacterial agent.
Disinfection	A process that is intended to kill or remove pathogenic microorganisms but which cannot usually kill bacterial spores.
Disinfectant	An agent that is used for disinfection.
DNA	Deoxyribonucleic acid; nuclear material which determines inherited characteristics and controls metabolism of living organisms.
Droplets	Rapidly sedimenting particles of liquid (>5 μm) expelled from the respiratory tract or water systems.
Droplet nuclei	Particles ($\leq$5 μm) which arise from dehydration of small airborne droplets and are capable of wide airborne dispersal.
D value	The time of exposure to heat or chemicals, or the dose of ionizing radiation, that effects a tenfold (decimal) or 90 per cent reduction in the number of viable cells in a microbial population.
Fomites	Inanimate objects, other than food, that may harbour and transmit microorganisms.
Fungicide	An agent that kills fungi and their spores.
Fungistat	An agent that inhibits fungal growth.
Germicide	A colloquial term, usually referring to chemical disinfectants; biocide or bactericide are recommended alternatives.
Heat penetration time	The additional time required for all of the articles in a steam or dry heat sterilizer to reach the selected sterilizing temperature after it has been reached in the chamber.
Heat shock	A sublethal heat treatment that may be applied to bacterial spores to kill residual vegetative forms or induce spore germination.
Holding time	The time for which all of the articles in a steam or dry heat sterilizer must be held at the selected sterilizing temperature.
Inactivation	Death of microorganisms, destruction of enzyme activity or 'neutralization' of the antimicrobial activity of a disinfectant.
Infection	Growth of microorganisms in the tissues of a host, with or without detectable signs of injury.
Infectious disease	The harmful result of infection by microorganisms.
Isolator	An enclosure for protecting germfree animals, susceptible persons, sterility testing procedures or products from microbial infection or contamination.
Laminar air flow (unidirectional)	System in which the entire body of air in a confined area moves with uniform velocity along parallel flow lines.
Pasteurization	A process that kills non-sporing microorganisms by hot water or steam at 65–100°C.
Pathogenic microorganism	A species that is capable of causing disease in a susceptible host.
Plenum	A chamber upstream from the air filters in a ventilation system.
Preservation	Prevention of microbial spoilage of foods, pharmaceuticals or industrial materials.
Preservative	A chemical agent used for preservation.
Pyrogens	Heat-stable substances in the cell walls of Gram-negative bacteria that cause a febrile reaction if introduced into the blood or tissues.
Relative humidity (RH)	The amount of water vapour in air, steam or other gaseous atmospheres, expressed as a percentage of the maximum amount that is possible at the existing temperature.
RNA	Ribonucleic acid; controls protein synthesis.
Sanitization	A process that reduces microbial contamination to a low level by the use of cleaning solutions, hot water or chemical disinfectants.
Spores (bacterial)	Thick-walled resting cells formed by certain Gram-positive bacteria (e.g. *Bacillus* and *Clostridium*), capable of survival in unfavourable natural environments and often highly resistant to heat and chemicals.
Spores (fungal)	Unicellular or multicellular reproductive cells, capable of survival in dry conditions with some resistance to chemicals but not highly resistant to heat.
Sporicide	An agent that kills bacterial spores.
Sterilant	An agent that kills all types of microorganisms.
Sterile	Term applied to organisms that are incapable of multiplication or articles that are free from living microorganisms.
Sterilization	A process that is intended to kill or remove all types of microorganisms, with an acceptably low probability of an organism surviving on any article.
Sterilization time	The time for which sterilizing conditions are maintained in a steam, hot air or gas sterilizer.
Tuberculocide	An agent that kills *Mycobacterium tuberculosis* and related acid-fast bacteria.
Vegetative bacterium	A bacterium that is in the growth and reproductive phase.
Viable microorganism	A microorganism that is capable of multiplication in favourable conditions.
Virucide	An agent that renders viruses non-infective.

ESSENTIAL PREREQUISITES FOR STERILIZATION AND DISINFECTION

The efficiency of sterilization and disinfection depends on:

1. Biocidal action
2. Effective contact between biocidal agent and the microorganisms
3. Appropriate biocidal agents and apparatus
4. Severity of treatment.

Biocidal action

Biocidal action implies death of microorganisms, as indicated by their failure to multiply in any situation. It must be distinguished from reversible inhibition of multiplication (biostasis), from which the organisms may recover on return to favourable conditions. Biocidal action is essential for sterilization and disinfection. A biocidal agent is one that is capable of killing microorganisms. The term is sometimes restricted to agents that kill all types of microorganisms but is also used in a less exact sense to imply that some organisms are killed. Biocidal action against microorganisms of a specified type is termed bactericidal, sporicidal, virucidal or fungicidal.

Effective contact

Effective contact between a biocidal agent and its microbial target requires penetration of the physical or chemical agent to all sites at which the organisms may be located.

Saturated steam

Steam under pressure reaches the outer surfaces of solid objects and penetrates into accessible cavities and packed cotton textiles if the air has been removed. It cannot penetrate into nonaqueous liquids and impervious solids. Effective contact involves condensation to water. The latent heat that is released brings the articles rapidly to the sterilizing temperature and the film of moisture ensures that conditions are optimum for biocidal action. Wrapping materials must be permeable to steam and also to the removal of air. In sterilizers that rely on gravity for the downward displacement of air by steam, the articles must be packed and loaded to facilitate drainage of the heavier air from trays, bowls, tubes and textiles. Flexible tubes should not be tightly coiled.

Gaseous chemicals

Sterilization by gas or gas plasma requires the efficient penetration of the load by the vaporized chemical agent. Ideally, the gas should be not only highly diffusible but also capable of passing through many different types of materials.

Dry heat

Dry heat sterilization does not involve penetration of vapours but the articles must be heated to the sterilizing temperature by conduction or convection. Metals are good conductors but glass and oily materials are poor conductors of heat.

Ionizing radiation

The penetrating power of sterilizing radiations depends on the type of radiation and the energy level. Electromagnetic gamma radiation is capable of penetrating deeply into large cartons containing materials for sterilization. Accelerated electrons have greater energy than gamma radiation but have less penetrating power because they are particulate.

Chemical disinfectants

Effective contact between the solutions and the articles to be disinfected depends on the nature of the articles and the condition of the microorganisms. Contact is unlikely to be achieved if the microorganisms are located in pores or crevices or are protected by hardened deposits of organic or crystalline material. The complex, lipid-rich cell walls of Gram-negative bacteria, especially *Pseudomonas* species, present a barrier to the entry of some bactericidal agents into the cells. The wetting power of disinfectants is enhanced by alcohol or detergents.

Table 1.1 Biocidal agents for sterilization

Agent	Applications	Apparatus
Saturated steam	Wrapped articles Unwrapped instruments and utensils Aqueous liquids	Prevacuum sterilizer, 134°C Downward displacement sterilizer, 132–134°C Downward displacement sterilizer, 121°C
Dry heat	Metal articles, glassware, oils	Hot air oven, 160°C
Gaseous chemicals	Heat-sensitive instruments and medical devices	Ethylene oxide, plasma or low-temperature steam and formaldehyde sterilizers
Ionizing radiation	Medical devices	^{60}Co installation or electron accelerator
Peracetic acid	Endoscopic instruments	Steris system

Table 1.2 Biocidal agents for disinfection

Agent	Applications	Apparatus
Hot water	Articles not required in sterile condition Decontamination of used articles Heat-sensitive instruments Anaesthetic apparatus Blankets and linen Mopheads Eating and drinking utensils	Washer/disinfector machines, 75–95°C
Low-temperature steam	Heat-sensitive instruments	Low-temperature steam and formaldehyde sterilizer (without the formaldehyde)
Ultraviolet radiation	Room air, water	Germicidal lamps
Formaldehyde, hydrogen peroxide vapour	Contaminated rooms, biological safety cabinets, isolators	Electrical vaporizer
Chemical disinfectants	Articles not required in sterile condition Decontamination of used articles Skin and mucous membranes	Suitable containers or dispensers

Appropriate agents and apparatus

Biocidal agents that are used for sterilization are listed, with main applications and types of sterilizers, in Table 1.1. Physical and chemical agents of disinfection are presented in a similar way in Table 1.2.

Steam sterilizers

Pressure steam sterilizers are specially designed for porous loads (comprising all wrapped articles), unwrapped instruments and utensils, or aqueous liquids. Prevacuum sterilizers, with mechanical air removal, are designed for efficient sterilization of porous loads. The downward displacement type may also be used but is more liable to error and the cycle is longer. Downward displacement steam sterilizers should be used for unwrapped instruments and utensils and also for bottled fluids. The provision of a spray-cooling system for fluids reduces the time required for sterilization and minimizes the deterioration of heat-sensitive ingredients.

Gas sterilizers

Sterilizers for heat-sensitive equipment are designed for the removal of air by mechanical evacuation, vaporization of the chemical agent (ethylene oxide, hydrogen peroxide or formaldehyde) and maintenance of the relative humidity required for biocidal action.

Dry heat sterilizers

Dry heat sterilization is usually carried out in hot air ovens with forced air convection. Direct flaming is used to sterilize some laboratory bench tools such as inoculating loops. Incineration of waste material is also a form of dry heat sterilization; the design of incinerators is critical as live microorganisms may escape with the effluent if burning is incomplete.

Radiation installations

Radiation sterilization is virtually restricted to industrial installations because of the complexity of the equipment and the essential safety precautions. A cobalt-60 (^{60}Co) gamma radiation source or an electron accelerator may be used.

Chemical disinfectants

Chemical disinfection does not require complex apparatus. Containers should be of suitable composition, shape and size and filled with sufficient solution to ensure that the articles are completely immersed and that cavities are free from trapped air. The selection of an appropriate disinfectant is based on its range and degree of bactericidal activity (determined by an approved method) and its compatibility with the articles to be disinfected and other materials, including the container, with which it may come in contact during use.

Bacterial filtration

The physical removal of bacteria from liquids and air is accomplished by filters of appropriate pore diameter and retention efficiency. Suitable filter holders and other accessories are required. Membrane filters which have an average pore diameter of 0.22 μm or 0.45 μm and act as mechanical sieves are most suitable for filtration of liquids. Fibrous filters have a greater bacterial load capacity but the flow rate is slow and the quality of the filtered solution may be affected by adsorption of solutes, alteration of pH or contamination by fibres. Fibrous filters in the form of packed columns or thin paper sheets, are commonly used for air filtration but hydrophobic membrane filters are

suitable for some applications. The fibrous sheets have a large surface area and are used in conventional or laminar flow ventilation systems; each sheet is pleated and all the edges are sealed into a frame to form a compact unit. HEPA (high-efficiency particulate air) filters are 99.97–99.997 per cent efficient for retention of particles with a diameter of 0.3 μm.

Severity of treatment

Heat sterilization processes are defined by time at a specified temperature. Recommended times for steam sterilization are 15 minutes at 121°C and 3 minutes at 132–134°C (at 103 kPa and 206 kPa above atmospheric pressure). These represent the minimum holding times for which the whole of the material treated must be held at the selected sterilizing temperature to kill the microbial contaminants. They are based on the resistance of *Bacillus stearothermophilus* spores to moist heat. For dry heat sterilization, a holding time of 120 minutes at 160°C is recommended.

Gas sterilization by pure ethylene oxide or plasma operates at a temperature of 55°C or below. With ethylene oxide, the gas must be removed by aeration so the total time for the process is 6 to 8 hours. No aeration is required in the plasma process. Sterilization times are 54 or 72 minutes for the Sterrad^{TM} 100S process, 43 minutes for the Sterrad 50 process and 1, 2 or 3 hours for the Abtox^{TM} Plazlyte^{TM} process.

A radiation sterilization process is described by a single value, the minimum absorbed dose. An absorbed dose of 25 kGy is commonly used in the commercial production of medical devices but it may be increased or decreased depending on the level of contamination of the articles or materials to be sterilized.

The efficiency of chemical disinfection depends on the concentration and the time for which the solution is in contact with the articles or surfaces to be disinfected.

THE MICROBIAL TARGET

The rational selection and correct performance of procedures that are intended to kill, remove or exclude harmful microorganisms requires knowledge

Table 1.3 Major groups of microorganisms

Group	Affiliates	Growth habits	Sources
Bacteria	Neither plants nor animals	Free-living or parasitic	Soil, water, organic materials, humans, animals, plants
Viruses	Subcellular particles	Obligate intracellular parasites	Human, animal, plant or bacterial hosts
Fungi (moulds and yeasts)	Some resemblance to plants, but not photosynthetic	Free-living or parasitic	Decaying organic matter, soil, fruit juices, plants, animals, humans
Protozoa	Animals	Free-living or parasitic	Soil, water, animals, humans
Algae	Green plants	Free-living	Sea, fresh water, soil

of their nature and distribution, their capability of survival in different conditions and their resistance to physical and chemical biocidal agents.

The term 'microorganism' embraces a wide range of primitive life forms; most of them are unicellular and all require the use of a light or electron microscope for observation. Microorganisms are widely distributed in outdoor and indoor environments, on the human skin and in the mouth, upper respiratory tract, large intestine and parts of the urogenital tract. They are rarely harmful in these situations but are likely to cause disease if they gain access to organs or tissues that are normally sterile. Despite their small size and primitive nature, microorganisms present a formidable challenge to the methods that are used to prevent or control the spread of infection. The major groups and some of the distinguishing characteristics, together with their relationship to higher forms of life, are listed in Table 1.3.

Bacteria

Structure and composition

The bacteria will be described in more detail than other microorganisms. They are neither plants nor animals; the single cells differ from these higher forms of life in that the nuclear DNA is not confined within a membrane and does not break up into chromosomes during cell division. Bacterial DNA is a single circular, tightly coiled molecule, bearing the genes that determine the characteristics and metabolic processes of the particular species. Bacteria also lack cytoplasmic particles

called mitochondria, which are sites of enzymes concerned with respiration and other metabolic activities in animal cells. The delicate cell membrane, composed of proteins and lipids, acts as a semi-permeable barrier, regulating the entry of essential nutrients and preventing loss of vital constituents from the cells. The nuclear material, cytoplasm and membrane are enclosed in a rigid cell wall whose composition is unique to bacteria. The wall contains a lattice-like compound called peptidoglycan which maintains the shape and integrity of the bacterium. A step in its synthesis is the specific target of the bactericidal action of the penicillin and cephalosporin (β-lactam) antibiotics.

Some bacteria have additional structures that are located outside the cell. Flagella are long, thin hair-like processes which cannot be seen by light microscope unless specially stained. They arise in the cell membrane and their external movement

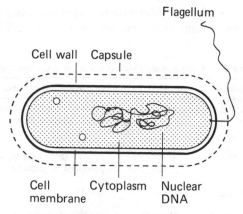

Fig. 1.1 Structure of a bacterial cell. Note: flagella and capsules are usually mutually exclusive.

confers motility on the bacterium. Other bacteria may have a capsule of viscous carbohydrate or protein material which can prevent the uptake of the organisms by phagocytic cells. Capsulated bacteria are usually non-motile. The structure of a bacterial cell is shown in Figure 1.1.

Morphology and staining

The term morphology embraces the shape, size and arrangement of bacteria as seen in tissues or in laboratory cultures. Variation in the shape of the cells is limited by their unicellular nature to two main types: spherical cocci (*sing.* coccus) and rod-shaped bacilli (*sing.* bacillus). The cocci are round or oval and approximately one micrometre (μm) in diameter. They may be arranged in clusters, chains or pairs but also occur singly. Bacilli exhibit greater variation as the cells vary in width (0.2–2.0 μm) as well as in length (2–10 μm). Spirochaetes are long cells (up to 20 μm) in which a thin strand of protoplasm is wound around an axial filament and enclosed in an outer sheath. Most of the basic bacterial forms recognized today were observed and drawn in the seventeenth century by the Dutch draper Antonie van Leeuwenhoek when he examined material from around the teeth with simple, high quality lenses which he made.

Clinical specimens and laboratory cultures containing bacteria are prepared for microscopic examination by spreading a sample thinly on a glass slide. The dried smear must be stained with a suitable dye to render the cells visible. Basic dyes, such as crystal violet, methylene blue and carbol fuchsin (red) serve this purpose by combining with the negatively charged bacterial cells. However, Gram's stain is routinely used for most purposes because it also differentiates between the Gram-positive and Gram-negative bacteria. The stain may be performed as follows:

1. Stain with crystal violet (30 seconds), rinse
2. Mordant with iodine solution (30 seconds), rinse
3. Decolourize with acetone (a few seconds), rinse
4. Counterstain with neutral red or dilute carbol fuchsin (30 seconds), rinse and blot dry.

Both groups of bacteria take up the purple stain. The Gram-positive species retain it when treated with acetone and appear purple when the slide is examined. Gram-negative species are decolourized by acetone and are counterstained red to render them visible. Tissue, pus, sputum and other material of human or animal origin also stain red.

The Gram stain reaction is attributable to differences in the structure and chemical composition of bacterial cell walls. The peptidoglycan in Gram-positive bacteria constitutes 50–100 per cent of the cell wall material and is a closely linked lattice which contracts on treatment with acetone, retaining the dye-iodine complex that has been formed within the cell. Gram-negative bacteria have only 5–10 per cent of peptidoglycan in their cell walls and the open lattice does not contract sufficiently to retain the purple dye (Salton, 1963; Beveridge & Davies, 1983). A comparison of important properties that differ in Gram-positive and Gram-negative bacteria is given in Table 1.4.

The genus *Mycobacterium*, which includes the species that causes tuberculosis, has a high lipid

Table 1.4 Comparison of Gram-positive and Gram-negative bacteria

Characteristic	Gram-positive bacteria	Gram-negative bacteria
Cell wall composition	50–100% peptidoglycan; polyalcohol and polysaccharide complexes	5–10% peptidoglycan; lipid-protein-polysaccharide complexes (pyrogens, or endotoxins)
Toxins	Potent, specifically acting exotoxins may be produced (diphtheria, tetanus, botulinum)	Non-specifically acting endotoxins (cell wall lipopolysaccharide)
Resistance to drying	Good	Poor
Susceptibility to chemical disinfectants and antibiotics	Susceptible to a wide range	Susceptibility restricted to a narrower range

content, including wax. It is stained by treatment with hot concentrated carbol fuchsin (red) or fluorescent auramine-rhodamine (golden) for 10 minutes. Species of *Mycobacterium* are termed acid-fast bacilli (a.f.b.) because they retain the primary stain on treatment with acid alcohol. Gram-positive and Gram-negative bacteria, tissue cells and tissue debris are decolourized and are counterstained with methylene blue or malachite green.

Growth and multiplication

In common with other living organisms, bacteria require sources of carbon, hydrogen, nitrogen, oxygen, sulphur and phosphorus for growth and reproduction. Water is also essential. Many bacteria have additional requirements for trace metals and vitamins. Certain soil bacteria which can utilize carbon dioxide and atmospheric nitrogen are essential for the continuation of life on earth because they convert these elements to forms that can be used by plants and animals. Most bacteria, including human and animal parasites, require organic carbon such as carbohydrate. Organic nitrogen, such as amino acids, is also commonly required. Most bacteria will grow on a suitable artificial culture medium in the laboratory. Basal media are prepared from meat extracts but added blood or serum may be required to isolate some pathogenic bacteria. Liquid media are solidified to a gel by the addition of agar for isolation of microorganisms in pure culture.

When a culture medium has been inoculated with material containing bacteria, it is incubated at the optimum temperature for the likely species (usually 37°C in medical bacteriology) and in the presence or absence of oxygen, as appropriate. Aerobic bacteria require oxygen for growth and strict anaerobes grow only in the absence of oxygen. Many bacteria grow in the presence or absence of oxygen; these are described as facultative. Incubation times for the development of bacterial colonies on an agar medium or of turbidity in a liquid medium range from less than 24 hours to several days. The relatively slow-growing *Mycobacterium tuberculosis*, the causative agent of tuberculosis, requires 3–6 weeks to produce visible growth.

The growth of bacteria is measured by the rate of multiplication because the cells alter little in size during the growth cycle. They multiply asexually by binary fission, a process in which a cell divides into two similar daughter cells. The DNA is replicated to provide a copy of the nuclear material for each daughter cell. The mother cell divides after a septum consisting of cell membrane and cell wall material has been formed across the centre of the cell. When a small number of cells of a fast-growing species of bacterium is inoculated in a suitable medium and incubated in suitable conditions, cell division typically occurs at 20 minute intervals doubling the population each time. The number of bacteria reaches a maximum at 10^8–10^{10} per millilitre of a broth culture; exhaustion of oxygen or an essential nutrient, or the accumulation of metabolic waste products slows and eventually terminates multiplication. Multiplication could be sustained indefinitely in living tissues if the bacteria are supplied with nutrients by the blood, which also removes their waste products. Termination may be brought about by the host defence mechanisms or antibiotic treatment.

Although bacteria are isolated as pure cultures in the laboratory for investigation and identification, natural populations are usually mixed. The type of nutrients and amount of moisture determine which types of microorganisms predominate in a given ecological situation. Non-pathogenic Gram-positive cocci and bacilli constitute the normal resident bacterial flora of the skin, but streptococci predominate in the mouth and Gram-negative bacilli in the bowel.

Bacterial spores

Bacterial forms that are not killed by boiling water have been a subject of research since their discovery a hundred years ago. The resistant spores have apparently evolved as a response to adverse conditions; each vegetative cell usually produces only one spore and only a small proportion of the cells in a population may sporulate. *Bacillus* (aerobic) and *Clostridium* (anaerobic) species are the main bacteria that have the capacity to produce spores; their natural habitat is the soil and they are disseminated by dust to indoor as well as outdoor environments. Diseases caused by spore-forming bacteria include anthrax, tetanus, gas gangrene and other wound infections. Botulism food poisoning is caused by *Clostridium botulinum*; if spores survive the food canning process they can germinate and grow in the anaerobic conditions within sealed cans containing non-acid foods, producing their lethal toxin.

The production of a spore commences with the formation of a membranous septum towards one end of the rod-shaped mother cell. The smaller compartment develops into a spore which contains a copy of the nuclear material. The DNA, cytoplasm, cell membrane and cell wall of the vegetative cell constitute the vital spore core which is reduced in volume by loss of water to the mother cell during maturation of the spore. The involvement of a low moisture level in the heat resistance of spores is discussed in Chapter 4, which also contains a diagram of a mature spore. The spore core is enveloped by a wide cortex and one or more outer spore coats. When the integuments have been completed the remains of the mother cell degenerate.

The return of a resistant spore to a vegetative cell is stimulated by conditions that are not always understood. The process is initiated by activation, which involves a change in the physical state of the spore components. Activation is brought about by chemicals in the natural environment but may be accomplished by sublethal heat or the addition of calcium and dipicolinic acid in the laboratory. Germination follows activation; uptake of water activates the spore enzymes, the integuments are broken down and heat resistance and other spore characteristics are rapidly lost. The outgrowth of a vegetative cell completes the process of germination.

Nomenclature

Each bacterium is given two official names. The first is the genus and starts with a capital letter; the second identifies the species. The proper name is italicized in books and published papers and is usually underlined in typed manuscripts. Colloquial names, such as staphylococci, streptococci, gonococci, coliform bacilli and tubercle bacilli, may be used but are not italicized and do not have capital letters. Subdivision of species, such as *Staphylococcus aureus* and *Salmonella* Typhi, is

Table 1.5 Nomenclature of bacteria (with examples of some genera and species mentioned in this book)

Group	Genus	Examples of species
Gram-positive cocci	*Staphylococcus*	*S. aureus, S. epidermidis*
	Streptococcus	*S. pyogenes*
	Enterococcus	*E. faecalis, E. faecium*
	Deinococcus	*D. radiodurans*
Gram-positive bacilli	*Corynebacterium*	*C. diphtheriae, C. jeikeium*
	Bacillus	*B. anthracis, B. strearothermophilus*
	Listeria	*L. monocytogenes*
	Clostridium	*C. perfringens, C. tetani*
Gram-negative cocci	*Neisseria*	*N. meningitidis, N. gonorrhoeae*
Gram-negative bacilli	*Escherichia*	*E. coli*
	Klebsiella	*K. pneumoniae*
	Proteus	*P. vulgaris, P. mirabilis*
	Salmonella	*S.* Typhi, *S.* Typhimurium
	Serratia	*S. marcescens*
	Shigella	*S. sonnei*
	Pseudomonas	*P. aeruginosa*
	Acinetobacter	*A. baumannii*
	Legionella	*L. pneumophila, L. micdadei*
Acid-fast bacilli	*Mycobacterium*	*M. tuberculosis, M. avium*
Spirochaetes	*Treponema*	*T. pallidum*
	Leptospira	*L. icterohaemorrhagiae*

unnecessary for the diagnosis of disease but is of assistance in tracing the source of an epidemic. Some representative genera and species of bacteria are listed in Table 1.5.

Contamination, infection and disease

Microorganisms that are present in situations where they are not multiplying are termed contaminants. Gram-positive bacteria and bacterial spores are common on dry surfaces and airborne particles because they are not readily killed by drying. Gram-negative bacilli, such as coliforms and pseudomonads, die rapidly in dry conditions but survive in damp or wet situations; they may multiply in water if it contains impurities that are adequate for growth.

Bacteria that are growing in a close association with another form of life are parasites. Some parasites exist in a stable relationship with their human host and constitute the normal flora of body surfaces and adjoining mucous membranes. These relatively harmless bacteria are termed commensals. Pathogenic bacteria can also be found in some healthy individuals, who are referred to as carriers (for example, of *S. aureus*, *S.* Typhi and *N. meningitidis*). Colonization by parasites constitutes infection. Disease is the harmful result of infection. A pathogenic microorganism is one that is capable of causing disease in a susceptible host. Opportunistic pathogens cause disease in individuals with immune deficiencies that are inherited or caused by certain diseases or by treatment with immunosuppressive or cytotoxic drugs. A wide range of bacteria can act as opportunistic pathogens including species of the Gram-negative genera *Pseudomonas*, *Acinetobacter*, *Serratia* and *Legionella*; Gram-positive bacteria such as *S. epidermidis*, *C. jeikeium*, *L. monocytogenes*; and the acid-fast *Mycobacterium* species. Persons infected with the human immunodeficiency virus (HIV) are particularly susceptible to infection by *M. avium* and *M. tuberculosis*.

Viruses

Structure and composition

Viruses are subcellular particles, termed virions. They were initially detected as infective agents that passed through bacterial filters. They cannot be seen by the ordinary light microscope but their shape and structure is revealed by the electron microscope. Virus particles range in size from 20–200 nanometers (nm) and may be brick-shaped, bullet-shaped, spherical, helical or icosahedral.

The infective component of the virion is the nucleic acid core; this may be DNA or RNA but they do not both occur in the same virus. The core is enclosed in a protein coat, the capsid, which determines the external shape of the particle. Viruses which have an outer lipid envelope are inactivated by organic solvents, such as ether, and many chemical disinfectants. The non-enveloped viruses are more resistant to chemical disinfectants. All viruses are killed by boiling water but the time required has not always been precisely determined.

Reproduction

Viruses are obligate intracellular parasites because they do not contain the enzymes required for their own replication. They multiply within specific host cells in animals, plants or bacteria. When a virus particle attaches to the surface of the host cell it is taken up into the cytoplasm, where its components are dismantled by the host cell enzymes. The liberated viral nucleic acid programs the host cell to synthesize new viral protein and nucleic acid which are then assembled to form new virus particles. These are liberated from the host cell. The lipid envelope, when present, is acquired from the membrane of the host cell. For one virus particle that enters the host cell, a large number may be discharged. Viruses survive for varying periods outside their host cells but cannot reproduce until they invade a new cell.

Nomenclature

A binomial system is not yet in use. Viruses are characterized by the type of nucleic acid (DNA or RNA), the presence or absence of a lipid envelope, or by the route of infection (respiratory or alimentary tract), or by an intermediate host, such as a species of insect. Some groups of viruses, with examples, are listed in Table 1.6.

Table 1.6 Nomenclature of viruses

Group	Nucleic acid	Lipid envelope	Diseases (examples)
Adenoviridae	DNA	Absent	Pharyngitis
Arenaviridae	RNA	Present	Lassa fever
Coronaviridae	RNA	Present	Colds
Hepadnaviridae	DNA	Absent	Hepatitis B
Herpesviridae	DNA	Present	Cold sores, genital herpes chickenpox/shingles
Orthomyxoviridae	RNA	Present	Influenza
Papovaviridae	DNA	Absent	Warts
Paramyxoviridae	RNA	Present	Measles, mumps
Picornaviridae	RNA	Absent	Hepatitis A, poliomyelitis, colds
Reoviridae	RNA	Absent	Gastroenteritis (including rotavirus infections)
Retroviridae	RNA	Present	Acquired immunodeficiency syndrome (AIDS)

Prions

The term 'prion' was introduced in 1982 to distinguish the transmissible agent causing scrapie in animals from viruses (Prusiner, 1989). Prions are unique, infectious agents composed largely of protein that resist inactivation by procedures which destroy or modify nucleic acids. All attempts to demonstrate the presence of nucleic acid in these agents have failed. Prions do multiply and whether or not a small amount of nucleic acid is present is uncertain.

Prions cause fatal neurological diseases in mammals. These diseases are termed transmissible degenerative encephalopathies (TDE). Scrapie is a neurodegenerative disease of sheep and goats and its agent provides a model for the study of prions and of their exceptional resistance to conventional methods of sterilization and disinfection. In cattle, this agent causes bovine spongiform encephalopathy (BSE), or 'mad cow disease'. BSE resulted from the feeding of scrapie-infected sheep meat to cattle in Britain. Kuru, Creutzfeldt-Jakob disease (CJD) and Gerstmann-Sträussler-Scheinker syndrome (GSS) are neurodegenerative diseases in humans caused by prions.

Familial CJD and GSS are the only human diseases known to be both infectious and genetic. The incubation period for prion diseases is prolonged, ranging from months to decades. The invariable clinical picture is slow progression until death, usually within a year of the first appearance of dementia.

Mycoplasmas, Chlamydiae and Rickettsiae

These organisms are intermediate in size between the bacteria and viruses (0.3–0.5 μm). They are related to bacteria because they contain both DNA and RNA, have the cell wall peptidoglycan that is characteristic of bacteria (except Mycoplasmas), multiply by binary fission and are susceptible to some broad-spectrum antibiotics. Although difficult to stain by any method, they are classed as Gram-negative. Mycoplasmas lack cell walls but can be grown on laboratory media. They cause atypical pneumonias, formerly thought to be viral in origin. Chlamydiae are obligate intracellular parasites because they cannot produce the energy that is necessary for growth and must derive it from the host cell. They are released as elementary bodies, which survive until they are taken up by another cell. The group includes organisms causing trachoma, inclusion conjunctivitis of the newborn, non-gonococcal urethritis, and psittacosis (a disease of birds which can be transmitted to humans). The rickettsiae are obligate intracellular parasites because they depend on the host cell for certain metabolic reactions and products. Rickettsial diseases in humans include typhus, scrub typhus and the spotted fevers. The life cycle generally involves a vertebrate and an invertebrate host. One species causes epidemic typhus, a human infection with an arthropod vector, the body louse.

Fungi

These ubiquitous organisms are usually saprophytes, growing on non-living organic matter. They are known principally as causes of spoilage in foods, textiles, painted surfaces and many other materials. However, some cause human and animal disease, especially in individuals whose resistance to infection is impaired.

Morphology

The filamentous fungi, commonly called moulds, are multicellular organisms with complex life cycles that involve the production of spores by sexual or asexual processes. The spores of terrestrial fungi are shed into the air in large numbers. Their primary function is reproduction of and dissemination of the species. They withstand dry conditions but are much less resistant to heat than are bacterial spores.

The yeasts are unicellular fungi. Some produce spores but they reproduce mainly by budding from the vegetative cells. Some yeasts form filaments in addition to single cells. In Gram-stained smears, yeasts are usually round or oval Gram-positive cells and about 5 μm in diameter (cf. spherical bacteria, 1 μm).

Conditions for growth

Fungi flourish in tropical and temperate climates. They are usually grown in the laboratory at 25–30°C but pathogenic species may grow better at 37°C. The filamentous fungi are strict aerobes but yeasts can grow aerobically or anaerobically. Glucose peptone agar and malt extract agar are commonly used culture media. Antibiotics may be added to the medium to facilitate the isolation of fungi from pathological specimens by preventing overgrowth by bacteria and common saprophytic fungi.

Fungal infections

Fungal diseases may be superficial or systemic, depending on the organism and the route of infection. Species of filamentous fungi belonging to the genera *Microsporum*, *Trichophyton* and *Epidermophyton* cause tinea, or ringworm, which is restricted to the skin, hair and nails but may occur at various body sites. The capsulated yeast, *Cryptococcus neoformans*, causes skin and lung infections and meningitis, especially in those with AIDS. The filament-forming yeast, *Candida albicans*, infects the skin and mucous membranes, causing oral and vaginal thrush and infections of the nail beds. It also causes serious blood-borne systemic infections such as endocarditis in intravenous drug users, as well as oesophagitis in patients with AIDS. Systemic fungal infections may involve the lungs, brain and kidneys. Aspergillosis is a mild or severe infection of the lungs, caused by species that are widely distributed in the environment. Tissue invasion by *Candida* or *Aspergillus* species frequently occurs in patients with terminal cancer. The conditions that predispose individuals to fungal infection cannot always be identified but they include HIV infection, extremes of age, diabetes, imbalance of the normal bacterial flora of the body by treatment with antibiotics, and treatment with steroids, cytotoxic agents or immunosuppressive drugs.

Protozoa

These single-celled forms of animal life occur in aquatic environments and in the soil as well as in animals and humans. They do not possess a rigid cell wall but may have an external skeleton of secreted minerals. Most are motile by means of hair-like processes (flagella or cilia) or by amoeboid movement. Some protozoa produce non-motile cysts which are resistant to drying and chemical agents. Protozoa causing human disease include *Trypanosoma* (sleeping sickness), *Trichomonas* (vaginitis), *Toxoplasma* (congenital brain damage and encephalitis), *Cryptosporidium* and *Giardia* (intestinal infection), *Pneumocystis* (pneumonia), and amoebae (contact lens infections, amoebic dysentery or meningoencephalitis). Patients with AIDS are likely to suffer from serious disease due to *Toxoplasma*, *Cryptosporidium* or *Pneumocystis*.

Algae

Although capable of photosynthesis, the blue-green algae (cyanobacteria) are true bacteria with endotoxins in their cell walls. Other algae (e.g. green and red algae) are primitive plants. The occurrence of dense growths or blooms of cyanobacteria in reservoirs, lakes and rivers presents problems, especially as some blue-green algae may produce hepatotoxins and neurotoxins. These toxins can kill livestock, dogs, birds and laboratory mice. They may also cause human illnesses such as skin reactions, conjunctivitis, vomiting, diarrhoea, atypical pneumonia and liver toxicity (Elder et al, 1993). Copper sulfate is effective in destroying the blooms. Diatoms are algae that contain silica in their cell walls.

REFERENCES

Beveridge T J, Davies J A 1983 Cellular responses of *Bacillus subtilis* and *Escherichia coli* to the Gram stain. Journal of Bacteriology 156: 846–858
Elder G H, Hunter P R, Codd G A 1993 Hazardous freshwater cyanobacteria (blue-green algae). Lancet 341: 1519–1520
Prusiner S B 1989 Scrapie prions. Annual Review of Microbiology 43: 345–374
Salton M R J 1963 The relationship between the nature of the cell wall and the Gram stain. Journal of General Microbiology 30: 223–235

FURTHER READING

Block S S (ed) 1991 Disinfection, sterilization, and preservation, 4th edn. Lea & Febiger, Philadelphia
Fleming D O, Richardson J H, Tulis J J, Vesley D (eds) 1995 Laboratory safety principles and practices. ASM Press, Washington DC
Murray P R, Baron E J, Pfaller M A, Tenover F C, Yolken R H 1995 Manual of clinical microbiology, 6th edn. American Society for Microbiology, Washington DC
Russell A D, Hugo W B, Ayliffe G A J (eds) 1992 Principles and practice of disinfection, preservation and sterilization, 2nd edn. Blackwell Scientific Publications, Oxford

2. Efficiency of sterilization

Sterilization is a process that is intended to kill all types of microorganisms. A particular article is either sterile or unsterile (an all or none state) but, when all of the items that are treated by a particular process are considered, there is always a chance that some contaminants may survive and a proportion of the articles will remain unsterile. An efficient process is one that has been designed to achieve an acceptably low proportion (e.g. one per million) of surviving microorganisms and unsterile items.

Efficiency is built into the design of the process by determining the severity of treatment (e.g. time of exposure at a specified temperature or dose of ionizing radiation) that is required to kill the types and numbers of microbial contaminants on the articles to be treated. The process must be validated by appropriate physical, chemical and biological tests and monitored regularly during routine operation to ensure that the intended conditions for sterilization are achieved throughout the materials to be sterilized and are maintained for an adequate time. This chapter deals with:

Designing the process
Testing the process
Testing the product.

DESIGNING THE PROCESS

The following information is required for calculation of the conditions that will sterilize the articles for which the process is intended:

1. Rate of biocidal action
2. Initial contamination level (bioburden)
3. Sterility assurance required.

Rate of biocidal action

Determination of death rates

The rate at which a biocidal agent reduces the number of viable cells in a microbial population is determined by counting the survivors in samples taken after graded exposures of a suspension of bacteria to heat, radiation or chemical vapour in specified conditions. The viable counts may be performed by preparing serial (e.g. tenfold) dilutions of each sample and spreading a volume (e.g. 0.1 ml) of each dilution (in duplicate) on nutrient agar medium. Each colony that develops on incubation represents a colony-forming unit (single cell or small clump) of viable bacteria. Plates yielding 25–250 colonies are counted and the viable count of the original suspension calculated as follows:

If 220 colonies grew from 0.1 ml of a 10^{-3} dilution, the count would be $220 \times 10 \times 10^3 = 2.2 \times 10^6$/ml.

If the initial count and the sample counts are plotted on a logarithmic scale against the exposure time and a line is drawn through the separate points, a death rate curve is obtained. A straight line represents a constant (logarithmic or exponential) death rate. Nonlogarithmic death rates are represented by curves which show initial or final lags in the killing rate.

The range of time or dose over which reliable counts can be obtained for preparation of a death rate curve limits the experimental determination of killing rates to a level of about 200 survivors per ml. Extrapolation of the death rate to lower survivor levels may be valid when the available curves do not deviate from linearity but extrapolation of nonlinear curves may result in an underestimate of the conditions required for sterilization.

Logarithmic death rate

A hypothetical series of viable counts, which shows that a constant proportion (not a constant number) of microorganisms is killed in each unit of time or dose, is presented in Table 2.1; the corresponding logarithmic curve is illustrated in Figure 2.1.

In this stylized example, a tenfold reduction in the number of survivors, corresponding to 90 per

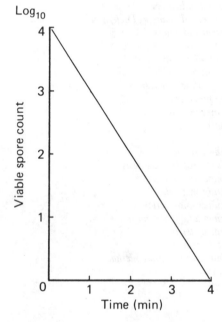

Fig. 2.1   Logarithmic (linear) death rate curve.

Table 2.1   Set of survivor counts illustrating logarithmic death rate

Time of exposure (min)	No. viable spores/ml (at commencement of time unit)	% Survivors killed (during each time unit)	% Killed (cumulative)
0	10 000	0	0
1	1 000	90	90
2	100	90	99
3	10	90	99.9
4	1	90	99.99
5	0.1 (1/10 ml)	90	99.999
6	0.01 (1/100 ml)	90	99.9999

cent kill, has occurred during each minute of exposure to the specified conditions. As the initial count was 10^4, the population would be reduced to the probability of a single survivor (10^0) in 4 minutes. Further reduction would be expressed as the probability of a microorganism surviving (e.g. 10^{-1}, 10^{-2}, and so on) as the duration or severity of treatment increases.

Nonlogarithmic death rates

A survivor curve that is nonlinear over part or all of its length indicates that the death rate is not constant. The deviations usually take the form of an initial or final lag; a curve that shows a lag at each end is described as sigmoid. Some common types of nonlogarithmic death rate curves are illustrated in Figure 2.2.

The anomaly in curve A is an initial increase in viable count. This is followed by a regular logarithmic killing rate. This type of curve is usually associated with heat-resistant bacterial spores, such as *Bacillus stearothermophilus*, which are activated for germination as they approach the sterilizing temperature. This results in early counts that are higher than the initial count obtained on the unheated spore preparation. The rate of activation exceeds the rate of killing until the peak of the hump has been reached; beyond this point, the killing rate increases until the true logarithmic rate

is established (Shull et al, 1963). If this type of curve were obtained for a non-sporeforming microorganism, it would suggest that clumped cells were being dispersed in the early stage of the killing process.

The flat shoulder in curve B, if obtained for a spore population, would indicate that the number of spores activated balances the number that are killed. A similar curve for non-sporing bacteria may be explained by clumping of the organisms; each clump registers as a single colony-forming unit until the last survivor in the clump has been killed and a logarithmic death rate may then become apparent.

Curve C shows the type of lag that is often observed when the death rate is slow (e.g. at a relatively low temperature or radiation dose, or when the bacteria are treated with a solution of chemical disinfectant). Terminal lags may be explained in various ways (Cerf, 1977). They might represent the combined logarithmic death rates of two or more species of microorganisms as shown individually by the dashed lines; the steeper part of the curve would correspond to a relatively sensitive population that was present in larger numbers initially, while the lag corresponds to a more resistant species. The latter would determine the outcome of the process although it may be a minor component of the original population. Evidence for this explanation was provided by Bond

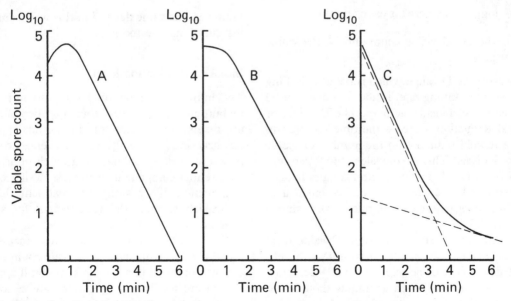

Fig. 2.2 Types of nonlogarithmic (nonlinear) death rate curves.

et al (1970) who studied mixed soil isolates containing heat-sensitive and heat-resistant spores. The separate killing curves were logarithmic but the nonlinear curve was reproduced when they were recombined.

Tailing curves are rarely accounted for by variation in the resistance of individual cells in a homogeneous population because the same curve is obtained if the survivors are cultured and re-tested. However, a true lag in the killing rate may occur if the biocidal agent causes a gradual change in the microorganisms that hinders its access to the cellular target. The hardening of the protein coat of a virus by progressive treatment with formaldehyde protects the nucleic acid core, preventing the desired loss of infectivity (Gard, 1957). However, the theoretical model of Davey (1990) indicates no significant delay in heat transfer to the centre of clumps of bacteria in fluid from possible shielding by the outer cells of the clumps.

D value

A quantitative expression of the death rate is required to describe the activity of a biocidal agent against different microorganisms, or to compare the resistance of different microorganisms to a particular agent. The inactivation rate coefficient k is applied to the death rate of microorganisms by use of the formula:

$$k = \frac{1}{t} \log_{10} \frac{N_o}{N_t}$$, where t is exposure time,

N_o is the initial viable count and N_t the viable count at time t.

However, the D value, which is based on killing time instead of killing rate, is now commonly used as a measure of biocidal activity. The D value, or Decimal Reduction Time, is the time required to effect a tenfold reduction in the number of viable microorganisms. This is equivalent to 90 per cent kill. When a D value refers to sterilizing radiation, it is expressed as a dose. The derivation of a D value from a logarithmic death rate curve is shown in Figure 2.3.

It is difficult to estimate a useful D value from a nonlogarithmic death rate curve unless the observed deviation can be explained and accounted for as, for example, when an initial shoulder or hump is followed by a logarithmic killing rate.

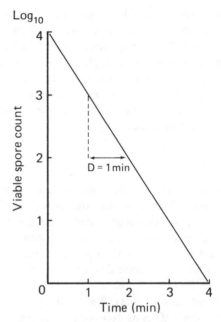

Fig. 2.3 Constant D value (Decimal Reduction Time) for a logarithmic death rate curve.

When the curve does not include a linear section of significant length, an average D value may be calculated from the equation (Stumbo, 1973):

$$D = \frac{t}{\log_{10} N_o - \log_{10} N_t}$$, where t is the relevant time, N_o is the initial viable count and N_t is the viable count at time t.

However, the value derived in this way from a tailing curve may be too low.

Initial contamination level

The initial contamination level (also termed the bioburden) refers to the total number of microorganisms on articles or in liquids prior to sterilization. Knowledge of the average contamination level of a manufactured batch of articles is an essential component of process design because it influences the severity of treatment that will be needed to meet the requirement for sterility assurance.

The number of microbial contaminants in a liquid can be estimated by the plate count method that was outlined in a previous section if appropriate culture media and conditions are selected. If the number is too low for accurate determination by this method, a sample of the liquid may be passed through a membrane filter. Colonies develop on the surface of the membrane when it is incubated in contact with an appropriate solid or liquid medium. Microorganisms on solid objects must be collected by immersion in, or rinsing with, a diluent, which may contain a suitable non-ionic dispersing agent. Counts are performed on the resulting suspension. Contamination levels are always likely to be underestimated because no single culture medium or set of conditions will grow all types of microorganisms.

It is not necessary to isolate and identify the types of contaminants in detail but it may be important to determine the highest level of resistance in the natural population. Bacterial spores are most resistant to heat but viruses, fungal spores and certain types of vegetative bacteria may have greater resistance to sterilizing radiation. The most resistant types or species in a population of natural contaminants can be isolated by submitting samples of the product to treatment of decreasing severity until some survivors are recovered. When a sterilization process is designed, it is generally assumed that all of the contaminants have the maximum resistance level although the most resistant types may constitute only about 1 per cent of the microorganisms in soil or dust.

Sterility assurance

Sterility assurance is expressed as a calculated probability that a microorganism may survive a sterilization process and that a corresponding proportion of treated articles may be unsterile. The level of sterility assurance required varies with the intended use of the articles. A likelihood that one article per million processed may be unsterile (10^{-6} probability of a surviving organism) is required for medical equipment that will be used in surgery or other aseptic procedures. A less rigorous requirement of 10^{-3} may be acceptable for devices that only come in contact with intact skin or mucous membranes. A more rigorous standard of 10^{-12} for the probability that a spore of *Clostridium botulinum* will survive is applied to the heat treatment of non-acid canned foods. A standard of 10^{-4} was the subject of international agreement for the sterilization of space exploration vehicles designed to seek evidence of extraterrestrial life on

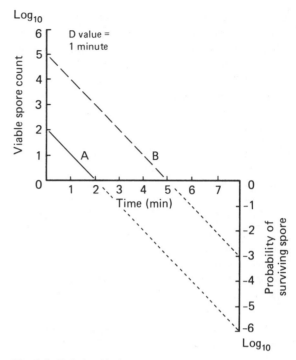

Fig. 2.4 Relationship between D value, initial contamination level and level of sterility assurance.

the planet Mars; this was considered adequate because fewer than 10 vehicles would be likely to land on the planet, intentionally or accidentally, in the foreseeable future.

Determination of sterilizing conditions

When the D value is constant, as in a logarithmic killing process, the initial contamination level is known, and the desired level of sterility assurance has been specified, conditions for sterilization can be calculated as shown in Figure 2.4.

The process involves determining the treatment that will reduce the presterilization bioburden to the single survivor level (10^0) and adding an additional 6 logarithms of microbial reduction. After the treatment, the probability of a nonsterile item will be, at most, one in a million. In this example, where the hypothetical D value is 1 minute, 6 minutes would be required to provide the desired safety margin. The articles in batch A, with a low contamination level of 100 organisms per item, will require 2 minutes to reach the single survivor level and those in batch B, with 10^5 organisms per item, will require 5 minutes to reach the single survivor level. Thus, those in batch B, which may have been manufactured in unhygienic conditions, will require a total of 11 minutes, compared with 8 minutes for batch A, to provide the required level (10^{-6}) of sterility assurance.

The following examples will serve to illustrate the application of the design calculation to sterilization practice.

1. Linen packs with a contamination level of 10^4 are to be sterilized by steam at 121°C. If the D value for *B. stearothermophilus* is 1.8 minutes at this temperature, the minimum holding time will be the sum of 7.2 minutes (4D) plus 10.8 minutes (6D), making a total of 18 minutes.
2. The D value of gamma radiation for spores of *Bacillus pumilus* is approximately 3 kilogray (kGy) and the proposed minimum dose is 25 kGy. This dose is equivalent to 8D and will be adequate for the sterilization of articles that carry no more than 100 microorganisms.
3. The heat treatment of non-acid canned foods of a type which is likely to be contaminated with spores of *C. botulinum* is based on a D value of 0.21 minutes at 121°C. If each can contains a single spore, 2.52 minutes (12 × 0.21) will be the minimum treatment required. In practice, this is extended to 4 minutes to ensure safety and keeping quality.

These examples underline the importance of minimizing initial contamination levels in order to ensure that requirements for sterility assurance are met. A sterilization process that has been designed for articles with a certain contamination level may be inadequate if the contamination level increases. This may occur as the result of a change in raw materials or factory hygiene. With medical devices and pharmaceutical products, a periodic assessment of contamination levels should be conducted in order to detect any increase above the level for which the process was originally designed. Surveillance of the raw materials and methods used in production plays an important part in drawing attention to the need for re-evaluation of contamination levels. Medical devices and pharmaceuticals that are manufactured and sterilized commercially are subject to regulations based on an official Code of Good Manufacturing Practice

(GMP). The codes provide guidelines for hygienic production, covering the quality of raw materials, cleaning and disinfection of the processing equipment and hygiene in the factory environment, including the provision of defined clean room conditions for aseptic filling of pharmaceuticals into the final containers. The health of employees is also included. Quality control procedures for sterile pharmaceuticals are also subject to the requirements of a national pharmacopoeia.

The contamination of raw materials depends on the type, source and the treatment used in their preparation. Plastic devices that are moulded by heat emerge from the machine in sterile condition but acquire a small number of microbial contaminants during assembly and packaging. On the other hand, starches and resins used as raw materials for pharmaceuticals may be so heavily contaminated that they require pretreatment to reduce the number of microorganisms before they are added to the formulation. Cotton gauze may also be heavily contaminated.

The regulations for commercial production are difficult to apply to sterilization within hospitals and laboratories because monitoring the initial contamination level of a wide variety of articles sterilized in relatively small numbers is impractical. Thorough cleaning (with disinfection if necessary) and careful handling are essential to minimize the bioburden before sterilization. Every effort should be made to provide the same standards of sterility assurance as are applicable to commercial sterilization of medical devices and pharmaceuticals.

TESTING THE PROCESS

The purpose of carrying out a sterilization process is to deliver the intended biocidal treatment to the whole of the material to be sterilized. Achievement of this objective depends on the design and performance of the sterilizing apparatus, the nature of the articles to be sterilized, and the methods used for packaging the articles and loading them into the sterilizing chamber. Physical, biological and chemical methods are used, as appropriate, to demonstrate correct performance of the sterilization cycle and to determine whether the prescribed conditions for sterilization have been achieved in the chamber and at the most challenging sites in the load of material to be sterilized. Responsibility for performance of the tests is shared between the operator of the sterilizer, the hospital maintenance engineer and, where appropriate, a highly trained authorised person (sterilizers). The assistance and advice of a microbiologist may be required in the performance and interpretation of biological tests and for evaluating the end result of a testing program (HTM, 1994).

Physical tests

Temperature and automatic process control test

Tests for the performance of steam and gas sterilizers involve observation of temperature, pressure and vacuum gauges and also of stage timers throughout an automatically controlled sterilization cycle. Temperature and pressure readings should be taken at least three or four times during the sterilizing stage of autoclaves and ovens (HTM, 1994). Recording charts should be examined carefully and kept until all other tests have been completed. Gauges and recorders should be calibrated at regular intervals against standard instruments.

Thermometric tests

Temperatures at selected sites in the chamber and within the load of a dry heat, steam or gas sterilizer are measured by thermocouples or alternative temperature sensors. Thermocouples consist of insulated leads containing two wires of different composition (e.g. copper constantan or nickel chromium/nickel aluminium) which are joined together at one end to form a temperature-sensitive junction. This end of the lead is passed into the chamber of a steam or gas sterilizer through a pressure-tight thermocouple port. Introduction through the door closure is unsatisfactory as it could create a leak and is likely to damage the wire. The tip of the lead is placed within the chamber at the most challenging site in a test pack or bottle of fluid. Care is taken to avoid creating an artificial path for access of steam during this procedure. The external end of the lead is connected to a temperature recorder. Thermocouples are also used in hot air ovens and special entry ports should be provided in this equipment as well.

At least two thermocouples are used in a test; one should be placed in the chamber drain of a steam sterilizer. Other sites in the chamber may also be monitored. The number of thermocouples to be placed in the load depends on whether a single test pack or several bottles of fluid in a full load are to be tested. Thermocouples provide the only means of determining the heat penetration time for packs and bottles in steam sterilizers or for containers in a hot air sterilizer. They are also used in determining temperature distribution in ethylene oxide sterilizers and the time taken for the selected operating temperature to be reached in the load.

Leak rate tests

Prevacuum steam sterilizers are tested at least once a week for the rate of air leakage into the evacuated chamber. The test is usually performed in the drying stage when all parts of the sterilizer are hot. The chamber should be evacuated to an absolute pressure of 5 kPa (50 mbar) or less. After the pressure gauge reading has stabilized, it should not increase by more than 134 Pa (1.3 mbar) per minute. It is important that permissible limits are not exceeded. The test is applicable to any sterilizer that uses vacuum to remove air from the load, e.g. low-temperature steam and formaldehyde sterilizers. For the latter, the vacuum leak rate should not exceed 50 Pa (0.5 mbar) per minute (HTM, 1994).

Measurement of radiation dose

A radiation sterilization process is described by a single parameter, the amount of energy absorbed by the material treated. Sterilizing doses are measured in kilogray (kGy). Dose distribution in the large load of material within the irradiation chamber is measured by placing small strips or cylindrical pieces of red, yellow or colourless Perspex at various sites. The Perspex darkens in proportion to the dose, which is determined by reading the colour change in a spectrophotometer or a white light photometer. Each batch of Perspex dosimeters must be standardized against a reference dosimeter. Dosimetry is repeated as required to monitor changes in dose rate which occur as the output of the ^{60}Co source decreases, or to determine the time required to deliver the prescribed dose to materials of different density.

Chemical indicators

Chemical indicators may be solutions or solids that are sealed in ampoules or dye patterns printed on small paper strips or directly on the outside of wrapping materials. The chemicals undergo a specified change in consistency or colour on exposure to a particular sterilizing agent. The indicators may be intended for strategic placement within test packs or for external use only. The main purpose of chemical indicators is the prompt detection of potential sterilization failures; no chemical indicator can prove that sterilization has occurred. A wide variety of commercially produced chemical indicators is available and care must be taken in their selection. The manufacturer should provide information concerning the intended purpose of the indicator and the nature and interpretation of the response (ISO 11140.1, 1995).

External indicators

External, or throughput, indicators are intended only to distinguish packs which have been through a sterilization cycle from those which have not been processed. They may reveal a gross equipment malfunction but do not confirm sterilizing conditions in the chamber or the load.

Paper bags, or pouches made from combinations of paper and plastic, are prepared commercially for use in steam or gas sterilization. They bear printed patterns which undergo a specified change in colour on exposure to the sterilizing agent. Adhesive tapes, such as 'autoclave tape' which are commonly used to fasten paper or cloth wrappings also incorporate a chemical indicator, usually as diagonal stripes which darken or change in colour during the sterilization process. Different types of external indicators are required for steam, dry heat and ethylene oxide sterilization. Adhesive discs which change colour during exposure to gamma radiation are fixed to the outer cartons and may also be provided on the shelf storage carton. They indicate that the packs have been irradiated but do not provide evidence of the dose.

Internal indicators

These indicators are designed for placement within test packs at sites that are likely to be least access-ible to penetration by steam or chemical vapours, or slowest to reach the sterilizing temperature in a hot air oven. They should be used only in conjunction with thermocouples and biological indicators. Different types of indicators are required for steam, dry heat, ethylene oxide, plasma and low-temperature steam and formaldehyde processes. The following types of chemical indicators are available for internal use:

1. Sealed tubes containing pellets which fuse and darken or change in colour when a specified minimum temperature is reached. Time is not included in the response.
2. Sealed tubes containing a liquid which changes colour. Such indicators are available for steam sterilization at 120°C (16 minutes) and 135°C (3 minutes). Other types respond to hot air sterilization at 160°C (60 minutes) and 180°C (16 minutes).
3. Paper strips impregnated with a single band of indicator or rectangular pieces bearing a pattern of spots which show a graded colour change. These indicators usually respond to time as well as temperature. Many brands are available for steam, dry heat, ethylene oxide and low-temperature steam and formaldehyde processes.
4. Integrators consisting of sachets containing a chemical which undergoes a progressive visible change along a wick at a defined rate. These multiparameter indicators provide an integrated response to defined combinations of temperature, time of exposure and the presence of steam. They can show the degree of under- or over-exposure on either side of a marked end point response and can indicate poor steam quality. Multiparameter indicators are available for steam or ethylene oxide processes. These indicators should not respond to dry heat. They may equal or surpass the challenge presented by biological indicators of both standard (enveloped) or self-contained types. Despite these advantages over other types of chemical indicators, integrators should not be used alone to prove that sterilization has been achieved. However, they can provide information about a range of potential problems (ISO 11140.1, 1995).

The user of chemical indicators may select a

type or brand by subjecting them to conditions of under- or over-exposure and by testing several samples of a product under the same conditions to assess the reproducibility of the response.

Air removal (Bowie-Dick) test

The Bowie-Dick test is only applicable to pre-vacuum (porous load) steam sterilizers. It was designed by Bowie et al (1963) to provide evidence of the complete removal of air from, and uniform steam penetration into, a standard test pack. It does not verify the temperature reached in the pack or the time for which it was maintained. It is the most sensitive test for residual air and daily performance of this test in all prevacuum steam sterilizers is mandatory (HTM, 1994). A more detailed description of the pack and its use is contained in Chapter 6. Briefly, the test pack is made up of a stack of folded cotton towels to a specified size and weight. The chemical indicator is made by laying autoclave tape, in the shape of a St Andrew's cross, on a sheet of white paper that is similar to the towels in its permeability to air and steam. Alternatively, manufactured sheets of the same size, incorporating an equivalent area of the temperature-sensitive indicator, may be used. The indicator is placed in the fold of a towel at the midpoint of the horizontal stack.

After the test cycle with the pack alone in the chamber, the indicator sheet is recovered and carefully examined to detect any sign of nonuniformity in the colour change. Any paler area, usually near the centre of the pack, denotes the presence of sufficient residual air to interfere with sterilization. It

may be necessary to match a corner of the indicator to the central area to detect small differences. If a fail result is obtained, the sterilizer must not be used until the cause has been found and corrected. Several brands of disposable substitutes for the standard towel pack are now available; they should be thoroughly tested before being adopted for routine use. The Bowie-Dick test is not applicable to downward displacement sterilizers as these operate a longer cycle during which time the indicator could be changed by the temperature of the heat penetration phase, despite the continuing presence of air.

Biological indicators

A biological indicator is a standardized preparation of bacterial spores on or in a carrier which serves to demonstrate whether sterilization conditions were met. The inoculated carrier is put up in a package which maintains its integrity and is designed to be of convenience to the user. Biological indicators may be used to monitor sterilizing conditions within test packs but the realistic nature of the tests must be weighed against the inherent variability of living microorganisms. They should not be used as the sole criterion of sterilization efficiency. A brief outline of the methods used in the preparation and standardization of biological indicators will assist understanding of their use and the significance of results. The species of spore-forming bacteria that are commonly used in the different sterilization processes are listed in Table 2.2. *B. stearothermophilus* and *Bacillus subtilis* subsp. *niger* may be combined in

Table 2.2 Species of spore-forming *Bacillus* used as biological indicators

Process	Species	Incubation temperature °C	Importance in test programme
Steam at high pressure	*B. stearothermophilus*	56	Low
Dry heat	*B. subtilis* subsp. *niger*	37	Low
Ethylene oxide	*B. subtilis* subsp. *niger*	37	High
Plasma	*B. subtilis* subsp. *niger*	37	High
Subatmospheric steam and formaldehyde	*B. stearothermophilus*	56	High
Gamma radiation	*B. pumilus* E601	37	Low

multi-purpose biological indicators. They are incubated at 56°C for sterilization by steam above atmospheric pressure or the subatmospheric steam and formaldehyde process. For sterilization by dry heat or ethylene oxide, they are incubated at 37°C.

Preparation

The bacterium is grown on a solid or liquid medium under conditions that produce a high yield of spores. The spores are harvested, treated to eliminate the remaining vegetative cells and washed until they are free from medium constituents and cell debris. The resistance of the suspension to the relevant sterilizing agent is determined and expressed as a D value. Minor variations between batches of spores can be adjusted by varying the number of spores inoculated onto each carrier. Water-soluble polymers, such as polyethylene glycol and methyl cellulose, may be added to the washed spores to bring the level of resistance to that of naturally occurring microbial contaminants (Doyle, 1971).

The suspension is inoculated on small strips or discs of absorbent paper or other suitable material and dried under controlled conditions. The number of spores per unit varies between 10^4 and 10^6. If two species are inoculated on to the same carrier, the full number of each is required. Two packaging methods are commonly used:

1. In the conventional method, each spore paper is placed in a transparent glassine (steam permeable) packet in which it remains during the test. The individual packets are placed in outer paper envelopes which may be divided into two compartments, one sealed and one open; a single unit in the sealed compartment is retained for incubation as untreated control and the two in the open compartment are used in the test.
2. Self-contained biological indicators are small, plastic capsules containing one spore paper and the culture medium in a thin glass vial. After the test cycle has been completed, the vial is broken by pressure on the outside of the capsule and the medium is released to engulf the spore paper. The unit is then incubated at the appropriate temperature.

The first method involves a slight risk of accidental contamination when the paper is transferred to culture medium in a separate container; however, contaminants will not significantly interfere because only B. stearothermophilus will grow above 50°C and B. subtilis subsp. niger may be recognized by the orange pigmentation of the growth.

When used in downward displacement steam sterilizers, self-contained biological indicators should be positioned with care to ensure that steam can gain access through the cap to the spore strip within the capsule. This is especially important with those steam sterilizers that operate a high-temperature process for a short exposure time. In these sterilizers, an improperly placed self-contained indicator can give a false positive result when thermocouple measurements indicate that the cycle is satisfactory. However, false positive results are less likely to occur in prevacuum sterilizers (Reich & Fitzpatrick, 1985; Fitzpatrick & Reich, 1986).

All biological indicators should be accompanied by the following information, on the label or in a separate brochure, as appropriate: name of manufacturer, lot no., microorganism, number of viable spores per unit, sterilization process, incubation temperature, storage condition and expiry date. Additional information about the method of preparation, acceptance criteria and quality control may be provided.

Standardization

The United States Pharmacopeia (1995) specifies the range of D values for spores which are used in the preparation of biological indicators; these are listed in Table 2.3.

Specially designed testing apparatus, termed Biological Indicator-Evaluator Resistometer (BIER) vessels, are used for evaluating the performance of biological indicators. For ethylene oxide, the timing begins with the rapid admission of the vaporized gas to the exposure chamber, after sterilization conditions have been met (ANSI, ST44). For steam under pressure, a dedicated steam generator is used and the timer is graduated to be read with the precision of one second (ANSI, ST45).

The aim of the test is to determine the maximum exposure that results in all of the samples showing growth and the minimum exposure that is required for all to be sterilized. The curve in

Table 2.3 Range of D values for standard spore cultures used as biological indicators for sterilization processes (from United States Pharmacopeia 1995)

Standard cultures	Sterilization process	Range of D values (min)
B. stearothermophilus ATCC[1] 7953, NCTC[2] 10007, NCIB[3] 8157	Steam above atmospheric pressure Subatmospheric steam and formaldehyde	1.5–3.0
B. subtilis subsp. niger ATCC 9372, NCIB 8058, NCTC 10073, NCIB 8649	Dry heat at 160°C Ethylene oxide	1.0–3.0 2.6–5.8

[1] ATCC = American Type Culture Collection, Rockville, Maryland, USA
[2] NCTC = National Collection of Type Cultures, London, UK
[3] NCIB = National Collection of Industrial and Marine Bacteria, Aberdeen, Scotland

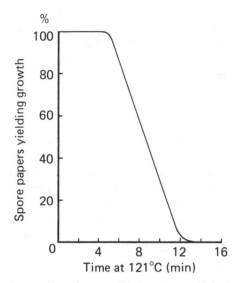

Fig. 2.5 A dose-response curve for *B. stearothermophilus* spore papers to steam at 121°C.

Figure 2.5 represents a hypothetical result for *B. stearothermophilus* indicators in steam at 121°C. There is a high probability of positive culture up to 5 minutes exposure and a high probability of negative results after 13 minutes. In the intermediate zone of partial survival, the proportion of negative cultures increases with the time of exposure. The inherent variability of response, even around the endpoint of 'complete kill', accounts for the observation that it is rare for biological indicators to provide the first warning of trouble (Smith, 1986).

A sensitive indicator would have a narrow zone of partial survival but no biological indicator is capable of giving a sharp end point. The aim is to ensure that the chance of obtaining a positive culture after exposure to adequate sterilizing conditions is extremely low. However, spores are not biological thermometers and it is inevitable that positive cultures will occasionally occur although the sterilizer has performed satisfactorily.

It has been recommended that biological indicators for use in ethylene oxide sterilizers should be standardized at a temperature above 50°C and a relative humidity close to 50 per cent (Oxborrow et al, 1983). The stability of biological indicators may be influenced by environmental temperature and relative humidity and the manufacturer's instructions should be strictly observed. The stated resistance must be maintained during storage until the expiry date. Reich & Morien (1982) demonstrated that storage at a relative humidity below 20 per cent decreases the resistance of *B. stearothermophilus* indicators to heat but increases the resistance of *B. subtilis* spore papers to ethylene oxide, so that they no longer conformed to the requirement of the United States Pharmacopeia. They recommended that storage of both types of indicators below 20 per cent or above 60 per cent RH should be avoided.

Incubation

After the sterilization cycle under test has been completed, the biological indicators are recovered and cultured, together with an unexposed control. A good quality nutrient broth, such as tryptone soya broth, is used. A pH indicator such as bromcresol purple is sometimes added so that early growth may be detected by acid production but it is necessary to demonstrate that the concentration of the indicator used does not inhibit germination of the spores (Cook & Brown, 1960). The temperature of incubation is 37°C for *B. subtilis* subsp.

niger and 56°C for *B. stearothermophilus*. A water bath is not recommended for incubation at the higher temperature but, if used, the culture bottles should be placed in fixed racks and the water level should not be so high that it can wet the screw caps. A thermostatically controlled metal block with cavities for the culture containers is the preferred option. The unexposed spore strip should yield growth in 24 hours and those that have been used in a test are likely to show growth within 3 days if they contain surviving spores. However, incubation should be continued for 7 days before a negative result is recorded. Shorter incubation times for the self-contained biological indicators are usually recommended by manufacturers.

Interpretation of results

The validity of the result of a biological indicator test is influenced by the number of units used. A result obtained with a single unit may be meaningless because there is a chance of obtaining a positive or negative culture at either end of the partial survival zone. If a single unit has a 1 in 10 chance of producing a positive culture despite exposure to sterilizing conditions, two units will reduce the probability of a false result to 1 in 100. As biological indicators provide the main method for testing the efficiency of sterilization by ethylene oxide, plasma and low-temperature steam and formaldehyde, up to 10 units are used in each cycle initially until confidence in the process has been established.

Testing programs

Qualifying tests

A combination of all the appropriate tests, including biological and chemical indicators, is required for validation of the process when a new sterilizer has been installed and on recommissioning after major repairs or modifications. The sterilizing department supervisor, trained maintenance engineers and a microbiologist may be involved in the performance and interpretation of the tests. They may be repeated at weekly, quarterly, half-yearly or yearly intervals as part of the planned maintenance (PM) program (see Ch. 14).

Routine tests

Routine tests are carried out to confirm efficiency in the day-to-day operation of the sterilizer. They must be convenient to perform so that they do not interfere with the production of sterile supplies but sensitive enough to give early indication of a fault. Temperature, pressure and vacuum readings may be sufficient in steam sterilization but the additional use of a biological indicator and test pack, at least once a week, is recommended for porous load sterilizers and for inclusion in every load that contains implantable devices (ANSI, ST46). Biological and chemical indicators are required in gas sterilization. The Bowie-Dick (air removal) test must be performed daily in prevacuum porous load sterilizers. A summarized testing program is set out in Table 2.4.

TESTING THE PRODUCT

The performance of sterility tests on a limited number of samples of the final product (pharmaceutical or medical device) is a less sensitive method for testing the efficiency of sterilization than are tests on the sterilization process, as described in the preceding section. However, sterility tests must be performed on pharmaceutical products that are sterilized in bulk by filtration and then filled aseptically into the final containers. Sterility tests also detect mechanical malfunctions, human error or the mix-up of sterilized and non-sterilized goods. The frequency of testing, or the number of samples tested, may be reduced when the initial contamination level of the product is known and it is sterilized by steam in a process that has been monitored by approved methods including biological indicators (United States Pharmacopeia, 1995).

Limitations of sterility tests

1. Number of samples
2. Culture methods
3. Antimicrobial action
4. Accidental contamination.

Number of samples

A batch or lot is a homogeneous collection of sealed containers or packages, prepared in such a

Table 2.4   Testing efficiency of sterilization (minimum requirements)

Type of sterilizer	Qualifying tests	Routine tests
Dry heat sterilizer	Sterilizer function Thermocouple test	Observation of temperature readings
Instrument or bottled fluid sterilizer	Sterilizer function Thermocouple test	Observation of temperature and pressure readings
Porous load sterilizer (prevacuum type)	Sterilizer function Leak rate test Bowie-Dick tape test Thermocouple test Chemical indicators } optional Biological indicators }	Observation of temperature, pressure and vacuum readings Leak rate test (weekly) Bowie-Dick tape test (daily) Biological indicator (weekly)
Low-temperature plasma sterilizer	Sterilizer function Biological indicator	Observation of cycle parameters Biological indicator (each cycle)
Ethylene oxide sterilizer	Sterilizer function Thermocouple test Biological indicator (essential)	Observation of temperature, pressure and vacuum readings Biological indicator (each cycle) Chemical indicator (each cycle)
Low-temperature steam and formaldehyde sterilizer	Sterilizer function Thermocouple test Biological indicator (essential)	Observation of temperature and vacuum readings Biological indicator (each cycle) Chemical indicator (each cycle)
Gamma radiation installation	Measurement of absorbed dose and dose distribution Biological indicator	Dosimetry (as required) Biological indicator (optional)

manner that the risk of contamination is the same for all of the items. It may be a single sterilizer load or the products of a continuous process, such as radiation sterilization, or an aseptic filling operation over a specified period. The sterility of a whole batch could be guaranteed only if all of the material was tested. In practice, the likelihood of all the items in the batch being sterile is determined by testing a sample containing a relatively small number of items. The sensitivity of a sterility test depends on the:

1. Per cent of contaminated items in the batch
2. Number of items tested.

The relationship between the per cent of unsterile items in the batch and the probability of accepting a contaminated batch as sterile when 10 or 20 items are tested is shown in Table 2.5. The quantity of a powder or liquid from each container that is tested also influences the sensitivity of the test. The amount or volume of material tested, and the sensitivity of the test, may be increased by use

Table 2.5   Relationship between per cent of contaminated items, number of items in the sample, and sensitivity of sterility tests

Unsterile items (per cent)	Probability of drawing 20 sterile items	Probability of drawing 10 sterile items
0.1	0.90	0.99
1.0	0.82	0.90
2.0	0.67	0.82
5.0	0.36	0.60
6.7	0.25	0.50
10.0	0.12	0.35

of the membrane filtration method for soluble powders and liquid products.

Ernst et al (1969) reported the results of 12 separate sterility tests on a batch of sterilized material in which 5 per cent of items had been subsequently inoculated. Each test was done on a sample of 20 items. Approximately 4 per cent of the 240 samples yielded positive cultures, but 7 of the 12 separate tests failed to detect the contamination. It is generally recognized that product sterility tests are reliable only for detecting a high per cent of unsterile items, such as might be expected from a faulty sterilization process.

Culture methods

No single medium or condition of incubation will recover all types of microbial contaminants. Thioglycollate broth, incubated at 32–37°C, is widely used because it will support the growth of anaerobic bacteria. It will also grow many aerobes and facultative anaerobes, but the low oxygen tension is unfavourable to *Bacillus* species if the bacteria are few in number and have been damaged by the treatment received (Doyle et al, 1968). Soybean casein digest medium is commonly chosen for growing fungi and bacteria that have a low optimum temperature range (20–25°C).

Antimicrobial action

Sterility tests are performed on antibiotics that have been sterilized by filtration and subsequently dispensed into the final containers, where they may be freeze-dried before sealing. Pharmaceuticals that are intended for repeated use also contain an antimicrobial agent, such as an organic mercurial, a phenol, a quaternary ammonium compound or chlorhexidine, to kill or inhibit the growth of contaminants that enter the product after the container has been opened. Antimicrobial action in the culture medium may be prevented by dilution of the samples, by chemical inactivation or by use of the membrane filtration method.

Solutions of penicillin are filtered and the membrane filter is washed with a diluent that contains an appropriate amount of the enzyme penicillinase. As inactivators are not available for other antibiotics, their removal must be accomplished by washing alone. Quaternary ammonium compounds and chlorhexidine may be inactivated by including lecithin and a nonionic detergent in the culture medium. Mercurial preservatives are inactivated by thioglycollate medium but not by soybean casein digest medium. Phenolic compounds, such as chlorocresol, may be added directly to the culture medium if the dilution factor is sufficient to inactivate them.

Accidental contamination

The accidental introduction of contaminants to samples, culture media or equipment during the performance of a sterility test results in false positive cultures which necessitate repetition of the test and may cause costly recalls of industrial products. Contamination cannot be prevented completely but the risk can be reduced to a very low level by suitable selection and training of staff, the provision of special outer wear (masks, gowns, headgear, overshoes and gloves) and an ultraclean environment in which particulate contamination is controlled and which is used in such a way as to minimize the introduction, generation and retention of particles. This necessitates the use of a laminar flow room or a Class II biological safety cabinet, located in a room with a clean air supply.

All equipment brought into the testing area must be sterile and the outer surfaces of the containers or packs to be tested should be chemically disinfected. Ethyl alcohol is commonly used because it leaves no residue. Containers that have been sealed under vacuum should be opened by piercing the rubber closure with a sterile hypodermic needle attached to a bacterial filter. Packages containing solid articles should be inspected for integrity before they are opened aseptically. The article is transferred to the culture medium with sterile forceps. Transfer forceps should not be sterilized by alcohol flaming because the temperature on the metal surface may be only 118°C although the air temperature 3 mm away is 205°C (Doyle & Ernst, 1969). Large or complex articles, such as dressings or intravenous sets, present an added risk of contamination if they must be dismantled or aseptically cut into pieces for testing.

The rate of accidental contamination in a testing laboratory may be estimated in the long term from the accumulated results of negative controls. Accidental contamination rates below 0.1 per cent can be achieved by skilled workers in favourable conditions.

Methods of testing

Direct method

Aqueous liquids and water soluble powders may be added directly to the culture media, but a preliminary test is required to determine whether they contain antimicrobial agents. The sample and culture medium are mixed in the usual proportions and inoculated with a small number of organisms that are sensitive to the antimicrobial agent. Failure to grow within 48 hours indicates a need to increase the volume of medium or decrease the amount of sample, within permitted limits, until growth is demonstrated. The direct method may also be used for devices that are small enough to be immersed in not more than a litre of medium. Larger devices may be dismantled or cut into pieces aseptically if this is feasible. Contamination of tubular devices is most likely to be detected if they are filled with sterile culture medium which is incubated in situ.

Membrane filtration method

This technique requires more elaborate apparatus and a high level of skill but it is the method of choice in most situations. It overcomes the problem of antimicrobial action in the culture medium because the membrane and the microorganisms retained on its surface can be washed thoroughly with a diluent or treated with an appropriate inactivator. Membrane filtration is also used for testing oily substances and large volumes of liquid, such as intravenous solutions or a diluent which has been used to recover microbial contaminants from large objects for enumeration.

Membrane filters of average pore diameter of 0.45 μm are used. Membranes with hydrophobic edges are required to avoid retention of antimicrobial substances between the sealing surfaces of the filter holder. Filtration apparatus with a closed reservoir and receiver is essential. The units should be sterilized by autoclaving with the membrane in place and the system must be tested for integrity before use (see Ch. 9). The membranes are wetted with a sterile diluent before the sample is filtered, except with oils for which a dry sterile membrane is required.

The liquid samples may be pooled and filtered through one membrane, which is divided aseptically for addition to each of the culture media. Alternatively, the pooled liquid may be divided into equal parts by an automatic pumping device and distributed to separate filter units. Self-contained sterility testing units, which are designed to reduce the incidence of false-positive results due to external contamination, are also available. After the test solution is filtered under pressure through a 0.45 μm filter with hydrophobic edge at the base of the unit, sterile broth medium is added to the growth chamber above the filter for the culture of any microorganisms on the filter surface. The air supply to the growth chamber is filtered through a small 0.45 μm hydrophobic air vent filter at the top of the unit (Eudailey, 1983).

Aqueous solutions and oils are filtered directly and the membrane is washed with a diluent containing polysorbate 80. Water soluble powders are dissolved in a suitable diluent, which is also used for washing the filter. Ointments are dissolved in isopropyl myristate which has been sterilized by filtration through a membrane of 0.22 μm average pore diameter (United States Pharmacopeia, 1995). Penicillin may be inactivated by the addition of a high concentration of penicillinase to the solution or a lower concentration to the diluent used for washing the filter.

Controls

Positive and negative controls should be included in each working session. Tests on 10 samples to which 10–20 bacteria have been added constitute a positive control, and a similar number of samples which have been sterilized by a severe process is used as the negative control.

All culture media must be tested for sterility by incubation under the conditions that will be used in the test. Growth-promoting ability must also be demonstrated by inoculation with fewer than 100 cells of recommended species of bacteria and yeasts. The membrane filtration method must be tested to demonstrate effective removal or inactivation of antimicrobial agents. Ten to 20 viable microorganisms are added to the final rinse and the membrane is cultured in an appropriate medium for each species used. Growth should be detected within 48 hours. Media that have been used in a sterility test should be incubated for 14 days; a number of the positive cultures may be missed if incubation is terminated after 7 days. An additional test for the ability of the media to support growth may be performed at the end of the normal incubation period by adding microorganisms and incubating for a further 48 hours. This is referred to as a 'stasis test'.

Results

The sample tested, and the batch it represents, passes the sterility test if no growth occurs in any culture vessel. If occasional growth is observed, repetition of the test may be permitted. The report on a sterility test cannot state that the whole batch is sterile; it demonstrates only that the incidence of contaminated units is below the level that the sampling system used is capable of detecting. The decision to accept a batch of sterilized material should be undertaken by a responsible microbiologist who understands the limitations of sample size. Sterility testing is laborious and requires a high level of skill. It should never be undertaken by persons, however well qualified, who lack the necessary training, equipment and environmental conditions. Neither should it be performed on an inadequate number of samples.

REFERENCES

ANSI/AAMI ST44 — 1992 BIER/EO gas vessels. American National Standards Institute, New York

ANSI/AAMI ST45 — 1992 BIER/Steam vessels. American National Standards Institute, New York

ANSI/AAMI ST46 — 1993 Good hospital practice: steam sterilization and sterility assurance. American National Standards Institute, New York

Bond W W, Favero M S, Petersen N J, Marshall J H 1970 Dry-heat inactivation kinetics of naturally occurring spore populations. Applied Microbiology 20: 573–578

Bowie J H, Kelsey J C, Thompson G R 1963 The Bowie and Dick autoclave tape test. Lancet i: 586–587

Cerf O 1977 Tailing of survival curves of bacterial spores. Journal of Applied Bacteriology 42: 1–19

Cook A M, Brown M R W 1960 Preliminary studies of the heat resistance of bacterial spores on paper carriers. Journal of Pharmacy and Pharmacology 12(Suppl): 116T–118T

Davey K R 1990 Equilibrium temperature in a clump of bacteria heated in fluid. Applied and Environmental Microbiology 56: 566–568

Doyle J E 1971 Sterility indicator with artificial resistance to ethylene oxide. Bulletin of the Parenteral Drug Association 25: 98–104

Doyle J E, Ernst R R 1969 Alcohol flaming — a possible source of contamination in sterility testing. American Journal of Clinical Pathology 51: 407–408

Doyle J E, Mehrhof W H, Ernst R R 1968 Limitations of thioglycolate broth as a sterility test medium for materials exposed to gaseous ethylene oxide. Applied Microbiology 16: 1742–1744

Ernst R R, West K L, Doyle J E 1969 Problem areas in sterility testing. Bulletin of the Parenteral Drug Association 23: 29–39

Eudailey W A 1983 Membrane filters and membrane filtration processes for health care. American Journal of Hospital Pharmacy 40: 1921–1923

Fitzpatrick B G, Reich R R 1986 Sterilization monitoring in vacuum steam sterilizers. Journal of Healthcare Materiel Management 4(5): 82–85

Gard S 1957 Chemical inactivation of viruses. In: Wolstenholme G E W, Millar E C P (eds) Ciba Foundation Symposium on the nature of viruses. Churchill, London, p 123

HTM 1994 Health Technical Memorandum 2010 Part 3: Validation and verification. Sterilization. NHS Estates, London

ISO 11140.1 1995 Sterilization of health care products — chemical indicators — Part 1: General requirements. International Organization for Standardization, Geneva

Oxborrow G S, Placencia A M, Danielson J W 1983 Effects of temperature and relative humidity on biological indicators used for ethylene oxide sterilization. Applied and Environmental Microbiology 45: 546–549

Reich R R, Fitzpatrick B G 1985 Flash sterilization. Evaluation of sterilization indicators in gravity steam sterilization cycles. Journal of Hospital Supply, Processing and Distribution 3(4): 60–63

Reich R R, Morien L L 1982 Influence of environmental storage relative humidity on biological indicator resistance, viability, and moisture content. Applied and Environmental Microbiology 43: 609–614

Shull J J, Cargo G T, Ernst R R 1963 Kinetics of heat activation and of thermal death of bacterial spores. Applied Microbiolgy 11: 485–487

Smith R F 1986 Sterile? The ten parameters of steam sterilization. Journal of Healthcare Materiel Management 4(4): 34–36, 38–39

Stumbo C R 1973 Thermobacteriology in food processing, 2nd edn. Academic Press, New York, ch 7, p 74–75

United States Pharmacopeia 1995 23rd rev. United States Phamacopeial Convention Inc, Rockville

3. Preparation and packaging for sterilization

Effective contact between the biocidal agent and the microbial contaminants is an essential prerequisite for sterilization. Access of the biocidal agent to all areas where the contaminants may be located depends on the types of articles and the methods of cleaning, wrapping and packing that are used to prepare them for sterilization. Packaging materials and package design are also important in the maintenance of sterility during storage and transportation of the sterilized articles and at the time when the packages are opened for use. The preparation of articles for sterilization will be discussed under the following headings:

  Cleaning and disinfection
  Packaging materials
  Package design
  Types of packs
  Closing and sealing
  Package testing
  Maintenance of sterility.

CLEANING AND DISINFECTION

The collective term 'decontamination' refers to the processes of cleaning and disinfection that are required, separately or in combination, to make used equipment which may be contaminated with pathogenic microorganisms safe to handle by persons who inspect, repair, pack or sterilize it for reuse. Cleaning removes organic and inorganic soiling materials and also many of the microbial contaminants which have been acquired during treatment of patients. It is especially important to remove Gram-negative bacteria before the pyrogenic substances which may be liberated from their living or dead cells are adsorbed on the surfaces of equipment or containers, from which it is difficult or impossible to remove them.

Cleaning is an integral part of the 'make-safe' process as it influences the efficiency of disinfection by heat or chemical agents and is also vital to the efficiency of the final sterilization process. The role of cleaning and disinfection in minimizing contamination levels prior to sterilization may be compared to the principles and methods of Good Manufacturing Practice (GMP) that govern the commercial production of sterile pharmaceuticals and medical devices. These are equally applicable to hospitals.

The main types of reusable equipment that are cleaned and disinfected in hospitals to prepare them for resterilization are surgical instruments, drills, bowls, other utensils made from metal or heat-stable plastic and a small number of reusable syringes. A central sterilizing department may incorporate a section for cleaning and disinfecting anaesthetic apparatus, respiratory therapy equipment, incubators and other complex equipment to prepare them for reuse without further treatment. Endoscopes, which may be required for immediate reuse, may be cleaned and disinfected in the department where they are used. Surgical linen is washed and disinfected in the laundry and delivered to the sterilizing department for packing and sterilization.

Cleaning and disinfection of domestic apparatus for patient care, such as bedpans, urinals and, when required, eating utensils which have been used by a patient harbouring a specified communicable disease such as tuberculosis, are carried out in equipment installed in the hospital wards. Microbiological laboratories also include a service area where reusable equipment and glassware are cleaned and disinfected prior to resterilization.

Risks and precautions

The risks posed by most pathogenic bacteria can be avoided by taking appropriate precautions in the transportation and cleaning of the contaminated equipment (Mitchell, 1974). *Mycobacterium* spp. and vancomycin-resistant enterococci merit special attention, as do antibiotic-resistant strains of *Staphylococcus aureus* and some types of Gram-negative bacteria. Opportunistic pathogens, such

as species of *Pseudomonas*, *Acinetobacter*, *Proteus* or *Klebsiella*, are unlikely to affect healthy persons, although they present a serious risk to hospital patients whose immunity to infection is naturally defective or therapeutically depressed.

Hepatitis B and hepatitis C viruses and HIV cause particular concern in hospitals and microbiology or pathology laboratories because they can be transmitted by blood or blood products. A minute quantity of blood may contain an infective dose of hepatitis B virus. Occasional but potentially serious hazards are associated with exposure to patients with viral haemorrhagic fevers or to neurological tissue from patients with Creutzfeldt-Jakob disease.

Certain basic precautions, such as protective clothing with gloves, eye protection and strong shoes should be observed as routine, along with education and training of workers in the avoidance of needle punctures and cuts from sharp instruments and the safe handling and disposal of contaminated materials. In the United Kingdom, the management of chemical and biological hazards has been legislated under the Control of Substances Hazardous to Health (COSHH) Regulations of 1994.

Agents for cleaning and disinfection

Cleaning solutions

Solutions containing nonionic or anionic detergents are used for cleaning. An appropriate enzyme (usually proteolytic) may need to be included to soften dried residues of blood and other body fluids. Detergents are surface-active agents that are characterized by frothing; however, excess frothing may be a disadvantage and does not contribute to the cleaning action of the solution. The selection of an appropriate type of cleaner for manual, mechanical or ultrasonic cleaning depends on the type of action required. A cleaner may emulsify fat, soften or dissolve blood, or bind calcium and magnesium ions in hard water or iron from a poor quality steam supply, thus preventing deposition of scale or rust on instruments. The properties that are desirable in a product for cleaning medical equipment and the types of products that are available have been described by Harrison et al (1990) and in AS 4187 (1994).

The product selected should be capable of preventing scaling and rusting of instruments, should not cause corrosion of stainless steel, titanium, tungsten carbide inserts (on cutting instruments) or brass or copper fittings used in mechanical cleaners. It should also be compatible with plastics and rubber. Excess foaming should be avoided and deposits from components of the cleaning solution should be easily removable by rinsing.

Cleaning agents may be supplied as powders or concentrated solutions, with clear instructions for dissolving the powder or diluting the liquid. The anionic or nonionic detergents are the principal components. Formulations may be characterized by pH and available alkalinity, in the form of sodium hydroxide, potassium hydroxide or silicates. Products with neutral pH (7–9) and negligible alkalinity are safe for use on most metals but are least effective in removing organic soil. Those with moderate pH (9–11) and low alkalinity have improved cleaning action but cause increasing harm to the protective chromium oxide layer on the surface of stainless steel. They may be slightly corrosive to aluminium, brass and copper unless corrosion inhibitors are included in the formulation. Products of high pH and high alkalinity must be used with caution for removal of heavy soil because harmful effects, such as scale and deposit formation, are increased. Their use should, be avoided if possible and contact should be restricted to a maximum of 10 minutes. Acid cleaners, based on phosphoric acid, are intended for rust removal but cannot stop active corrosion sites. Their use should also be avoided, if possible, or restricted to a short period of time.

Disinfectants

Thermal disinfection by hot water is achieved if the surface temperature of the instruments is 80°C or more for 2 minutes (minimum) or 75°C for 10 minutes (AS 4187, 1994). This usually occurs in the final rinse after cleaning instruments in a mechanical washer/disinfector or an ultrasonic cleaner. Instrument washer/sterilizers, which operate at 121°C, are not recommended because their cleaning efficiency varies and the coagulated (baked) blood or other biological material which they produce is difficult to remove.

Chemical disinfectants, such as quaternary ammonium compounds (QACs) or synthetic phenols which are formulated with compatible detergents, may be used for the precleaning of instruments in the department where they have been used or for manual cleaning in the Sterile Services Department (SSD). QACs or phenolic disinfectants may help to reduce the bioburden but they are ineffective on soiled articles. When on-site disinfection is carried out to make instruments, such as endoscopes, safe for immediate reuse, 2 per cent (w/v) activated glutaraldehyde is recommended; thorough rinsing to remove residual disinfectant is essential.

Equipment and methods

Used equipment may be cleaned by the following methods:

1. Precleaning
2. Manual cleaning
3. Mechanical cleaning
4. Ultrasonic cleaning.

Precleaning

Regardless of whether a manual, mechanical or ultrasonic cleaning method will be used, gross soil should first be removed by rinsing with cold water, a detergent solution or a detergent/disinfectant formulation. If blood or exudates have dried or hardened, soaking in a warm solution of an enzymatic cleaner is required. The preliminary treatment may be carried out in the department where the equipment was used or on arrival in the SSD. Direct dispatch to the SSD in closed, leakproof containers is usually recommended. On-site treatment may contribute to the spread of infection via nurses' hands. Prerinsing or soaking does not involve mechanical agitation.

All equipment that consists of more than one part must be separated into its components before cleaning; the parts should be kept together (e.g. in a basket) for reassembly.

Manual cleaning

Although cleaning by hand is both labour and time intensive, it is still widely practised for cleaning delicate articles, such as fine cutting instruments, endoscopes and dental handpieces, which must be dismantled and cleaned by specially trained staff. Jugs, bowls, trays and rigid containers for surgical instruments may also be cleaned manually unless an appropriate machine is available.

A system of two, preferably three, sinks is required for manual cleaning: one for washing with the aid of a soft bristle brush; the second for the first rinse with tap water; the third for a final rinse with distilled or deionized (softened) water. Rinsing may be done by immersing or spraying. A concentrated neutral anionic detergent, which may contain additives to minimize adverse effects on the skin in the event of splashing, is suitable; low- or high-foaming products may be used but the latter should be avoided if subsequent mechanical or ultrasonic cleaning is to be carried out. Highly caustic detergents are unsuitable for manual cleaning and abrasive pads or powders must not be used. Manual cleaning may also include the use of a detergent/disinfectant and may even be preceded by steam sterilization if there is concern about the possible presence of HIV or hepatitis viruses. However, subsequent treatment with an enzyme preparation may then be required to remove coagulated blood.

Workers who carry out manual cleaning should be trained in avoidance of needle punctures or cuts from sharp instruments. Recommended protective attire includes a waterproof apron, rubber gloves (strong enough to resist punctures or cuts) and eye and face protection from splashing (AS 4187, 1994). Non-slip shoes, strong enough to protect against injury by dropped articles, should be worn. These items should be changed whenever the worker leaves the SSD.

Some laboratory equipment is cleaned manually. Screw caps, cotton wool plugs and coagulated material must be removed from bottles and other containers before they are placed in a washing machine. Pipettes may be rinsed by a water jet at the sink; they are difficult to clean if they have been soaked in a disinfectant which precipitates protein. Phenolic formulations, which have a high detergent content, and sodium hypochlorite solutions are suitable. Glassware that is difficult to clean with detergent or is required for critical tests, such as microbiological assays, may be cleaned by soaking in chromic acid. Detergents that have a high level of bacteriostatic activity should not be used for cleaning culture bottles and tubes because adsorbed residues may inhibit the growth of microorganisms.

Mechanical cleaning

Specially designed machines, termed washer/disinfectors, are available for cleaning instruments and utensils, complex equipment, such as anaesthetic breathing circuits and flexible fibreoptic endoscopes, and laboratory glassware. With the possible exception of washer/disinfectors for endoscopes, the machines are installed in the SSD. Some washer/disinfectors clean baskets of instruments by impingement (forced spraying) from fixed or rotating arms in a closed chamber. This is a batch process. Tunnel washers perform a continuous process in which articles on a moving belt proceed through a series of chambers. Machines for cleaning and disinfecting anaesthetic equipment are fitted with water jets to distribute the cleaning solution and rinsing water to the external and internal surfaces of corrugated tubes, connectors, valves and rebreathing bags. Bottle washers include supports for the bottles, when inverted. BS 2745.1 (1993) specifies general requirements for washer/disinfectors. BS 2745.3 (1993) gives specific requirements for machines used for equipment other than human waste containers and laundry. AS 2711 (1993) specifies requirements for washer/disinfectors for respiratory apparatus.

Modern washer/disinfectors are controlled by microprocessors that provide program flexibility. They also offer automatic program selection, based on sensor recognition of the contents of the load, and digital display of maintenance requirements.

A washer/disinfector cycle includes the following stages (AS 4187, 1994):

1. Cold water rinse
2. Warm water wash, with cleaning agent
3. Hot water rinse, with disinfection (e.g. 80–85°C for 2 minutes)
4. Drying by radiant heat or hot air.

Ultrasonic cleaning

Articles for ultrasonic cleaning are immersed in a

suitable detergent and subjected to ultrasonic vibration for a few minutes. This method is similar in efficiency to manual and mechanical cleaning methods but does not remove stains, except those which are caused by the presence of boiler additives in steam sterilizers. Ultrasonic vibration at the frequency used for cleaning does not kill microorganisms and infective aerosols may be produced unless the lid of the tank is tightly closed during operation. If the articles have not been previously disinfected, the wearing of protective clothing is recommended.

Ultrasonic cleaning is generally used as a supplement to manual or mechanical cleaning (e.g. for weekly treatment of hinged instruments) or to clean delicate tubes and other hollow instruments such as special syringes and needles. Articles made from stainless steel or polypropylene are most suitable for ultrasonic cleaning but glass, polytetrafluoroethylene (Teflon®) and chromium plate may also be treated. However, flaking may occur if the metal plating has been damaged, exposing underlying carbon steel to corrosion. The method is unsuitable for cystoscopes because the lens cement may be loosened. It also causes damage to cutting instruments with tungsten carbide inserts. Rubber and polyvinyl chloride (PVC) cannot be cleaned ultrasonically because these materials absorb the vibrations. Dissimilar metals should not be included in the same load. Rusting or pitted instruments should not be included in loads for ultrasonic cleaning because the condition may be spread to other metalware in the load.

Ultrasound is energy in the form of a wave motion which is above the maximum level of audible sound (16 kHz). An electronic generator converts ordinary alternating electric current to oscillations (expansions and contractions) of the desired frequency in a bank of transducers which are mounted externally on the bottom of the cleaning tank. The oscillations are transmitted to the cleaning solution in the tank as ultrasonic vibrations which produce alternating phases of low and high pressure. This results in a process termed cavitation; the tiny bubbles of vaporized liquid which are created in the low-pressure phase expand until they implode violently in the succeeding high-pressure phase. The resulting shock waves dislodge soil from the surfaces and crevices of the

articles placed in the cleaning fluid. Two types of transducers — magnetostrictive and electrostrictive — may be used. The former operate at the lower frequency of 20–25 kHz, which has greater imploding power. The latter, operating at 40–90 kHz, are equally reliable, have greater penetrating power and make less noise (Detwiler, 1989).

An ultrasonic cleaner usually consists of two tanks. The cleaning tank is provided with a tightly fitting lid to prevent the escape of infective aerosols and audible sound. The bank of transducers under the floor of the tank must be removable for replacement. The second tank may perform successive stages of post-rinsing and drying. The wire loading basket or tray should be 2.5 cm from the sides of the tank, where cavitation intensity is low. The detergent must be carefully selected, in accordance with advice from the manufacturer of the cleaner, and should be effective at a low concentration because ultrasonic vibration may enhance any corrosive effect. A neutral or alkaline, low-foaming detergent is suitable; foam is undesirable because it settles on instruments when they are removed from the tank. If a high-foaming detergent has been used for preliminary manual cleaning, the articles must be rinsed thoroughly before transfer to the ultrasonic cleaner. Hollow instruments and suction tubes can be precleaned with an alkaline detergent, if necessary, and rinsed with cold water.

Power to the tank should be turned on for 20 minutes after filling in order to expel dissolved air, which decreases the effect of cavitation by introducing non-condensable gases into the bubbles. The cleaning solution is heated to 45–55°C; higher temperatures prevent cavitation by producing large vapour-filled pockets instead of minute bubbles. The basket is loaded with instruments to a depth of about 76 mm and carefully placed in the tank to avoid reintroducing air into the liquid. All instruments should be disassembled if possible and hinges or box joints should be opened. Heavy instruments are placed in a bottom layer, with fine cutting instruments in the top one. Special trays may be used for microsurgery instruments. One tray per cycle is sufficient; two will reduce cleaning efficiency. The time of treatment ranges from 3–6 minutes but 5 minutes is usually sufficient; extended times are likely to redeposit the soil unless scum is removed by an overflow system. The water used for post-rinsing may be heated to 90°C, which assists subsequent drying of the instruments. Tubes and cannulae should be jet flushed. The tank should be emptied daily, or more often if the quality of cleaning deteriorates (Detwiler, 1989). If the instruments are stained by an alkaline detergent, they may be treated with a dilute citric acid solution (Weymes, 1973). The instruments may be lubricated by dipping the basket in an oil-in-water emulsion lubricant before drying.

Drying

Instruments and other equipment that have been cleaned manually, mechanically or by ultrasonic treatment should be dried quickly to prevent corrosion and stains. Hot air drying is commonly used; the process may be carried out as the terminal stage in a washer/disinfector cycle, or in specially designed drying cabinets which cater for tubing of different diameters.

Inspection, lubrication and repair

Routine inspection of articles for efficiency of cleaning and for need of repair or lubrication are important steps in the preparation of articles for sterilization. If instruments remain soiled after manual or mechanical cleaning, ultrasonic treatment might be successful. All metalware should be free from corrosion because a damaged surface prevents proper cleaning and protects microorganisms from contact with the sterilizing agent (Meredith, 1977). Instruments should be examined for alignment of jaws, tight closure of ratchets, sharpness of blades and points, and correct stiffness of hinges and joints.

The need for lubrication should be assessed carefully because many instruments, especially those with box joints, do not require oiling if they are perfectly clean. Grinding to loosen stiff joints should be unnecessary if the instruments are maintained in good condition and are dipped, after cleaning, in an oil-and-water emulsion lubricant which may contain an antimicrobial agent (Ryan & Romey, 1989). This permits access of steam to the surfaces and facilitates cleaning after use by decreasing the adherence of soil. The same type of emulsion may be applied to dental and surgical drills before steam sterilization but supplementary lubrication of the dried instruments with sterile oil may be required.

The person in charge of assembly and packaging should check the condition of the articles and ensure that they will be sterilized by the most suitable method. Equipment that withstands steam or dry heat sterilization should not be treated by a low temperature gaseous process. Laundered surgical linen should be inspected for freedom from stains, loose fibres and holes. Stains may be caused by oil, rust or bleaching agents but the cause is sometimes difficult to identify. Loose fibres (lint) result from laundering linens with cloth or paper towels that have been carelessly discarded into laundry bags. The significance of holes caused by towel clips during an operation is difficult to assess. All items in which holes have been detected should be rejected but a high rejection rate may overload the laundry facilities. Holes may be repaired with adhesive patches, which are satisfactory if the edges do not lift off. Any hole that is detectable when the material is held against strong daylight or a glass-topped table which is lit from below can provide a passage for microorganisms. Linen that has been packed for sterilization should not be placed in a hot sterilizing chamber until the cycle is due to be started. Articles and wrapping materials to be sterilized by ethylene oxide should also be protected from dehydration while awaiting sterilization.

PACKAGING MATERIALS

The aim of packaging is to protect sterilized articles against recontamination until they are used. The requirements of a packaging material include:

1. Permeability to air, steam and gaseous sterilants (does not apply to dry heat or ionizing radiation)
2. Resistance to penetration by microorganisms
3. Resistance to punctures and tears
4. Suitability for moulding, closing and sealing
5. Freedom from loose fibres and particles
6. Freedom from toxic ingredients and non-fast dyes
7. Compatibility with sterilizing agent

8. Compatibility with contents under the proposed sterilizing conditions.

Closely woven cotton fabric, bleached kraft paper, drapable creped paper and paper combined with transparent plastic film to form a 'window pack' are commonly used in hospital sterilization processes because they are permeable to air, steam and chemical vapours. They do not provide an absolute bacterial barrier but are satisfactory for short term storage of sterilized packs if they are kept in a clean and dry condition. Medical grade paper is free from loose particles but liberates fibres if sealed packs are opened by tearing, cutting or by opening a fibre tear seal. Aluminium foil, aluminium tubes, and canisters made from aluminium, steel or copper are used for dry heat sterilization in hot air ovens. Glass and autoclavable plastic containers of a quality that does not liberate particles are used for water and parenteral solutions. A wide variety of synthetic materials is used for industrial packaging of medical devices. The types of packaging materials that are suitable for different sterilization processes are listed in Table 3.1. Before use, packaging materials should be allowed to equilibrate at room temperature (18–22°C) and at a relative humidity of 35–70 per cent for a minimum of two hours. Equilibration is especially important for large textile packs as a desiccated pack may prevent adequate steam penetration and lead to superheating (ANSI, ST46).

Cotton fabrics

Woven cotton material, such as unbleached calico (muslin in the United States) and newer cotton/polyester blends, are used for heavy packs that are sterilized in prevacuum or downward displacement steam sterilizers. They are less efficient as bacterial barriers than is kraft paper but are more resistant to tearing and will maintain sterility for several weeks in clean, dry storage conditions. Two layers of cloth or one of cloth and one of drapable paper, separately removable, should always be used. The cloth wrappings should be freshly laundered.

Papers

Papers including bleached kraft paper and newer

Table 3.1 Selection of packaging materials for sterilization

Process	Suitable packaging material
Steam sterilization	Papers Cellulose/synthetic wraps Cotton, cotton/polyester cloths Sterilizable cellophane Window packs (paper and heat-stable plastic) Perforated rigid containers with bacterial filters Glass containers for liquids (plastic containers for liquids sterilized commercially)
Dry heat sterilization (hot air oven)	Metal canisters Aluminium foil Glass tubes, bottles
Ethylene oxide sterilization	Paper and plastic (combined in window pack), papers Perforated rigid containers with bacterial filters
Low-temperature steam and formaldehyde process	Paper Cloth
Low-temperature plasma-based sterilization	Non-woven polypropylene wrap (e.g. Kimguard™ and Spunguard™) Tyvek® (spun polyethylene) Tyvek®/Mylar pouches
Abtox™Plazlyte™ plasma system	Paper Cotton (muslin)[1]

[1] Used only in the longest (3 h) cycle

wraps combining cellulose and synthetic fibres are commonly used packaging material for steam, dry heat and gas sterilization in hospitals. They are permeable to steam, air and chemical vapours and provide an effective bacterial barrier if the packs are stored in clean, dry conditions for relatively short periods. Paper absorbs hydrogen peroxide so is unsuitable for use in the Sterrad™ sterilization system in which hydrogen peroxide is used to generate plasma. It can be used in the Abtox™ Plazlyte™ system because the plasma is generated from an inert gas mixture. The impregnation of paper with resins improves its wet strength and water repellency without affecting permeability to sterilizing vapours and air. Such treated paper is often laminated to plastic film or metal foil.

Bleached kraft paper and the cellulose/synthetic medical wraps are the principal types used for hospital packaging procedures. Plain white paper is used for bags but creped paper, which has good draping quality and is not noisy to handle, is preferred for wrapping linen, instrument trays, and ward procedure packs. Bags may be made entirely from paper, or a web of paper may be joined to a web of transparent plastic film to produce a 'window pack'.

Standards, e.g. BS 6254 (1989) and BS 6255 (1989) for creped and plain papers and AS 1079 Part 2 (1994), apply to the quality of wrapping paper for use in sterilization. Physical properties which are subject to specification include weight (grammage), dry and wet bursting strength, dry and wet breaking load, water repellency, surface absorbency and draping quality. Chemical properties include the pH of the water extract and the content of chlorides and sulphates. The penetration of particles which are 0.5 μm or less in diameter may be determined by tests using a chemical dust, such as dioctyl phthalate or sodium chloride. Microbiological tests are more difficult to standardize.

Metals and metal containers

Aluminium foil may be used as a wrapping material for large articles, such as surgical drills, which are sterilized by dry heat. However, the foil tends to collapse around the article and pinholes may be produced where it creases. Of course, aluminium foil wrapping is impervious to steam and gaseous sterilizing agents. Metal canisters, which are made from aluminium, copper or stainless steel and are round or square in cross section, are used for holding glass pipettes (either graduated or Pasteur pipettes) for sterilization by dry heat. Metal containers with perforated lids and floors, which are lined by filter material, were used formerly in the Bowie-Dick test for air removal from textile packs in prevacuum steam sterilizers. However, because of the likelihood of overpacking, the routine use of such perforated metal containers for the sterilization of textiles generally has never been recommended.

Reusable rigid container systems

A new generation of reusable rigid containers which serve as a packaging method for the steam sterilization of large sets of surgical instruments has recently emerged. They are made from ferrous metals, aluminium, high-density polymers, or metal and plastic in combination (ANSI, ST33). The containers are generally rectangular, the size depending on the instrument set for which they are intended. They have perforations in both lid and base, or in the lid only if usage is restricted to prevacuum sterilizers or ethylene oxide processes which operate a vacuum in the cycle. The perforated panels are lined with steam permeable, high-efficiency filter material, which is firmly held in place on their inner surfaces by a retainer frame. Pressure-gradient valves which expand and open in the sterilizing stage and close during the postvacuum and cooling stage may be fitted as an alternative to perforations. A removable wire basket or perforated loading tray is part of the assembly.

The containers should be properly loaded in terms of density of the metalware to avoid problems of moisture retention and the need for increased drying times (Kneedler & Gattas, 1988). After each use, the containerized packaging system should be disassembled and cleaned by washing with a mild detergent, either manually or in a washer/disinfector machine. After sterilization, the containers can be conveniently stacked for storage without the threat of damage to their contents or contamination due to puncturing or tearing.

These reusable rigid container systems have gained wide acceptance for the sterilization of instruments. Advantages of the systems include time savings, ease of storage and protection of instruments, particularly delicate microsurgical instruments (Kneedler & Gattas, 1988). Published guidelines for the selection and use of reusable rigid sterilization container systems are available (ANSI, ST33).

Glass

Glass tubes, closed with non-absorbent cotton wool plugs or crimped foil caps may be used for dry heat sterilization of glass syringes and needles in a hot air oven, but they are poor conductors of heat. Needles should be supported so that the tip does not contact the wall of the container. Glass bottles, vials and ampoules are used for steam sterilization of aqueous liquids and lidded jars for dry heat sterilization of oils. Glass containers are unsuitable for gas sterilization because they are impermeable to vapours. They are inappropriate for radiation sterilization unless darkening of the glass is desired.

Synthetic materials and laminates

Synthetic non-woven polymers (plastics) are widely used, as flexible films and moulded containers, for industrial sterilization of medical devices by ionizing radiation and ethylene oxide. Flexible or semi-rigid plastic is also used for water and aqueous solutions that are sterilized commercially by heat. Plastics provide an absolute barrier to dust and microorganisms, permitting indefinite storage of sterile products if the seals are intact and the packaging material is free from pinholes, punctures and tears. They are robust, transparent and can be heat sealed. However, some materials are unstable to heat or to ionizing radiation.

Polyethylene (polythene)

Although polyethylene is heat-labile, it is widely used for small devices and dressing packs which are sterilized industrially by ethylene oxide or ionizing radiation. Ethylene oxide vapour will pass through a 0.076 mm thickness of low-density polyethylene by dissolving in the film and eluting from the inner surface (Ernst, 1973). However, the impermeability of polyethylene to air and water vapour makes it unsuitable for hospital use except as part of a composite pack with a web of permeable paper or as wraps for plasma sterilization.

High-density polyethylene is spun as a fine continuous fibre and bonded by heating to produce grades of paper-like material which is permeable to air and vapours (Marotta, 1981a). It is commonly referred to by the brand name Tyvek®. Although porous, it is water repellent and provides a satisfactory bacterial barrier for dry articles. It presents some problems in sealing and printing, but these may be overcome by the application of heat-seal lacquer coatings and by the use of inks which are not oil-based. Lacquered Tyvek® may be sealed to a transparent polyethylene/polyester laminate to make peelable pouches. As Tyvek® is expensive, it is used mainly as breathable lidding material for blister packs or as a peelable insert in a web of transparent material. A strip may be used to form a breathable seal by joining the edges along one side of a pack. Tyvek® has a tendency to electrostatic attraction of dust and fibres; an antistatic grade is unsuitable for sterilization because it is likely to contain pinholes.

Polyester

Oriented polyester film withstands steam sterilization. It is commonly used as a laminate with polyethylene, in which the polyethylene presents a heat-sealing surface and the outer layer of polyester provides a good printing surface.

Polyvinyl chloride (PVC)

PVC has low stability to heat and ionizing radiation. It absorbs a large amount of ethylene oxide which combines with phthalate plasticizer, from which it elutes very slowly under ambient conditions. However, suitable grades are widely used to make moulded bases for blister packs.

Polypropylene and polycarbonate

These heat-stable plastics are extensively used, separately or laminated together, as flexible, semi-rigid or rigid containers for heat sterilization of water and aqueous solutions. A laminate of nylon and polypropylene has also been used (Weymes, 1971). Polypropylene may also be laminated with aluminium foil for packaging wet or oily materials such as skin swabs and wound dressings. Polypropylene film is impermeable to ethylene oxide, moisture and air.

Nylon

Nylon film is heat stable and permeable to steam but is unsuitable for use as a wrapping material in prevacuum and downward displacement steam sterilizers because retention of air delays steam penetration and may cause the packs to burst. It is not stable to irradiation.

PACKAGE DESIGN

The number of layers of packaging material, the type of pack (two-dimensional or three-dimensional), the method of sealing and provision for extracting the articles aseptically are the principal features of package design. Although sterilization processes are designed to reduce the probability of an unsterile article to 1 in 10^6, this level of sterility assurance may be seriously compromised by careless opening of packs. The package should be designed to minimize the chance of contamination during opening and removal of the contents.

Number of layers

Individual product package

Individual products which are produced commercially may be enclosed in a single layer of wrapping material, or they may be double-wrapped to reduce the likelihood of contamination when the package is opened to remove the contents (Speers & Shooter, 1966; Hughes et al, 1967). The outer wrap is sealed and provides the bacterial barrier. The inner wrap, which is unsealed, acts as a protective cover during the removal of the article. Moulded plastic shields which cover hypodermic needles, the opening of syringe barrels and connections of intravenous administration sets perform the role of inner wraps as well as giving physical protection. Double wrapping is strongly recommended for urinary catheters, intravenous cannulae and other equipment that will be used in an aseptic environment, such as an operating room or a protective isolation unit (Duncan, 1972). It is unfortunate that the cost of double wrapping may defeat its purpose (Lewis, 1972; Rutter, 1972). If single-wrapped products are purchased to save money, they should be stored in the shelf carton or a clear plastic dust cover until they are used. Single wrapping is adequate for Ryles tubes, oesophageal and suction tubes, urine bags, mouth toilet and rectal examination sets, which do not penetrate to the blood stream or sterile tissue.

Surgical instrument and dressing packs that are sterilized in hospitals are wrapped in two separate layers of paper or cloth; the inner layer provides a sterile field when the pack is opened on table or tray in the operating room.

Ancillary packaging

In commercial production, cardboard cartons of appropriate thickness are commonly used as ancillary packaging for sterile goods. The individual packaged products may be packed in shelf storage cartons, each containing a relatively small number of articles. Several cartons are then enclosed in transport cartons, which must withstand predictable risks arising from pressure, rough handling or accidental dropping (Nyström, 1973). All layers of packaging material may be applied prior to industrial sterilization by ethylene oxide or gamma radiation. The transport container, which is soiled and contaminated in the outside environment, should be removed before the contents are taken into a storage area for sterile equipment.

TYPES OF PACKS

The wide variety of package designs may be grouped in three categories:

1. Wrapped packs
2. Formed bags and pouches
3. Moulded blister packs.

Wrapped packs

The sheets of paper and cloth which are used to wrap textile and instrument packs in hospitals may be folded in two different ways. In the parcel fold or square wrap used for large packs, the contents are placed parallel to the edges of the wrapping sheets, which are folded to overlap the centre line. The edges are turned back to facilitate aseptic opening. The ends are then turned in and folded, one over the other. Large packs are tied with cord. An envelope wrap or diagonal fold is suitable for small packs, such as wound dressing trays and ward instrument sets. The pack is placed diagonally and slightly off centre on the wrapping sheet. Three folds are made by bringing the corners to the centre and each corner is turned back to provide a flap for opening. The larger fold is then brought over the top and tucked in, with a corner protruding.

Two wrapping sheets are used in the typical double-wrapping procedure to ensure protection of the contents. Each sheet may consist of two double-thickness woven wrappers, two non-woven wrappers, or a combination. The packs are first wrapped with one sheet and then the other in sequence giving a parcel within a parcel. The outer wrap is fastened, usually with autoclave indicator tape, and labelled. Large packs may be tied with cord. The two methods of wrapping packs are illustrated for the inner wraps only in Figure 3.1.

Bags and pouches

Paper bags may be gussetted to facilitate filling and to separate the broken edges when the article is removed. The glued joints must be as strong as the paper. The bottom of the bag should be folded twice, with each fold glued and a peelable seal may be provided at the top. A protruding lip or thumb cut assists filling. Window packs that are made by sealing plain or treated paper to a transparent plastic film are used in hospitals as well as in industry. They may be cut from a continuous roll and sealed at both ends, or they may be supplied individually with a peelable seal at one end.

Flat pouches for industrial sterilization may be constructed entirely from plastic films, or from a combination of paper and plastic or paper and metal foil, depending on the sterilization process and the intended use of the article. When a single type of film is used, the package may be formed from a cut length of lay-flat tubing, or from a flat piece of film which is folded and sealed along three edges. When webs of different material are used, the four edges are sealed (Powell, 1973).

Laminates of polyester, nylon or cellulose are suitable for dry articles. Plain or treated paper or spun-bonded polyethylene (Tyvek®) is used for one side of the pack if permeability to air, moisture and ethylene oxide is required. Wet devices, such as impregnated sponges or skin swabs, wound dressings, sutures in alcohol, gels and solutions, must be packaged in materials that are proof against leaching or leaking and are solvent and grease resistant, chemically inert and capable of being sealed through a film of the liquid or grease (Marotta, 1982a). Aluminium foil, laminated with plastics such as polypropylene,

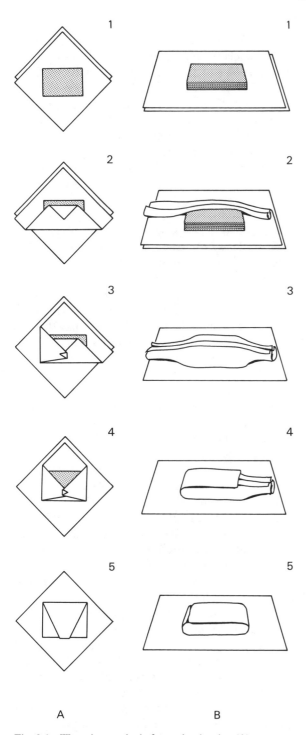

Fig. 3.1 Wrapping methods for packs showing (A) envelope fold or diagonal wrap and (B) parcel fold or square wrap. Inner wraps only illustrated; steps 1–5 are repeated for outer wraps (© 1988 Association for the Advancement of Medical Instrumentation).

polycarbonate, nylon, polyethylene or polyester, may be used for swabs, dressings and sutures. An inner layer of pinhole-free polyester is essential for swabs soaked in a povidone-iodine disinfectant because iodine attacks aluminium. A package made from a film and foil laminate, sealed to a polyethylene/ metallized polyester laminate, is resistant to puncturing and suitable for gels. Polypropylene/ polycarbonate laminates have been used as containers for sterilizing water. Transparent, flexible packaging is widely used for intravenous solutions; it has the advantage that air, which may introduce microbial contaminants, is not drawn in as the container empties.

When two-dimensional packs are used for solid articles, sufficient material must be used to ensure that the article does not break through the seal if, for example, a carton is dropped during transport. The extra material adds to the cost of packaging and increases the storage space required.

Blister packs

Blister packs are used industrially to accommodate solid articles in the minimum amount of material. Tubular semi-rigid packs are used for urinary catheters. The most common form of three-dimensional pack is a moulded tray, conforming to the shape of the contents, with flanges that are sealed to a flat lid. The trays may be made from PVC, polystyrene, polyester, acrylic or cellulosic material. These materials may be laminated to polyethylene to provide a heat-sealing surface. The lid is made from coated Tyvek® or treated paper when permeability to air and vapours is required. Advantages of three-dimensional packs are avoidance of stress on the seal, economy of material and decrease in storage space. However, an inner wrap cannot be accommodated (Lewis, 1972; Powell, 1973). The industrial use of blister packs has increased as automated packaging methods have been developed.

CLOSING AND SEALING

Packs that are wrapped in hospitals are fastened with autoclave tape and may also be tied. Paper bags which are not provided with heat-sealing surfaces should be closed by turning in the corners, folding the open edges three times and fastening with autoclave tape; a piece at the centre of the fold is sufficient. Staples must never be used because they perforate the packaging material. Heat sealing is performed by pressing the lacquered surfaces between heated plates; the temperature, pressure and contact time must be accurately set and controlled. Creases may result in faulty seals. Gussetted bags may be difficult to seal because the thickness across the sealing area is uneven. When paper is heat-sealed to polyethylene film, the plastic melts and flows into the paper. Paper to paper and paper to plastic seals may release fibres when opened. These can cause adverse reactions if they gain access to human tissues (Marotta, 1983).

A wider variety of sealing methods is used for industrial packaging. The seals may be plain or they may be crimped parallel with the edge of the pack or at right angles to it. Channels may develop in the seal if the crimping plates are not perfectly aligned. Peelable seals facilitate opening and are less likely to disturb microorganisms on the surface of the pack but the flaps that are provided for opening should be folded or fastened together to prevent access of dust to the sealing area (Powell, 1973). However, a double wrapped pack provides better protection for its contents than does a peelable pack made from a single layer of wrapping material. The strength of a peelable seal is a compromise between maintenance of package integrity and ease of opening. The effect of the sterilization process on the seal must be taken into account. Heat seals are weakened during steam sterilization but usually return to the normal condition on cooling. Sterilization by ethylene oxide, plasma or radiation does not have a significant effect on seals.

Most peelable seals are of the non-fibre tear type, made from combinations of lacquered or latex coated paper, plastic films, coated metal foil and laminates. Tyvek® must be coated for heat sealing to other types of material and cannot be sealed above 150°C because it has a low melting point. It produces a non-fibre tear seal and is commonly used as lidding for blister packs. Polyethylene film and polyethylene/polyester laminates seal readily to many materials, polyethylene acting as the sealant. Polypropylene, polycarbonate and nylon are suitable sealants for aqueous dressings which are sterilized by steam at 120–

124°C. Special resin coatings are required for sealing aluminium foil packs containing wet skin-cleansing swabs, antiseptic dressings or vaseline gauze. Solvent-resistant, peelable adhesives are used for packs containing sutures in alcohol.

Different methods are used to make breathable seals for packs that are impermeable to ethylene oxide (Marotta, 1981b); however, package integrity may be compromised. A strip of fibrous material may be incorporated in the sealing area, or the unsealed edges may be joined externally by a strip of Tyvek®, which may be peeled off to open the pack. Syringes are sometimes packaged in moulded plastic containers, closed by overlapping caps which are spot welded at one point to the base. These cannot be recommended because the maintenance of sterility depends on a tortuous path to the interior of the pack and the effectiveness of the system cannot be proven.

Sealed packs should always be inspected for integrity before they are opened. Faults in fibre tear seals might not be detected before opening unless one web is transparent (Marotta, 1982b).

PACKAGE TESTING

The essential function of a package as a barrier to dust and microorganisms may be lost for a variety of causes which include:

1. Use of poor quality or unsuitable packaging material
2. Failure to establish and maintain the integrity of the pack
3. Lack of provision for opening aseptically.

The functions of physical protection, identification of the contents and labelling with instructions for use must also be taken into account when assessing the efficiency of packaging.

Medical grade paper is manufactured to specifications for physical and chemical properties, resistance to air flow and penetration by chemical dusts. Standards are also available for paper bags (BS 6257, 1989; AS 1079 Part 3, 1994) and for flexible packaging systems (AS 1079 Part 4, 1988) for sterilization for medical use. Specifications cover types and dimensions, materials and construction, marking and labelling, and performance standards including impact resistance, tensile strength, process stability and seam and seal integrity. The tests that are described below are concerned with the performance of porous packaging materials as bacterial barriers, the detection of pinholes and the integrity of sealed packs.

Tests for bacterial penetration (Schneider, 1980)

The paper and other porous wrapping materials that are used for steam or gas sterilization processes must be permeable to air, steam and the chemical vapour. Effectiveness as a bacterial barrier cannot be deduced from airflow measurements. Tests for penetration by chemical dusts, such as sodium chloride with an average diameter of 0.6 μm or dioctyl phthalate (DOP) particles with an average diameter of 0.3 μm, are most reliable. Microbiological methods have been described but the conditions are difficult to standardize and they suffer from problems of reproducibility. Some tests involve inoculating a bacterial culture on one side of the material to be tested and placing the other side in contact with a solid or liquid culture medium for a specified time. The medium is then incubated to detect growth. The sample may be placed between Rodac plates; one is inoculated with the test organism and the other is incubated to detect growth. In a similar method, the sample is mounted on the rim of a wide-mouth bottle containing nutrient broth and the bottle is inverted to place the sample in contact with an agar plate. In a more elaborate method, a bacterial aerosol is drawn through the sample at a specified velocity and the bacteria that pass through are collected on a membrane filter for culture and counting. Per cent penetration is calculated from the density of the aerosol and the volume that passed through the paper.

Tests in actual storage conditions are time consuming, extending to weeks or months. Sterilized packs are placed in dusty, draughty conditions and penetration is detected by culturing cotton wool swabs that were placed inside the wrapping material. A simulated storage test in which the material is placed over the mouth of a bottle containing nutrient broth and stored in adverse conditions is also prolonged.

Tests for pinholes

A pinhole in porous material, such as paper or spun-bonded polyethylene, is any aperture that is larger than the normal range of pore diameter. Any opening is significant in non-woven plastics and metal foil. Pinholes are caused by fold lines or creases in paper and metal foil; they are unlikely to occur when two layers of material are laminated together because the chance of holes at the same place in both layers is remote.

Pinholes in aluminium foil can be detected by holding the sample over a strong light beam in a darkened room. If an electric discharge is applied to films with a low moisture content, the openings can be detected by sparks. Other methods involve passage of a dye solution through the sample to a piece of white paper underneath, or of ammonia to a filter paper impregnated with ferrous ferrocyanide; the filter paper turns white.

Tests for package integrity

Physical, chemical and microbiological tests for package integrity are designed to reveal a variety of faults. Fifty per cent of faults have been attributed to poor sealing due to faulty equipment or the use of incompatible materials. Seals may break if insufficient material has been used to make the pack or if cartons are dropped during transportation. Punctures, tears or pinholes in the packaging material may be caused by unprotected sharp or rough edges within the pack or by stress during filling. Most of the tests for integrity of sealed packs involve destruction of the pack and can only be carried out by selecting samples for testing.

Limit testing, or testing for an acceptable value short of destruction, has been suggested as an alternative to destructive testing. However, the drawback is that the procedure may weaken the package leaving it with insufficient strength to withstand subsequent handling abuse. For destructive testing, the conditions of testing should simulate actual stresses of use and the selection and size of the sample and analysis of results should be statistically based (Hirsch, 1981).

A break in the bacterial barrier, such as a faulty seal, a hole or a tear, can usually be detected by inspection. The person who intends to use the article should always inspect the pack before opening it. Physical tests for integrity may be carried out in the following ways (Powell, 1973):

1. A waterproof pack is squeezed under water
2. The pack is placed in a vacuum desiccator; it should distend on evacuation and return to normal when atmospheric pressure is restored
3. A solution of dye is injected into a plastic pack, the hole is sealed and the outside surface is inspected for stains. A similar type of test using carbon black has been used to test the corners of paper packs (Thompson, 1969).

Microbiological tests may be carried out by immersing the packs in a bacterial suspension or tumbling them in a closed vessel containing a bacterial aerosol; after disinfection of the exterior surfaces, the pack is opened aseptically and the contents are cultured.

MAINTENANCE OF STERILITY

The contents of sterilized packs may become recontaminated during transport, storage or removal for use. Causes of recontamination include damage to the packaging material, broken seals, unclean storage conditions and unsatisfactory methods of opening the packs.

Transport

Commercial products may be transported over short distances by the manufacturer but public transport by land, sea or air must be used for distribution to country, interstate or international destinations. Hazards that could lead to contamination include rough handling, accidental dropping and gross soiling of the containers.

Within hospitals, trolleys, service lifts, passenger lifts or ducted systems may be used for distribution of sterile supplies to the departments where they are used. Closed trolleys or sterilized boxes should be used unless the articles are contained in shelf storage cartons or plastic dust covers.

Storage

Packs from steam sterilizers should be cooled on open mesh shelves to prevent wetting of porous wrapping material by condensate. Equipment that has been sterilized in the hospital is transferred directly to a special store that is free from dust, draughts and dampness. Sudden temperature changes, which cause air movement that could carry microorganisms through porous material, should be avoided. The packs should be handled, as little as possible, by staff with clean, dry hands. Commercially sterilized supplies may be kept in the same store after they have been removed from the outer transport containers in a nonsterile area (see Ch. 14).

Storage facilities in operating rooms, wards and diagnostic departments should conform to the same standard of hygiene as is practised in the central store. Cupboards are superior to open shelves, as shown in Table 3.2. Packs which are placed in drawers may be damaged. Shelf storage cartons or plastic dust covers should be retained until the articles are taken to the place where they will be opened for use.

Duration of sterility

Hospital staff enquire frequently about the duration of shelf life for sterile articles. There is no simple answer to this question because efficiency of packaging, amount of handling and conditions of transport and storage are more important than is the time that has elapsed since sterilization. Studies on the maintenance of sterility under normal storage conditions are time consuming and involve testing a large number of packs. However, the studies by Standard et al (1971, 1973), summarized in Table 3.2, show that one layer of crepe paper provides the same duration of sterility as do two layers of cloth, and that storage life may be prolonged indefinitely if an impervious dust cover is used. Although prediction of a meaningful shelf life for packaged equipment is not feasible, it is good hospital practice to avoid prolonged storage by ensuring rotational use. This may be achieved by organizing the distribution of supplies to prevent unnecessary hoarding. A small number of packs, containing emergency equipment that is rarely required but must always be available, may be kept for several months if they are placed in impervious dust covers after sterilization.

Table 3.2 Storage life of dressing packs (Standard et al, 1971, 1973)

Types of wrappings	Storage conditions	Duration of sterility (days)
Single cotton fabric[1]	Open shelves	3–14
	Closed shelves	14–21
Double cotton fabric	Open shelves	28–56
	Closed shelves	56–77
Single creped paper	Open shelves	28–49; >63
	Closed shelves	>63; >91
Single cotton cloth plus single paper	Open shelves	77–98
Single cotton cloth with polyethylene bag	Open shelves	>9 months

[1] A single wrapper of cotton fabric consisted of two layers stitched together at the edges

REFERENCES

ANSI/AAMI ST33 — 1990 Good hospital practice: guidelines for the selection and use of reusable rigid sterilization container systems. American National Standards Institute, New York
ANSI/AAMI ST46 — 1993 Good hospital practice: steam sterilization and sterility assurance. American National Standards Institute, New York
AS 1079.2 Part 2 1994 Packaging of items (sterile) for patient care. Non-reusable papers — for the wrapping of goods undergoing sterilization in health care facilities. Standards Australia, Homebush, NSW
AS 1079.3 Part 3 1994 Packaging of items (sterile) for patient care. Paper bags — for single use in health care facilities. Standards Australia, Homebush, NSW
AS 1079.4 Part 4 1988 Packaging of items (sterile) for patient care. Flexible packaging systems — for single use in hospitals. Standards Association of Australia, Sydney
AS 2711 1993 Washer/disinfectors for respiratory apparatus. Standards Australia, Homebush, NSW
AS 4187 1994 Code of practice for cleaning, disinfecting and sterilizing reusable medical and surgical instruments and equipment, and maintenance of associated environments in health care facilities. Standards Australia, Homebush, NSW
BS 2745.1 Part 1 1993 Washer-disinfectors for medical purposes. Specification for general requirements. British Standards Institution, London
BS 2745.3 Part 3 1993 Washer-disinfectors for medical purposes. Specification for washer-disinfectors except those

used for processing human-waste containers and laundry. British Standards Institution, London

BS 6254 1989 British Standard specification for creped sterilization paper for medical use. British Standards Institution, London

BS 6255 1989 British Standard specification for plain sterilization paper for medical use. British Standards Institution, London

BS 6257 1989 British Standard specification for paper bags for steam sterilization for medical use. British Standards Institution, London

Centers for Disease Control 1987 Recommendations for prevention of HIV transmission in health-care settings. Morbidity and Mortality Weekly Report 36 (Suppl 2S): 3S–18S

Centers for Disease Control 1988 Update: Universal precautions for prevention of transmission of human immunodeficiency virus, hepatitis B virus and other bloodborne pathogens in health-care settings. Morbidity and Mortality Weekly Report 37: 377–388

Detwiler M S 1989 Ultrasonic cleaning in the hospital. Journal of Healthcare Materiel Management 7(3): 46–48, 50

Duncan M H 1972 Double-wrapping — is it really necessary? Part VI. Journal of the Association of Sterile Supply Administrators 1 (2): 12–14

Ernst R R 1973 Ethylene oxide gaseous sterilization for industrial applications. In: Phillips G B, Miller W S (eds) Industrial sterilization : international symposium, Amsterdam, 1972. Duke University Press, Durham, ch 12, p 181

Harrison S K, Evans W J Jr, LeBlanc D A, Bush L W 1990 Cleaning and decontaminating medical instruments. Journal of Healthcare Materiel Management 8 (1): 36–42

Hirsch A 1981 Packaging forum. Is this test necessary? Medical Device & Diagnostic Industry 3 (4): 14–15, 63

Hughes K E A, Drewett S E, Darmady E M 1967 The risk of contamination of sterile dressings packed in paper bags. British Hospital Journal and Social Service Review 77: 764–765, 781

Kneedler J A, Gattas M 1988 A study of sterilization containers. Journal of Healthcare Materiel Management 6(4): 24–28, 30

Lewis C 1972 Double-wrapping — is it really necessary? Part V. Journal of the Association of Sterile Supply Administrators 1(2): 9–12

Marotta C 1981a Tyvek: 'wonder' material of sterile packaging. Medical Device & Diagnostic Industry 3 (5): 18–20

Marotta C 1981b Vented flexible packaging. Medical Device & Diagnostic Industry 3 (9): 33–34

Marotta C 1982a High-barrier packaging for wet devices. Medical Device & Diagnostic Industry 4 (1): 21–22

Marotta C 1982b Tamper-evident packaging. Medical Device & Diagnostic Industry 4 (7): 18, 54

Marotta C D 1983 Particulate contamination in packaging materials. Medical Device & Diagnostic Industry 5 (1): 20, 22–23

Meredith H G 1977 Corrosion of surgical instruments. Journal of the Association of Sterile Supply Administrators 6 (1): 6–8, 10–11

Mitchell E 1974 Merits or otherwise of sterilising theatre and other instruments prior to handling by staff of CSSD/TSSU, Part 1. Journal of the Association of Sterile Supply Administrators 3 (2): 5–6

Nyström B 1973 Handling sterile products in the hospital. In: Phillips G B, Miller W S (eds) Industrial sterilization: international symposium, Amsterdam, 1972. Duke University Press, Durham, ch 20, p 359

Powell D B 1973 Packaging of sterile medical products. In: Phillips G B, Miller W S (eds) Industrial sterilization: international symposium, Amsterdam, 1972. Duke University Press, Durham, ch 5, p 79

Rutter B 1972 Double-wrapping — is it really necessary? Part IV. Journal of the Association of Sterile Supply Administrators 1 (2): 6, 8–9

Ryan P, Romey S 1989 Instrument 'milk': the controversy continues. Survey on instrument lubrication. Journal of Healthcare Materiel Management 7 (6): 26–28, 32–34, 36

Schneider P M 1980 Microbiological evaluation of package and packaging-material integrity. Medical Device & Diagnostic Industry 2 (5): 29–37

Speers R Jr, Shooter R A 1966 The use of double-wrapped packs to reduce contamination of the sterile contents during extraction. Lancet ii: 469–470

Standard P G, Mackel D C, Mallison G F 1971 Microbial penetration of muslin- and paper-wrapped sterile packs stored on open shelves and in closed cabinets. Applied Microbiology 22: 432–437

Standard P G, Mallison G F, Mackel D C 1973 Microbial penetration through three types of double wrappers for sterile packs. Applied Microbiology 26: 59–62

Thompson R E M 1969 Testing the seals of paper packs. British Hospital Journal and Social Service Review 79: 1397–1398

Weymes C 1971 Sterilisation of water for topical use in plastic bags. British Hospital Journal and Social Service Review 81: 1553, 1555, 1557

Weymes C 1973 The Scottish scene and the present position of sterile supply in the United Kingdom. Journal of the Association of Sterile Supply Administrators 2 (2): 26–27

4. Principles of heat sterilization

Heat is generally regarded as the most reliable, readily available and economical method of sterilization for materials that are stable to temperatures above 121°C in wet conditions or above 160°C in dry conditions. The time required for sterilization decreases as the temperature is raised and many different combinations of temperature and time are equivalent in lethality. A set of parameters can be selected, therefore, that will achieve sterilization with minimum damage to heat-sensitive materials.

This chapter deals with the following topics:

Moist and dry heat
Mechanisms of biocidal action
Heat resistance of microorganisms
Factors influencing heat resistance
Design of heat sterilization processes.

MOIST AND DRY HEAT

The terms moist heat and dry heat, as applied to sterilization processes, refer to the moisture levels in the heating environment and the microbial cells. Moisture level is not identical with water content; it refers to the free, available water in a gaseous or liquid system. Moisture levels in air, steam or other gaseous environments are defined by relative humidity (RH). This is the water vapour content at a given temperature, expressed as per cent of the saturation content at that temperature. The RH scale ranges from zero to 100 per cent.

$$\% \text{ RH} = \frac{\text{actual water vapour content}}{\text{maximum at existing temperature}} \times 100$$

The moisture level of aqueous liquids is expressed as water activity (a_w):

$$a_w = \frac{\text{vapour pressure of solution}}{\text{vapour pressure of pure water}}$$

A_w values are always less than unity because the vapour pressure of solutions is less than that of pure water. If a_w values are multiplied by 100, they correspond to relative humidity; thus water activities of 0.2, 0.4 and 1.0 are equivalent to relative humidities of 20, 40 and 100 per cent respectively. Microbial protoplasm is a concentrated solution of organic and inorganic substances. The water activity within living cells cannot be measured directly but is assumed to be equivalent to that of the liquid in which the microorganisms are suspended or the relative humidity of air or other gases in their immediate gaseous environment.

The term moist heat is restricted to the condition of moisture saturation in the microorganisms and the heating environment. This exists when the organisms are in equilibrium with pure water or saturated steam. The term dry heat implies the absence of liquid water from the heating environment; it may refer to any moisture level from zero to just below saturation.

MECHANISMS OF BIOCIDAL ACTION

All types of microorganisms can be killed by moist or dry heat at a temperature appropriate to their level of resistance. This broad spectrum of biocidal action suggests that death is the result of physical or chemical changes that result in denaturation of major cell constituents, such as proteins or nucleic acids. Denaturation of proteins involves the rupture of bonds that maintain their coiled polypeptide chains in the configuration which is essential for specific functions, such as enzyme activity. Denaturation may lead to coagulation or precipitation.

Evidence for coagulation of proteins as the major cause of thermal death in microorganisms has been obtained by comparing the influence of moisture on the temperature required for protein denaturation and enzyme inactivation in vitro with its influence on the temperature required for biocidal action. Lewith (1890) observed that the temperature at which egg albumin coagulated in 30 minutes increased from 56°C in excess water to 74–80°C, 145°C and 160–170°C as the water content was reduced to 25 per cent, 6 per cent and finally zero. The protection of a purified enzyme (luciferase) against inactivation by heat was demonstrated by Chappelle et al (1967), who found that it retained 40 per cent of its activity when heated to 135°C for 36 hours in a gel under conditions of low moisture and oxygen content. These effects are similar to the influence of moisture on the biocidal action of heat. Bacterial spores are killed rapidly at 121°C in saturated steam but the temperature must be increased to 160°C for a comparable death rate in dry conditions. Additional support for protein denaturation as the major mechanism of thermal death is provided by the similarity of the activation energies of the two processes (Rosenberg et al, 1971). Nucleic acids are also denatured by moist heat (Brannen, 1970) but coagulation of cytoplasmic proteins and the resulting inactivation of enzymes is probably sufficient to account for thermal death in the presence of moisture. At extremely low moisture levels, coagulation is replaced by other processes including oxidative destruction.

Most of the information about the biocidal action of heat has come from studies on bacterial spores at rapidly lethal temperatures. The primary cellular target cannot be determined in these conditions, but Allwood & Russell (1967) demonstrated initial damage to the cell membrane during sublethal heat treatment of *Staphylococcus aureus* in water at 50–60°C. Impairment of the essential function of the membrane as a semipermeable barrier resulted in the leakage of amino acids, nucleic acid constituents and other essential metabolites from the cells. This eventually resulted in death of the bacteria from loss of vital constituents but they recovered if they were transferred to favourable growth conditions before the loss was too great. Studies on cells of *Bacillus cereus* (Silva & Sousa, 1972) with the aid of electron microscopy confirmed that sublethal heat treatment affected the structure of the cell membrane. When the temperature was raised above 60°C, coagulation occurred throughout the cytoplasm and the action was biocidal. The production of single-strand breaks in the DNA of *Enterococcus faecalis* by sublethal heat treatment (Andrew & Greaves, 1979) and of bacterial spores by lethal heat treatment (Grecz & Bruszer, 1981) has been described.

HEAT RESISTANCE OF MICROORGANISMS

Vegetative microorganisms

Vegetative bacteria, including *Mycobacterium tuberculosis*, are generally killed rapidly in hot water (65–100°C). *E. faecalis* has the highest resistance among the common species but a Gram-negative bacterium, *Thermus aquaticus*, grows in thermal springs at 70°C (Brock & Freeze, 1969). Similar heat-tolerant, non-sporing bacteria have been isolated from hospital hot water supplies (Pask-Hughes & Williams, 1975). The heat resistance of salmonellae in foods increases with decreasing water activity but varies with the strain and species of *Salmonella* and its growth conditions as well as the nature and composition of the food. *Salmonella* Senftenberg strain 775W, which was originally isolated from dried eggs, is particularly noted for its resistance to moist heat (Baird-Parker et al, 1970; Goepfert et al, 1970). *Listeria monocytogenes* is more heat-resistant than are the common serotypes of salmonellae and many other non-sporing, food-borne pathogens but it is not as resistant to heat as is *Salmonella* Senftenberg 775W. Cooking food to an internal temperature of 70°C for 2 minutes will destroy *L. monocytogenes*. Pasteurization will also kill *L. monocytogenes* in milk but the margin of safety is greater for vat pasteurization at 62.8°C for 30 minutes than it is for high temperature short time (HTST) pasteurization at 71.5°C for 15 seconds (Mackey & Bratchell, 1989). Although legionellae prefer water at warm temperatures, they are readily inactivated by moist heat. The D values for species of *Legionella* at temperatures of 60, 70 and 80°C range from 1.3 to 10.6, 0.7 to 2.6 and 0.3 to 0.7 minutes (Stout et al, 1986).

Most viruses and fungi are also killed at temperatures in the range of 65 to 100°C but boiling or autoclaving is recommended for the inactivation of viruses in association with blood and tissues, e.g. hepatitis B virus and HIV. Since HIV is inactivated by moist heat at 60°C for 30 minutes (Cuthbertson et al, 1987), these viruses are probably killed by boiling water within a few minutes but a period of 20 minutes of boiling is recommended (World Health Organization, 1988). Dry-heating at 60°C or 68°C for 72 hours inactivates HIV in freeze-dried concentrates of coagulation factor; dry-heating at 80°C for 72 hours inactivates hepatitis C virus in the freeze-dried concentrates (Colvin et al, 1988). Although heating at 134°C for 18 minutes in a prevacuum steam sterilizer has been recommended for the inactivation of the Creutzfeldt-Jakob agent in brain tissue (Kimberlin et al, 1983), recent findings indicate that this regime might not completely inactivate the agent (Taylor et al, 1994). Currently, 136°C for 1 hour is being used (Taylor, 1996).

Amoebic cysts of the parasite *Acanthamoeba polyphaga*, which causes infection in contact lens wearers, also require temperatures of 65°C or more for inactivation by moist heat. Kilvington (1989) reported D values of 3.75 minutes at 65°C and 30 seconds at 70°C for a strain of *A. polyphaga* isolated from a case of keratitis. He found that moist heat at 56–60°C was ineffective even after a contact time of 60 minutes.

Bacterial spores

Temperatures exceeding 100°C are usually required to kill bacterial spores but the level of heat resistance varies widely according to the species. Spores of *Clostridium botulinum* type E, *Bacillus anthracis* and *Clostridium perfringens* are relatively sensitive. Most pathogenic species, including *Clostridium tetani*, produce more resistant spores. The highest resistance occurs in thermophilic species, such as *Bacillus stearothermophilus*. Types of microorganisms are grouped in Table 4.1 according to their relative resistance to moist heat.

Resistance also varies with pH, e.g. Davey (1993) reported that *C. botulinum* spores in neutral food (pH 7) require a sterilization time five-fold that for acid food. He described a general procedure for predicting sterilization times in foods which accounts for the effects of pH.

It is difficult to make valid comparisons for dry heat resistance from published reports because the moisture level at which the tests were carried out has not always been known. However, Bond & Favero (1975) obtained D values of 2.5 hours at 150°C and 139 hours at 125°C for spores of a resistant *Bacillus* sp. (ATCC 27380) from soil.

Mechanisms of heat resistance

The mechanisms underlying the high resistance of

Table 4.1 Resistance of microorganisms to moist heat

Grades of resistance	Types of microorganisms (examples)
Extremely susceptible	Non-sporing bacteria (including *M. tuberculosis*) Viruses (not protected by biological material) Moulds and yeasts (vegetative growth stages)
Moderately susceptible	Viruses (with blood or tissue) Mould spores Group D enterococci (e.g. *E. faecalis*)
Slightly resistant	Spores of: *B. anthracis* *C. botulinum* type E *C. perfringens*
Moderately resistant	Spores of: *B. subtilis* *C. botulinum* type A *C. tetani*
Highly resistant	Spores of: *B. stearothermophilus*
Extremely resistant	Prions (e.g. Creutzfeldt-Jakob agent)

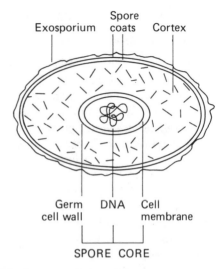

Fig. 4.1 Structure of a bacterial spore.

1981). This indicates that, although water is unequally distributed among spore structures, the a_w level within spores is about 0.7.

A concise account of spore structure, chemical composition and certain developmental aspects, along with theories on mechanisms of water distribution and heat resistance, follows. Figure 4.1 is a simplified diagram of a mature spore.

Exosporium

An exosporium is not present in all species. It may be loose-fitting or closely adherent to the underlying spore coats and consists mainly of protein. Its presence is not required for heat resistance and no other function has been assigned to it.

Spore coats

Electron microscopy reveals a complex structure of at least three layers, with a striated pattern in the centre. The coats consist mainly of proteins, with smaller amounts of carbohydrates, lipids and phosphorus-containing material. They are resistant to proteolytic enzymes and serve to protect the cortex against enzymic destruction by lysozyme (Koshikawa et al, 1984).

Cortex

The cortex is the most prominent of the layers that surround the spore core, occupying a wide zone

bacterial spores to heat and other biocidal agents have been the subject of speculation and experimental studies since they were discovered a century ago. Nevertheless, how spores become, and remain, resistant to heat is still not understood (Warburg et al, 1986). The refractility of mature spores provided an early indication that their resistance to heat and lack of metabolic activity might be associated with a low water content. Measurement of the water content of the spore cores, or protoplasts, of 28 strains of seven *Bacillus* spp. gave a range of 28 to 57 per cent w/w on a wet weight basis. Heat resistance of the spores increased with increasing protoplast dehydration. However, although dehydration is the major determinant of thermoresistance, spore resistance also increased as the temperature at which sporulation occurs increases and as protoplasts are remineralized with calcium (Beaman & Gerhardt, 1986). A water activity of 0.73, corresponding to a water content of 28 per cent, was shown to provide extracted spore enzymes with the same stability against heat inactivation as exists in the intact spore (Warth, between the coats and the germ cell wall. The electron microscope does not reveal any structure when the spore is intact but a network of fine fibres is revealed by a special staining method when the cortex swells during germination or as a result of artificial disruption of the spore. Swelling does not cause outward expansion of the cortex but the inner surface, adjacent to the germ cell wall, becomes densely folded. The principal component of the cortex is a peptidoglycan which is unique in its structural composition in that the glycan chains are loosely cross-linked (Popham & Setlow, 1993). The porous cortex is assumed to contain most of the spore water. The lytic enzymes that break down the peptidoglycan during spore germination may be the only proteins in the cortex. The cortex is essential for heat resistance, which does not develop until its formation is at least 90 per cent complete (Imae & Strominger, 1976).

Spore core (protoplast)

The central region of the spore is the spore core, or protoplast, which contains a full complement of the macromolecular constituents of the living cell; that is, nucleic acids, ribosomes, enzymes and lipids. These make up 50–60 per cent of the dry weight of the core. The other core components are low molecular weight substances, e.g. small acid-soluble proteins (SASP) that differ from proteins in vegetative cells. All of the dipicolinic acid (DPA), a compound that is unique to the bacterial spore, is located in the core (Leanz & Gilvarg, 1973). DPA is considered to be closely associated with cations in the spore core, particularly calcium. However, mineral uptake tends to precede DPA synthesis and minerals and DPA can be extracted separately from spore cores. The spore core is already dehydrated before synthesis of DPA or of the cortex begins. Any remaining water in the spore core is probably displaced by the dipicolinic acid, which can constitute up to 15 per cent of the dry weight of the spore.

The result of the severe dehydration is likely to be an amorphous, immobile matrix in which the concentrated, molecular components are tightly packed, together with a small amount of water in the bound state. Beaman & Gerhardt (1986) postulate that the lower limit of protoplast water of

28 per cent w/w corresponds to a threshold concentration at which the remaining water is held in a bound state. The immobility accompanying the severe dehydration in the vital spore core is associated with dormancy of the spore and with resistance to physical and chemical agents.

Regulatory mechanisms

The significance of DPA in the establishment or maintenance of heat resistance has received much attention. A consistent relationship between the amount of DPA in the spore and the degree of resistance has not been found; different species, or different types within a species, may contain similar amounts of DPA but vary widely in heat resistance (Murrell & Warth, 1965). Studies of mutant spores have also given equivocal results; a strain of *B. cereus* which lacked DPA was resistant although the resistance was readily lost (Hanson et al, 1972) whereas a strain of *Bacillus subtilis* which lacked DPA was not heat resistant unless supplied with exogenous DPA (Balassa et al, 1979).

A role for spore coats in thermal resistance of spores was proposed by Gorman et al (1985), who found that damage to, or removal of, the spore coats reduced the thermoresistance of spores of *B. subtilis* NCTC 10073, although the effect was not of great magnitude; the spores retained their refractility and full complement of DPA. In contrast, Senesi et al (1992) reported that spores of *B. cereus* NCIB 8122 that had been chemically depleted of their spore coats showed no decrease in heat resistance; these spores also retained their refractility and full complement of DPA.

Heat resistance is more closely associated with the cortex, which contains no DPA (Leanz & Gilvarg, 1973). Warburg et al (1986) have isolated and investigated heat-sensitive mutant spores of *B. subtilis* which retained their normal DPA content and showed no abnormality other then visibly defective cortices when examined by electron microscopy. The main role of the cortex appears to be the maintenance of the heat resistance after it has been established in the spore core. However, theories for an active role in the attainment of protoplast dehydration, by the squeezing out or drawing away of water from the spore core, have also been proposed.

The first theory involving a contractile cortex (Lewis et al, 1960) was abandoned when the expanded, water-filled structure of the peptidoglycan polymer was established. A similar fate has overtaken the proposal of Gould & Dring (1975) that a high osmotic pressure in the cortex, attributed to a surplus of electronegative groups on the peptidoglycan polymer and the mobile potassium ions that counterbalance them, might draw water away from the core, which is assumed to have a low osmotic pressure. Osmotic pressure has been ruled out as a major control mechanism because the calculated osmotic pressure in the cortex would only reduce the water activity in the core to about 0.97 — far short of the level of 0.73 that is required in vitro to stabilize the spore enzymes to the heat treatment which they withstand in the intact spore (Warth, 1981).

The physicochemical structure of the peptidoglycan polymer in the cortex is the focus of a theory proposed by Warth (1978), which is based on evidence that the cortex does not expand outwards when the spore is disrupted. The concept of a pressure exerted in a particular direction was first presented by Alderton & Snell (1963). The interpretation is that the outward expansion is restricted because the parallel orientation of the glycan chains to the cortex surface results in pressure being exerted towards the inner zone. However, Popham et al (1995) found that the protoplast water content was unaltered in a mutant spore in which the peptidoglycan was highly cross-linked. This indicates that protoplast dehydration is not dependent on pressure exerted by mechanical activity in a loosely cross-linked, flexible peptidoglycan.

Methods of determining heat resistance

Heat resistance is usually expressed as a D value, which is the time at a specified temperature that effects a tenfold reduction of the viable cells in a homogeneous microbial population. Thermal death times (TDT), referring to some other level of reduction, may be used but the degree of reduction must be specified. In tests for heat resistance, all conditions that may influence the resistance must be controlled before and during the heat treatment. The culture medium and conditions of incubation that are used to detect or enumerate survivors also influence the result. In the test, heating and cooling times must be reduced to a minimum, ideally to zero, so that the lethal action of heat is restricted to the temperature of the test. D values and thermal death times are read from a death rate curve, prepared by plotting viable counts on samples taken after increasing times of heat treatment.

Moist heat resistance

Resistance to moist heat at temperatures above 100°C may be investigated by mixing methods or by indirect heating methods. In the former, small volumes of suspensions of microorganisms are mixed with much larger volumes of preheated substrates; whereas, with the indirect methods, a physical barrier such as the wall of a capillary tube exists between the heating medium and test sample (Brown, 1994).

Wang et al (1964) developed a continuous flow device for mixing spore suspensions and preheated water, with flash cooling by expansion into a cooling chamber. Kooiman & Geers (1975) mixed small volumes of suspensions (e.g. 0.1 ml) with much larger volumes of buffer solution (e.g. 10 ml) in screw-capped, thin-walled tubes, which were heated in a glycerol bath and transferred to iced water after set time periods. Stumbo's resistometer (Stumbo, 1973) is a mechanical device for transferring samples to and from an ice bath. In Stumbo's technique, small volumes of suspensions (e.g. 0.01 to 0.02 ml) are introduced into steam at high temperatures for short exposure times from 0.1 second. The technique of Mallidis & Scholefield (1985), in which capillary tubes are heated in a solid aluminium block, is representative of the indirect heating methods. The holes in the block are filled with glycerol to facilitate heat transfer to the capillary tubes. A simple mathematical correction can be applied to compensate for the effect of 'come up' time.

Dry heat resistance

In tests for dry heat resistance, the microorganisms must be preconditioned to a specified moisture level and maintained at that level during the heat treatment. The microorganisms may be preconditioned by placing them in a tightly closed vessel, such as a desiccator, above a salt solution with the appropriate vapour pressure. For the heat treatment, they may be sealed into tubes with the correct amount of water for maintenance of the moisture level. The tubes are heated in a water or oil bath. Alternatively, the test organisms may be dried on metal strips or glass coverslips in small open cans where they will be severely desiccated during heat treatment on a thermostatically controlled hot plate or beneath an infrared heater. Heating in superheated steam may be used for determining dry heat resistance. Temperatures 40–50°C higher are needed to kill spores in superheated, as opposed to saturated, steam (Brown, 1994).

Recovering survivors

A culture medium that is normally adequate for the species of microorganism might contain substances that inhibit heat-damaged survivors (Roberts, 1970). Inhibitory substances can sometimes be removed or inactivated by the addition of powdered starch or finely divided charcoal to the medium (Stumbo, 1973; Labbe, 1979). Reducing the incubation temperature from 37°C to 32°C for mesophils, or from 50°C to 45°C for thermophils, also increases the number of survivors recovered. Sometimes it is necessary to stimulate the germination of surviving spores by adding calcium dipicolinate (Ca DPA) to the recovery medium (Riemann & Ordal, 1961).

FACTORS INFLUENCING HEAT RESISTANCE

The biocidal action of moist and dry heat is influenced by a variety of conditions that may alter the resistance of the microorganisms or protect them from effective contact with the lethal agent. The conditions that are used to grow vegetative cells or produce spores exert their effects prior to heating but the major influences operate during the heat treatment.

Conditions of growth or sporulation

It is generally accepted that differences in the physiological age of vegetative microorganisms and in the composition of the growth medium influence resistance. However, the reports indicate variation in the direction as well as the extent of the changes. The temperature at which spores are produced has a more predictable effect. Thermophils and most mesophils produce their highly resistant spores in the upper part of the growth temperature range but the resistance of *Clostridium* spores may be enhanced when they are produced below the optimum growth temperature.

Temperature

The time required to kill microorganisms decreases as the temperature is raised. The influence of temperature is described by a temperature coefficient, such as the z value. The z value is equal to the change in temperature that brings about a tenfold change in the D value. It is usually read from a linear thermal resistance curve, as in Figure 4.2. The range and generally accepted averages of z values for bacterial spores in moist and dry heat are given in Table 4.2. A low z value corresponds to a large influence of temperature, and vice versa.

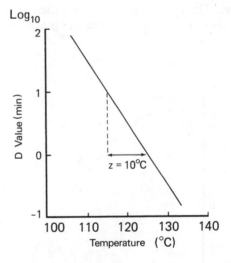

Fig. 4.2 Influence of temperature on the time required for sporicidal action (thermal resistance curve).

Table 4.2 z values for bacterial spores in moist and dry heat (Molin, 1992)

z Value	Moist heat	Dry heat
Range	7–24°C	10–60°C
Average[1]	10°C	21°C

[1] Widely accepted values

Moisture

The water activity of bacterial protoplasm is equivalent to that of the liquid in which the micro-organisms are suspended or to relative humidity if the environment is gaseous. The relationship between the moisture level and heat resistance of bacterial spores was demonstrated by Murrell & Scott (1966) and their findings are represented by the curves in Figure 4.3.

The different species used in the study varied widely in their resistance at 100 per cent moisture saturation (a_w 1.0). Curve A is typical of species which are relatively susceptible to moist heat and curve B represents more resistant species. As the moisture level was reduced, all of the species increased in resistance to reach a maximum between a_w 0.2 and a_w 0.4. At this intermediate range of water activities, the differences in resistance of the various species were minimal. As the moisture level decreased below a_w 0.2 (20 per cent saturation), the resistance of the spores declined but it remained above the level associated with full saturation. The relative resistance of different species is occasionally reversed during the transition from

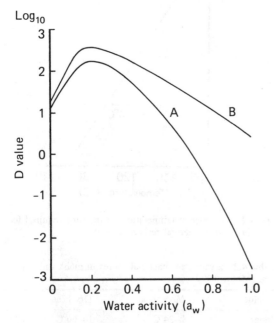

Fig. 4.3 Influence of water activity on the heat resistance of bacterial spores
Curve A: a species relatively susceptible to moist heat
Curve B: a species highly resistant to moist heat.

Table 4.3 Influence of water activity on the heat resistance of *B. subtilis* subsp. *niger* spores embedded in impermeable methylmethacrylate polymer (Angelotti et al, 1968)

Water activity prior to embedding (a_w)	D value, 135°C (min)
0.1	59.5
0.2	73.5
0.4	88.7
0.6	67.4
0.8	36.0
0.9	10.9

the intermediate moisture level to severe desiccation. This occurs with *B. stearothermophilus* and *B. subtilis*, the former being more resistant to moist heat and the latter more resistant to dry heat. This difference underlies the selection of these species for use as biological indicators of sterilization efficiency by steam and dry heat respectively. The findings of Murrell & Scott (1966) were confirmed by Angelotti et al (1968), who determined D values for spores of *B. subtilis* subsp. *niger* which were preconditioned to various water activities and then embedded in water-impermeable plastic blocks for heat treatment. Angelotti's results are shown in Table 4.3.

The heat resistance of non-sporing bacteria and yeasts is influenced by water activity in a similar manner. The effects are highly significant in the heat treatment of foods and other materials that have a low water activity because they contain a high concentration of sugar or salt.

Hydrogen ion concentration (pH)

Spores that are highly resistant to moist heat at pH 7 may be killed rapidly in an acid medium. In food canning, products are divided into groups according to the degree of acidity. Non-acid foods (pH >4.5), such as meat and vegetables, are processed at 121°C to ensure that the chance of a spore of *C. botulinum* surviving the treatment is reduced to 10^{-12}. However, acid products (pH 4.5 or below), such as tomatoes, could be processed at 100°C with similar assurance of sterility.

Alderton & Snell (1963) demonstrated a reversible change in the resistance to moist heat of spores produced by *B. stearothermophilus* and *Bacillus megaterium* that depends on interchange between hydrogen ions and calcium ions in the spore integuments prior to heating. In a subsequent study (Alderton et al, 1964), spores of *B. megaterium* were converted to the more sensitive hydrogen form by immersion in mineral acid (pH 4) at 25°C for 4–5 hours. Reversion to the resistant state occurred when they were transferred to an alkaline solution containing calcium. The transition required several days at ambient temperature in the calcium-containing solution but occurred in 1–2 hours at 50–60°C. The determinations of heat resistance were carried out in a neutral, calcium-free medium. Similar results have been reported by Ando & Tsuzuki (1983) for *C. perfringens* type A.

Associated materials

Microorganisms may be associated with many different materials in their natural environments. These include blood, tissue, food, sugars, salts, lipids, crystalline deposits and garden soil. The protection of microorganisms by associated material may be caused by delay in heat penetration but is usually attributable to the influence of the material on the moisture level. High concentrations of sugar or salt affect the resistance of vegetative bacteria, spores and yeasts by lowering the water activity of the suspending medium. La Rock (1975) compared the heat resistance of spores in an anhydrous oil to their resistance in the same oil after incorporation of 0.02 and 0.1 per cent water. The death rate curves obtained in the anhydrous oil had a broad shoulder which was reduced in width by 0.02 per cent and abolished by 0.1 per cent water content. The results showed that a decrease in resistance occurred as the amount of water increased. Molin & Snygg (1967) also showed that addition of water to oils decreased the resistance of bacterial spores and found that the type of oil influenced resistance in a way that could not be entirely explained by reduced heat conductivity of lipids or their water content.

Sodium nitrate, sodium nitrite and sodium chloride, which are used as curing salts, appear to exert their main effect subsequent to heat treatment by inhibiting the germination of surviving spores. Briggs & Yazdany (1970) showed that aerobic spore-formers are increasingly sensitized to sodium chloride in the recovery medium by increasing heat damage. They proposed that the increase in salt sensitivity contributes to the stability of canned foods containing sodium chloride.

DESIGN OF HEAT STERILIZATION PROCESSES

Different temperature-time combinations which are equivalent in lethality may differ in their effects on the materials to be treated. These differences should be investigated when a process is designed for articles or solutions containing heat-sensitive ingredients. The first decision to be taken is whether steam sterilization or some form of dry heat treatment is appropriate. Secondly, a favourable temperature-time combination should be selected. Finally, a choice between maintaining the whole of the material at the selected temperature for a specified time, or calculating the lethality of the heating and cooling stages and subtracting this from the holding time at a fixed temperature may be made.

Heat-stable materials

The sterilization time for articles or liquids that withstand the usual moist or dry heat sterilization processes is the sum of the penetration time and

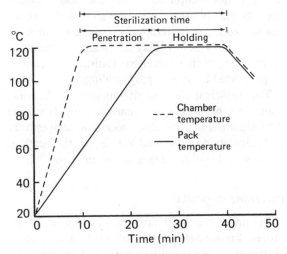

Fig. 4.4 Sterilization, penetration and holding times in steam sterilization at 121°C

the holding time. The penetration time is variable, depending on the nature and the bulk of the material. The holding time, for which the whole of the material must be held at the sterilizing temperature, depends on the temperature of the process. The relationship between sterilization time, penetration time and holding time for a textile pack in a steam sterilization process is shown by the temperature profiles in Figure 4.4.

Heat-sensitive materials

Rubber, synthetic polymers and many types of solutions deteriorate when they are subjected to conventional sterilization processes because they suffer unnecessary damage or deterioration during prolonged heating and cooling periods. Solutions for injection or intravenous administration, microbiological culture media and canned foods contain ingredients that may lose biological activity, nutrient quality or palatability. The heat-sensitive substances include drugs, antibiotics, sugars, proteins and vitamins.

Deterioration can sometimes be reduced or prevented by better management of the sterilization cycle. Many rubber articles withstand sterilization at 134°C in a prevacuum steam sterilizer because air is removed before the chamber and load are heated to the sterilizing temperature, whereas they deteriorate after treatment at 121°C in a downward displacement jacketed sterilizer because air removal is not completed before the load becomes hot. Some pharmaceuticals can be stabilized against oxidation by removal of headspace air from the containers before they are sealed. Caramelization of sugars in intravenous solutions is reduced or prevented by rapid spray cooling.

The principal method of minimizing deterioration of heat-sensitive material involves the determination of a suitable processing temperature and calculation of the total lethality of the heating, holding and cooling stages of the process.

Processing temperature

Selection of the most favourable temperature requires knowledge of the different temperature coefficients for sporicidal action and for deterioration of a critically heat-sensitive component of the

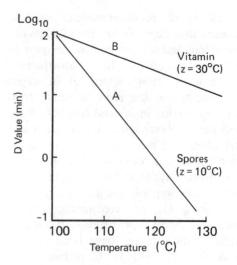

Fig. 4.5 Influence of temperature on the death rate of bacterial spores with a z value of 10°C and on the rate of deterioration of a heat-sensitive food constituent with a z value of 30°C.

material to be treated. Curve A in Figure 4.5 describes the effect of increasing temperature on the D value of bacterial spores with a z value of 10°C and curve B represents a heat-sensitive substance with a z value of 30°C. In this example, the margin between achievement of sterility and the occurrence of deterioration increases as the temperature is raised because the rate of sporicidal action is accelerated more than is the rate of deterioration. The opposite situation would exist if the z value for the biocidal action were higher than that for the adverse reaction.

Practical application of this approach is limited by the difficulty of isolating and identifying the critically heat-sensitive ingredient of complex materials, such as microbiological culture media and foods. Further, the potential benefit of a high temperature-short time treatment might not be realized in a batch sterilization process because extended heat penetration and cooling times could outweigh the advantage of a decrease in holding time. An increase in the holding time, as distinct from the penetration time, would be required if the volume per container of a given liquid were increased. If 100 ml contained 10 microorganisms, treatment equivalent to 1D value, to reach the level of a single survivor, plus an additional 6D would reduce the chance of survival to 10^{-6}. How-

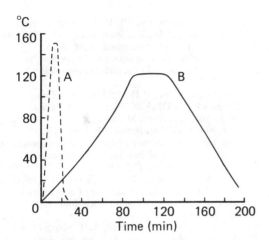

Fig. 4.6 Comparison of heating profiles of aqueous liquids in (A) a continuous process operated at 150°C and (B) a batch process at 121°C.

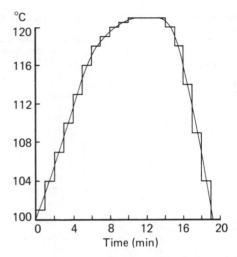

Fig. 4.7 Hypothetical temperature profile of a canned food, divided into 1 minute intervals for calculating the lethality of all temperature-time combinations (F_o value).

ever, if each container held 10 litres (1000 microorganisms), it would require 3D + 6D to provide the level of sterility assurance that was achieved when the same liquid was dispensed in smaller unit volumes.

The deterioration of heat-sensitive liquids that is caused by prolonged heating and cooling times and extended holding times is greatly reduced if a continuous heat treatment process can be used. This is only practicable in a large scale operation, where a homogeneous, non-viscous liquid is rapidly heated and cooled by a heat-exchange system; in these circumstances full advantage can be taken of using the combination of temperature and time that provides the widest margin between the rates of sporicidal action and product deterioration. The difference between the heating profiles of a batch and a continuous process is shown in Figure 4.6.

Method of integrated lethality

The relative sterilizing capacities of heat processes are compared by means of integrated lethality, designated by the symbol F. Comparisons are based on a unit of time of 1 minute of heating. If the recommended treatment (F) for non-acid canned foods is 4 minutes at 121°C, the time for which the product must be held at this temperature may be reduced by converting all temperature-time combinations during the heating and cooling stages to equivalent time at 121°C.

The total is then subtracted from the holding time of 4 minutes at the maximum temperature.

The lethality of a process is calculated from the heating profile of the product, which has been obtained by placing a thermocouple at the centre of a can at the slowest heating site in the sterilizer and recording the temperature continuously throughout the heat treatment. A hypothetical heating profile is shown in Figure 4.7, where it has been divided into separate segments, each representing a temperature that is assumed to have been maintained for 1 minute.

Different mathematical methods are used for converting the lethality of the heating and cooling times to equivalent times at the reference temperature of 121°C. The simplest method is the use of a Lethal Rate Table (Stumbo, 1973), which permits 1 minute at each temperature to be converted directly to a fraction of a minute at 121°C. The hypothetical data contained in Figure 4.7 have been subjected to this procedure and the result shows that the recommended holding time of 4 minutes at 121°C can be reduced by 3.74 minutes if the lethality of the heating and cooling stages is taken into account (Table 4.4).

The symbol F_o designates the lethality of a steam sterilizing process expressed in terms of equivalent time in minutes at a temperature of 121°C with reference to microorganisms with a z value of 10°C. F_o is used on the assumption that

Table 4.4 Use of Lethal Rate Table to calculate total heat treatment

	1 min at °C	Equivalent time at 121°C (min)
Heating	100	0.001
	104	0.002
	107	0.007
	110	0.022
	113	0.062
	116	0.168
	118	0.348
	119	0.486
	120	0.683
	120.5	0.824
Cooling	120	0.683
	118	0.348
	114	0.087
	109	0.014
	104	0.002
	100	0.001
	Total	3.74

the challenge microorganisms in the product to be sterilized have the same z value as the average for bacterial spores in moist heat. The calculation of F_o takes into account the sterilizing effects of temperatures below and above 121°C for microorganisms with a z value of 10°C, converting them into equivalent time values at 121°C. A recommendation for an F_o value of 20 minutes at 121°C for a culture medium to be used in a sterility test allows the treatment to be delivered in the manner that is least detrimental to its growth-promoting quality. Recommended F_o values may be influenced by the heat sensitivity of the material, the size of the containers and volume of material in each and the economics of the process. Modern electronically controlled sterilizers provide evidence that a given load has received heat treatment equivalent to the F_o value desired (Industrial Pharmacists Group, 1980).

REFERENCES

Alderton G, Snell N 1963 Base exchange and heat resistance in bacterial spores. Biochemical and Biophysical Research Communications 10: 139–143

Alderton G, Thompson P A, Snell N 1964 Heat adaptation and ion exchange in Bacillus megaterium spores. Science 143: 141–143

Allwood M C, Russell A D 1967 Mechanism of thermal injury in Staphylococcus aureus 1. Relationship between viability and leakage. Applied Microbiology 15: 1266–1269

Ando Y, Tsuzuki T 1983 Mechanism of chemical manipulation of the heat resistance of Clostridium perfringens spores. Journal of Applied Bacteriology 54: 197–202

Andrew M H E, Greaves J P 1979 Production of single strand breaks in the DNA of Streptococcus faecalis after mild heating. Journal of General Microbiology 111: 239–242

Angelotti R, Maryanski J H, Butler T F, Peeler J T, Campbell J E 1968 Influence of spore moisture content on the dry-heat resistance of Bacillus subtilis var. niger. Applied Microbiology 16: 735–745

Baird-Parker A C, Boothroyd M, Jones E 1970 The effect of water activity on the heat resistance of heat sensitive and heat resistant strains of salmonellae. Journal of Applied Bacteriology 33: 515–522

Balassa G, Milhaud P, Raulet E, Silva M T, Sousa J C F 1979 A Bacillus subtilis mutant requiring dipicolinic acid for the development of heat-resistant spores. Journal of General Microbiology 110: 365–379

Beaman T C, Gerhardt P 1986 Heat resistance of bacterial spores correlated with protoplast dehydration, mineralization, and thermal adaptation. Applied and Environmental Microbiology 52: 1242–1246

Bond W W, Favero M S 1975 Thermal profile of a Bacillus species (ATCC 27380) extremely resistant to dry heat. Applied Microbiology 29: 859–860

Brannen J P 1970 On the role of DNA in wet heat sterilization of micro-organisms. Journal of Theoretical Biology 27: 425–432

Briggs A, Yazdany S 1970 Effect of sodium chloride on the heat and radiation resistance and on the recovery of heated or irradiated spores of the genus Bacillus. Journal of Applied Bacteriology 33: 621–632

Brock T D, Freeze H 1969 Thermus aquaticus gen. n. and sp. n., a nonsporulating extreme thermophile. Journal of Bacteriology 98: 289–297

Brown K L 1994 Spore resistance and ultra heat treatment processes. In: Gould G W, Russell A D, Stewart-Tull D E S (eds) Fundamental and applied aspects of bacterial spores. Blackwell Scientific Publication, Oxford, p 67S

Chappelle E W, Rich E Jr, MacLeod N H 1967 Prevention of protein denaturation during exposure to sterilization temperatures. Science 155: 1287–1288

Colvin B T, Rizza C R, Hill F G H et al 1988 Effect of dry-heating of coagulation factor concentrates at 80°C for 72 hours on transmission of non-A, non-B hepatitis. Lancet ii: 814–816

Cuthbertson B, Rennie J G, Aw D, Reid K G 1987 Safety of albumin preparations manufactured from plasma not tested for HIV antibody. Lancet ii: 41

Davey K R 1993 Extension of the generalized sterilization chart for combined temperature and pH. Lebensmittel-Wissenschraft und Technologie 26: 476–479

Goepfert J M, Iskander I K, Amundson C H 1970 Relation of the heat resistance of salmonellae to the water activity of the environment. Applied Microbiology 19: 429–433

Gorman S P, Scott E M, Hutchinson E P 1985 Thermal resistance variations due to post-harvest treatments in Bacillus subtilis spores. Journal of Applied Bacteriology 59: 555–560

Gould G W, Dring G J 1975 Heat resistance of bacterial endospores and concept of an expanded osmoregulatory cortex. Nature 258: 402–405

Grecz N, Bruszer G 1981 Lethal heat induces single strand breaks in the DNA of bacterial spores. Biochemical and Biophysical Research Communications 98: 191–196

Hanson R S, Curry M V, Garner J V, Halvorson H O 1972 Mutants of Bacillus cereus strain T that produce thermoresistant spores lacking dipicolinate and have low levels of calcium. Canadian Journal of Microbiology 18: 1139–1143

Imae Y, Strominger J L 1976 Relationship between cortex content and properties of Bacillus sphaericus spores. Journal of Bacteriology 126: 907–913

Industrial Pharmacists Group 1980 Sterilisation: need for new approach. Pharmaceutical Journal 224: 41–43

Kilvington S 1989 Moist-heat disinfection of pathogenic Acanthamoeba cysts. Letters in Applied Microbiology 9: 187–189

Kimberlin R H, Walker C A, Millson G C et al 1983 Disinfection studies with two strains of mouse-passaged scrapie agent. Journal of the Neurological Sciences 59: 355–369

Kooiman W J, Geers J M 1975 Simple and accurate technique for the determination of heat resistance of bacterial spores. Journal of Applied Bacteriology 38: 185–189

Koshikawa T, Beaman T C, Pankratz H S, Nakashio S, Corner T R, Gerhardt P 1984 Resistance, germination, and permeability correlates of Bacillus megaterium spores successively divested of integument layers. Journal of Bacteriology 159: 624–632

Labbe R G 1979 Recovery of spores of Bacillus stearothermophilus from thermal injury. Journal of Applied Bacteriology 47: 457–462

LaRock P A 1975 Effect of water on the thermal death of a hydrocarbon bacterium in a nonaqueous fluid. Applied Microbiology 29: 112–114

Leanz G, Gilvarg C 1973 Dipicolinic acid location in intact spores of Bacillus megaterium. Journal of Bacteriology 114: 455–456

Lewis J C, Snell N S, Burr H K 1960 Water permeability of bacterial spores and the concept of a contractile cortex. Science 132: 544–545

Lewith S 1890 Ueber die Ursache der Widerstandsfähigkeit der Sporen gegen hohe Temperaturen. Ein Beitrag zur Theorie der Desinfection. Archiv für Experimentelle Pathologie und Pharmakologie 26: 341–354

Mackey B M, Bratchell N 1989 A review. The heat resistance of Listeria monocytogenes. Letters in Applied Microbiology 9: 89–94

Mallidis C G, Scholefield J 1985 Determination of the heat resistance of spores using a solid heating block system. Journal of Applied Bacteriology 59: 407–411

Molin G 1992 Destruction of bacterial spores by thermal methods. In: Russell A D, Hugo W B, Ayliffe G A J (eds) Principles and practice of disinfection, preservation and sterilisation, 2nd edn. Blackwell, Oxford, ch 18B, p 499

Molin N, Snygg B G 1967 Effect of lipid materials on heat resistance of bacterial spores. Applied Microbiology 15: 1422–1426

Murrell W G, Scott W J 1966 The heat resistance of bacterial spores at various water activities. Journal of General Microbiology 43: 411–425

Murrell W G, Warth A D 1965 Composition and heat resistance of bacterial spores. In: Campbell L L, Halvorson H O (eds) Spores III. American Society for Microbiology, Ann Arbor, p 1–24

Pask-Hughes R, Williams R A D 1975 Extremely thermophilic Gram-negative bacteria from hot tap water. Journal of General Microbiology 88: 321–328

Popham D L, Illades-Aguiar B, Setlow P 1995 The Bacillus subtilis dacB gene, encoding penicillin-binding protein 5*, is part of a three-gene operon required for proper spore cortex synthesis and spore core dehydration. Journal of Bacteriology 177: 4721–4729

Popham D L, Setlow P 1993 The cortical peptidoglycan from spores of Bacillus megaterium and Bacillus subtilis is not highly cross-linked. Journal of Bacteriology 175: 2767–2769

Riemann H, Ordal Z J 1961 Germination of bacterial endospores with calcium and dipicolinic acid. Science 133: 1703–1704

Roberts T A 1970 Recovering spores damaged by heat, ionizing radiations or ethylene oxide. Journal of Applied Bacteriology 33: 74–94

Rosenberg B, Kemeny G, Switzer R C, Hamilton T C 1971 Quantitative evidence for protein denaturation as the cause of thermal death. Nature 232: 471–473

Senesi S, Freer G, Batoni G, Barnini S, Capaccioli A, Cercignani G 1992 Role of spore coats in the germinative response of Bacillus cereus to adenosine and its analogues. Canadian Journal of Microbiology 38: 38–44

Silva M T, Sousa J C F 1972 Ultrastructural alterations induced by moist heat in Bacillus cereus. Applied Microbiology 24: 463–476

Stout J E, Best M G, Yu V L 1986 Susceptibility of members of the family Legionellaceae to thermal stress: implications for heat eradication methods in water distribution systems. Applied and Environmental Microbiology 52: 396–399

Stumbo C R 1973 Thermobacteriology in food processing, 2nd edn. Academic Press, New York

Taylor D M 1996 Exposure to, and inactivation of, the unconventional agents that cause transmissible degenerative encephalopathies. In: Molecular medicine: prion diseases. Humana Press, Totowa, New Jersey, ch 6, p 105–118

Taylor D M, Fraser H, McConnell I et al 1994 Decontamination studies with the agents of bovine spongiform encephalopathy and scrapie. Archives of Virology 139: 313–326

Wang D I-C, Scharer J, Humphrey A E 1964 Kinetics of death of bacterial spores at elevated temperatures. Applied Microbiology 12: 451–454

Warburg R J, Buchanan C E, Parent K, Halvorson H O 1986 A detailed study of ger J mutants of Bacillus subtilis. Journal of General Microbiology 132: 2309–2319

Warth A D 1978 Molecular structure of the bacterial spore. In: Rose A H, Morris J G (eds) Advances in Microbial Physiology 17: 1–45

Warth A D 1981 Stabilization of spore enzymes to heat by reduction in water activity. In: Levinson H S, Sonenshein A L, Tipper D J (eds) Sporulation and germination. American Society for Microbiology, Washington, p 249–252

World Health Organization 1988 Guidelines on sterilization and high-level disinfection methods effective against human immunodeficiency virus (HIV). WHO AIDS Series 2. World Health Organization, Geneva

5. Sterilization by dry heat

Dry heat sterilization refers to a variety of methods, in which the only common factor is the absence of liquid water from the heating environment. The dry condition actually embraces a wide range of moisture levels, from just above complete dryness to just below full saturation. The relationship between moisture levels, expressed as the relative humidity of a gaseous heating environment, or the corresponding water activity of the microbial cells, and heat resistance has been explained in Chapter 4 (Fig. 4.3). Dry heat sterilization is usually carried out towards the lower limit of the humidity scale, where the resistance of bacterial spores is about 100 times less than that at the peak level which occurs at 20–40 per cent saturation. More severe treatments are required if the organisms are at an unfavourable moisture level and cannot gain or lose water during the heating process.

The need for dry heat sterilization in hospitals declined sharply with the introduction of single-use syringes and needles that are sterilized commercially by radiation or ethylene oxide. However, the method is applicable to the sterilization of reusable glass syringes, needles, delicate cutting instruments, surgical drills, articles made from non-stainless steel, and oily materials. Dry heat sterilization is used extensively in microbiological laboratories for routine production of dry sterile glassware.

The following sources of dry heat and radiant energy will be discussed in this chapter but most attention will be paid to hot air sterilization:

Hot air
Microwave radiation
Conducted heat

Direct flaming
Incineration.

SUSCEPTIBILITY OF MICROORGANISMS

Species of sporing bacteria differ in their resistance to dry heat to a lesser extent than they do to moist heat. However, reported D values vary widely because, although the importance of specifying the moisture level is now appreciated, it was not always known or controlled during the tests.

The resistance of non-sporing microorganisms at water activities in the upper part of the humidity scale (e.g. 0.9–0.95) is of considerable importance in food canning and food preservation but is not particularly relevant to the sterilization of medical and laboratory equipment by dry heat.

Heat resistance tests that were carried out in connection with research on dry heat sterilization of spacecraft components containing electronic elements revealed a range of D values from less than 5 minutes to 58 minutes at 125°C (Bond et al, 1971); D values up to 5 hours have been reported in closed heating systems (Pflug, 1970) and a particularly resistant species of *Bacillus* (*B. xerothermodurans*) had a D value at 125°C of 139 hours (Bond et al, 1973; Bond & Favero, 1977).

FACTORS INFLUENCING EFFICIENCY OF STERILIZATION

Temperature

The time required for sterilization varies inversely with temperature, as in moist heat sterilization. However, dry heat sterilization is conducted in the higher temperature range of 160–180°C.

Temperature coefficients (z values) for spores range from 14°C at high environmental humidity to 55.5°C in a hot dry gas at a high flow rate (Fox & Pflug, 1968); values are usually between 15–30°C, e.g. the z value for *Clostridium sporogenes* in the temperature range of 105–120°C is 16.2°C (Pflug & Holcomb, 1991).

Moisture levels

The efficiency of dry heat sterilization depends on the initial moisture level of the microbial cells and the direction and extent of changes that may occur during the heat treatment by exchange of water between the microorganisms and the heating environment. Heating systems may be characterized as open or closed.

Open systems

An open system is one in which there is no limit to water transfer between the microorganisms and their environment. When the organisms are directly exposed to hot dry air in a large oven, they will lose intracellular water and reach a very low moisture level. The water activity in an open system is not constant and its adjustment may be hindered if the contaminated articles are enclosed in material that is not fully permeable to water vapour.

Closed systems

In closed systems, the microorganisms are isolated from the main heating environment by material that is impermeable to water vapour. They may be in a partly closed situation, represented by a small, impervious container or a closely wrapped film of aluminium foil. They may also be trapped in an air bubble within an impervious solid. In these situations, the microorganisms exchange moisture with the limited space around them until the levels are equalized. The final level depends on the initial levels in the cells and the air space and on the volume of the space. It may be predicted by calculation if this information is available.

The less common situation of a completely closed system occurs when microorganisms are embedded in direct contact with an impervious solid, with no surrounding space available for transfer of water. The resistance of the microorganisms is therefore determined by their initial moisture level, which is maintained during the heat treatment, and it will be very high if this happens to be about 20–40 per cent saturation. Encapsulation of spores of *Bacillus subtilis* subsp. *niger* in crystals of calcium carbonate was associated with a ninefold increase in their resistance to dry heat at 121°C (Doyle & Ernst, 1967). Closed systems are encountered when dry heat is used to sterilize impervious solids or anhydrous oils in depth.

D values in closed systems are about 10 times those that apply to open systems (Pflug, 1970). Microorganisms that are trapped between closely mated surfaces, which are common in space exploration vehicles, are in a partly closed system but their resistance is closer to levels encountered in open systems than to those associated with completely closed systems (Pflug, 1970; Simko et al, 1971).

Gaseous atmosphere

Experiments conducted in open systems at 160°C have revealed no significant differences between air, oxygen, carbon dioxide, nitrogen and helium (Pheil et al, 1967). D values for spores of *B. subtilis* 5230 at 160°C fell within the range 1.4–1.7 minutes and minor variations were attributed to differences in the humidity of the gases obtained from the cylinders. Fox & Pflug (1968) reported that the D value of these spores increased as gas flow rates increased, particularly for nitrogen. This was attributed to its very low water content and the more rapid desiccation of the spores.

APPLICATIONS OF DRY HEAT STERILIZATION

The main advantage of dry heat sterilization is its ability to penetrate solids, nonaqueous liquids and closed cavities. Lack of corrosion is also important in the sterilization of non-stainless metals and instruments with fine cutting edges. Disadvantages are the high temperature and the long time required for sterilization.

Glassware and metalware for which dry heat is the preferred method of sterilization include non-stainless and fine cutting instruments, syringes, hollow needles, test tubes and pipettes. Dry heat provides a method of sterilization for heat-stable powders (e.g. therapeutic drugs), waxes and non-aqueous liquids. Nonaqueous liquids include Vaseline (petrolatum), paraffin, Vaseline or paraffin gauze dressings, eye ointment bases, oily injections, silicone lubricant and pure glycerol. The boiling points of the nonaqueous liquids must be higher than the sterilizing temperature selected.

Rubber, plastics and substances that will vaporize or ignite at the sterilizing temperature do not withstand dry heat sterilization. Glycerol containing water should not be sterilized in a hot air oven because there is a risk of explosion.

HOT AIR STERILIZATION

Dry heat (hot air) sterilization is carried out in electrically heated ovens with mechanical air convection. Darmady & Brock (1954) reported that electrically heated ovens in which temperature distribution depends only on gravity convection are unsatisfactory because variations of 9–28°C were observed. Detailed specifications for sterilizing ovens with mechanical convection and automatic controls are provided in Health Technical Memorandum 2010 (HTM, 1994) and in the Australian Standard, AS 2487, 1981, and ANSI, ST40.

Design of sterilizing ovens

An electric heating unit is installed in the air duct leading to the chamber at a location that ensures uniform heating of the air. The non-pressurized chamber should be insulated against heat loss, and provision for the entry of 12 thermocouples is required. There may be one door at the front or a door at each end to permit removal of the sterilized load into the appropriate storage area. The chamber should be fitted with shelves for separating the layers of packs or containers. An interconnected electrical heater and fan unit circulates hot air between the shelves, passing it horizontally over the load through perforations in the side wall.

The controls include an overheat cut-out mechanism, which is designed to shut off the heating should the temperature in the chamber of the sterilizer exceed 200°C, and a sterilizing stage timer that returns to zero if power is disconnected. It should not re-start automatically because a decision must be made on whether to continue the process or start again from the beginning. Door operation is subject to controls that prevent a cycle being started if the door is not locked and prevent the door from being opened while a cycle is in progress. Where the sterilizing oven is fitted with doors at each end, interlocks should be provided to prevent both doors being opened together.

The recommended indicators include an indicating thermometer and process chart recorder. The separate temperature sensing elements should be placed where they will not interfere with loading but be close enough to give similar readings of temperature. Indicator lights should show when the power is switched on, the sterilizing process is in progress and when the process had been completed. In the event of a faulty cycle, an alarm should call attention to the interruption. The door should remain locked until the automatic cycle is started manually by a designated responsible person. While ovens equipped for an automatic cycle are now recommended, manual operation is acceptable; the door may be locked by a key and access should be restricted to the person in charge of the process. Equipment on modern ovens includes electronic program controllers and blowers for rapid cooling of the load by filtered air.

Packing and loading

A single layer of wrapping material should be used. Kraft paper bags are acceptable for some laboratory equipment but aluminium foil and aluminium containers are recommended for small instruments in hospitals. Aluminium tubes and oval canisters closed with crimped foil caps have been designed for small instruments (Darmady et al, 1963). Hinged instruments and forceps may be closed. Heavy instruments should be supported in a metal cradle to facilitate heating by conduction. Delicate instruments, such as cataract knives, should also be supported to guard against physical damage. Loading must not interfere with the air circulation in ovens.

Metal canisters are used in laboratories for unwrapped graduated and Pasteur pipettes. Large glass tubes are also used for Pasteur pipettes, swab sticks and similar articles. Foil caps and lids are often preferred for closure of these tubes because cotton wool sheds fibres.

Sterilization process

The oven may be preheated to the sterilizing temperature before loading, or it may be loaded when cold. The sterilization cycle includes the following stages:

1. Heating the chamber to the selected sterilizing temperature
2. Sterilizing the load
3. Cooling the load.

The oven and its heating system should be designed to reach the sterilizing temperature in the range 160–180°C within a specified time, e.g. 45 minutes from starting time for a cold chamber with no load (AS 2487, 1981). The sterilizing stage starts when this has been achieved and the sterilization time is the sum of:

a. Heat penetration time
b. Holding time.

The duration of the sterilization cycle is governed mainly by the penetration and holding times. The penetration time varies widely with the nature of the substances and their containers and the material composition, size and complexity of the articles and equipment to be sterilized by dry heat. Powders and oils have particularly long penetration times because they are poor conductors of heat. Some heating times for different quantities of powder and Vaseline, adapted from Perkins (1969), are shown in Table 5.1.

Table 5.1 Times required for powders and oils to heat from room temperature to 160°C in a hot air oven (Perkins, 1969)

Material	Quantity in jars	Time (min)
Powder	28 g	80
	112 g	115
Vaseline	28 g	110
	112 g	165

Holding times recommended in the United Kingdom (British Pharmacopoeia, 1993) are now in accord with those used in the United States (Perkins, 1969). These are shown in Table 5.2. For certain preparations, e.g. some oils, a lower temperature and longer time may be necessary, e.g. 150°C for 150 minutes (Perkins, 1969).

The heat penetration time for each type of load should be determined during commissioning and added to the appropriate holding time, as given in Table 5.2.

Table 5.2   Holding times in dry heat sterilization

Temperature °C	Time (min)
160	120
170	60
180	30

Testing efficiency of sterilization

The manufacturer of dry heat sterilizers conducts the thermometric test for a full load which is the basic performance test. This type of test need not be repeated unless the sterilizer fails to meet the requirements of the thermometric test for performance qualification. However, an automatic control test to demonstrate that the operating cycle functions correctly according to the instruments fitted to the sterilizer must be performed initially (HTM, 1994).

In the thermometric test for a full load, two thermocouples are placed in contact with the sensors for the temperature indicator and temperature recorder of the sterilizer; other leads are placed in jars containing 100 ml each of silicone oil or an equivalent heat-stable, non-volatile test liquid. The jars are distributed at five strategic positions per shelf among empty jars. In the performance qualification test, thermocouples are placed in packs in a representative but challenging load. Three placements are made in each of three positions: the slowest and the fastest to reach the sterilizing temperature and the slowest to cool to 80°C. These positions are predetermined. One thermocouple is also placed in the usual chamber position. Thus, 10–12 thermocouples are used in each of these performance tests.

The major criteria for satisfactory performance tests are that the sterilization temperature and holding time match specifications; the temperature overheat does not exceed 2°C; the temperatures registered by the thermocouples in contact with the temperature sensors of the sterilizer are within 1°C of the readings of the sensors; the temperatures measured in the loads are within 5°C of that of the chamber recorder and the latter does not drift by more than 2°C (HTM, 1994).

Other tests include a chamber overheat cut-out test to show that the temperature will not exceed 200°C when the oven is heated with the temperature control inactivated. An air filter integrity test is conducted on the high efficiency particulate air filters which are fitted to ovens that use fanned filtered air to cool the load.

Whereas performance qualification testing is undertaken on an annual basis, a simplified test for performance requalification is carried out quarterly. In this simplified version, three thermocouples are used — two for the temperature sensors and one for the item in the load that is the slowest to reach the temperature for sterilization (HTM, 1994).

Biological indicators of *B. subtilis* subsp. *niger* should be used at least weekly to monitor the sterilization of loads (ANSI, ST40; AS 4187, 1994). Internal chemical indicators of the integrator type are used for monitoring each load and external indicators are used on packages to show that they have been processed (ANSI, ST40).

MICROWAVE RADIATION

Microwaves are electromagnetic waves characterized by long wavelengths. Their range of wavelength, frequency and energy is given in Table 8.1 (see Ch. 8). Although microwave radiation offers a convenient means of rapid heating, its role in sterilization and disinfection remains a relatively minor one.

Killing action

A microwave oven typically produces electromagnetic waves of 2450 mHz frequency giving an electric field which alternates rapidly at 2450 million times per second. This form of energy interacts with ions and molecules and most efficiently with dipolar molecules, such as water, to generate heat. However, a problem with microwave ovens is the uneven distribution of the heat generated. Because of the irregular heating, even non-sporing bacteria such as *Salmonella* Typhimurium (Lindsay et al, 1986) and *Listeria monocytogenes* (Lund et al, 1989) can survive in chicken cooked for recommended times in microwave ovens, unless a standing time after cooking is allowed for heating by conduction. Lund et al (1989) also showed that, after 38 minutes of cooking in a 650 W microwave oven, the temperature range within a sample of chicken stuffing was as much as 26°C (52–78°C).

Microwaves are capable of killing bacterial spores in the dry state provided that the spores are exposed to a sufficiently high temperature for an adequate time. For example, a temperature of 137°C for 48 minutes will inactivate 10^5 spores of *B. subtilis* subsp. *niger* ATCC 9372 (Jeng et al, 1987). By accurately measuring temperatures and matching the rate of heating in a microwave oven to that in a convection hot-air oven through automated computerized control, Jeng et al (1987) showed that the kinetics of spore inactivation were the same for both ovens. From these findings, they deduced that the sporicidal activity of microwaves is due solely to the heat produced and that any nonthermal effects are insignificant. However, the findings of a more recent study on the effects of microwaves on the cellular integrity of *Mycobacterium bovis* dried on scalpel blades indicated that an additional, as yet unexplained, nonthermal effect does operate (Rosaspina et al, 1994).

Applications

The use of microwave ovens has been advocated as a practical and cost-effective method for sterilizing urinary catheters in the home (Douglas et al, 1990). Kindle et al (1996) concluded from their studies that heating infant milk feeds in a microwave oven to the point of boiling is a convenient and rapid method of decontamination. They showed that exposure to microwaves effectively destroyed or greatly reduced the numbers of different bacteria added to the infant milk formulae, e.g. *Escherichia coli*, *Enterobacter sakazakii*, *Klebsiella pneumoniae*, *Pseudomonas aeruginosa* and *Staphylococcus aureus*, as well as the yeast, *Candida albicans*, and the vaccine strain of poliomyelitis virus.

Another application in the medical area is to the treatment of infectious medical wastes. In a variation of the mechanical-chemical disinfection procedure, the medical waste is shredded, compacted, sprayed with water and disinfected by the heat produced by microwaves from a microwave generator (Block, 1991).

Although the major problem associated with the use of microwave ovens for sterilization is uneven heating, their use may be inappropriate or inconvenient for other reasons as well. Latimer and Matsen (1977) pointed out that the lack of pressurization within the oven precludes its use in the sterilization of newly prepared culture media, which would tend to boil over and lose water volume. Furthermore, their attempts at sterilizing dry, wrapped materials resulted in charring and ignition of the cloth and paper wrappings. However, they did find that a 5 minute exposure to microwave irradiation (600 W) provided a feasible and rapid method of decontaminating small volumes of culture media in a clinical microbiology laboratory.

Similarly, Sanborn et al (1982) used a 3 minute exposure for the decontamination of plastic tissue culture vessels. Precautions such as the inclusion of a beaker of water as a heat sink were required to prevent melting of the plastic. The procedure permitted limited recycling of the plastic culture vessels with economic benefit.

A modified 750 W microwave oven has been used for the sterilization of moistened or wetted dental instruments or equipment (Rohrer & Bulard, 1985, Young et al, 1985). The modifications consisted of the installation of a holding device that rotated the articles for sterilization through three dimensions of space and the inclusion of radar absorbent material (RAM). The purpose of the three-dimensional rotating device is to expose all surfaces of the articles to microwave radiation, thereby preventing the development of 'cold spots'. The RAM serves to absorb radiation reflected back by metal objects which would otherwise damage the microwave generator (magnetron).

STERILIZATION BY CONDUCTED HEAT

Small metal or glass articles may be heated rapidly if they are placed in direct contact with a metal block on a thermostatically controlled hot plate (Darmady et al, 1958). Cavities bored in the block can accommodate equipment of appropriate size and shape, while small instruments may be placed in a shallow covered tray recessed into the top surface. When the hot plate was preheated to 190°C, the instruments reached 180°C in 23 minutes. A holding time of 7.5 minutes was added.

Conducted heat, in the form of oil baths, has been used in dental surgeries for disinfection of conventional handpieces, and containers of heated glass beads are sometimes used for chairside disinfection of the small reamers and broaches that are used for debridement of root canals.

An instrument sterilizer which uses superheated glass beads is available for the sterilization of small metal instruments such as forceps, scalpels, needles and biopsy punches. Insulation prevents the outer casing of the sterilizing unit from becoming too hot for handling while the glass beads in the internal well are heated to a temperature of about 250°C. A special glass cup with a lid is placed on the glass beads in the heating well for holding smaller articles such as depilation needles during sterilization. The sterilizer requires an initial heating-up period of 18 minutes or more and monthly replacement of the special glass beads. The instruments for sterilization must be clean and dry before insertion into the bed of heated glass beads.

Sterilization times recommended by the manufacturers, e.g. 45 seconds, were found to be inadequate for the sterilization of articles on which a suspension of sporing bacteria (e.g. *Bacillus cereus*, 2×10^8 per ml) had been allowed to dry in the presence of protein, such as bovine serum, as shown in Table 5.3. The findings also illustrate the reduced efficiency of heat conduction by air to small articles in the glass cup and underline the need for decontamination and cleaning of instruments before sterilization in a heated bead sterilizer.

Table 5.3 Survival of a dried, protein-containing suspension of *Bacillus cereus* on articles in a heated-bead sterilizer[1]

Articles tested	Growth after heating times (min)			
	1	3	5	10
Instruments				
Forceps	+	−	−	−
Scissors	+	+	−	−
Articles in cup				
Lancets	+	+	+	−
Paper clips	+	+	+	−

[1]Data provided by Agnes Tan, Microbiological Diagnostic Unit, University of Melbourne

Forrester & Douglas (1988) also reported that the heating time recommended by the manufacturer of a glass bead sterilizer was inadequate for sterilization. They showed that the sterilizer failed to kill a load of 10^5 spores of *Bacillus stearothermophilus* ATCC 7953 which were dried on endodontic reamers in the presence of blood after 60 seconds of exposure. A period of 50 seconds was required to kill a load of 10^5 *Staphylococcus aureus* NCTC 6971 under the same conditions. In addition, they found a considerable variation in temperature within the chamber from a minimum of 185°C to a maximum of 215°C.

STERILIZATION BY FLAMING

Sterilization by direct flaming is limited to wire loops that are used for inoculating bacterial cultures. The loop is held in the flame of a bunsen burner until it becomes red hot. Precautions must be taken to avoid spattering of unsterilized material from the loop as it is heated. Electrically heated loop incinerators are now commonly used; they are especially suitable for use in biological safety cabinets or enclosures where anaerobic conditions are maintained. A support for the handle of the loop, which frees the hands for other operations during sterilization, has been described by Gordon & Davenport (1973). They also advised that handles should be insulated to guard against the possibility of electric shock if the loop comes in contact with the heating element.

The practice of flaming transfer forceps, glass rods, the outer surface of sterilized pipettes, and the mouths of culture tubes or bottles does not guarantee sterilization or protection against airborne contaminants because the temperature is too low and the time is too short. These limitations apply also to the method of dipping forceps, hypodermic needles or glass spreaders in ethyl alcohol and burning it off. Evaporative cooling lowers the temperature at the surface of the instrument to 118°C although the air temperature a short distance away may be 205°C (Doyle & Ernst, 1969). Furthermore, the alcohol may be contaminated with bacterial spores which resist killing at the surface temperature so that it can actually be a source of contamination in bacterial counts and sterility testing. The suspicion of many microbiologists that flaming the mouths of test tubes and bottles when opening them to transfer cultures is a waste of time receives support from an investigation by Brunker & Fernandez (1972), who found no significant difference in contamination rates between containers that were flamed and those that were not flamed.

A small hot air heater designed to replace naked flames in dental surgeries has been used for the rapid sterilization of endodontic reamers. The heater is conical in shape with a small nozzle at its apex from which a stream of hot air at a temperature of about 490°C emerges. Contaminated reamers held horizontally by forceps in the air stream at a distance of 2–4 mm above the nozzle were sterilized in 5 seconds (Forrester & Douglas, 1988).

INCINERATION

Combustible waste

Much of the waste material that is generated in hospitals and microbiological laboratories is contaminated with large numbers of microorganisms, including recognized and opportunistic pathogens. Hospital waste and certain types of laboratory waste materials, such as those from animal units, are incinerated but the efficacy of incineration cannot be taken for granted. Vegetative and sporing bacteria have been found in solid residues and gaseous effluents from incinerators. An investigation by Barbeito & Gremillion (1968) showed that an air temperature of 371°C in the firebox and 196°C in the brick lining with retention time of 26.5 seconds were required to kill spores of *B. subtilis* subsp. *niger* when they were mixed with dry animal bedding in a single-chambered incinerator.

Siting, design and operation of incinerators

High-efficiency incineration facilities for medical wastes may be located in hospital premises but are preferably located in industrially-zoned areas, off-site from hospitals and away from residential and adjacent buildings (Bennett, 1988; NHMRC, 1988). Designated vehicles are required for the collection and transport of wastes to the incineration plant as well as on-site facilities for its reception and short-term storage.

The incinerator should be designed for controlled, fuel-powered, high-temperature destruction of large volumes of waste, including plastics, with minimal emission of potentially harmful gaseous effluents. For efficient combustion, a two-stage process is used involving a primary and a secondary combustion chamber with the latter operating at the higher temperature. Since incomplete combustion is associated with the emission of potentially toxic gases, temperature controllers and recorders should be fitted to both combustion chambers to ensure that they operate at the specified temperatures (BS 3316 Part 1, 1987). The incinerator is also equipped with appropriate devices for the control of gaseous emission. These include afterburners for thermal oxidation of gases in the effluent and absorbers and scrubbers for the removal of acid gases and particulate matter from the effluent. Equipment for the measurement of smoke density and gases such as carbon monoxide and oxygen in the effluent are also required to monitor proper operation and performance (BS 3316 Part 2, 1987, Schifftner, 1990).

In operation, it is important that adequate temperatures and residence times for complete combustion are reached in the primary and secondary chambers. The primary chamber operates at a temperature above 800°C while a temperature of at least 1100°C for a minimum period of one second is recommended for combustion in the secondary chamber (Bennett, 1988). Exceeding the design capacity of an incinerator by overloading may also result in incomplete destruction and unwanted emissions. Automatic loading is the preferred method. All parts of the loading machine should be fully guarded and operators should be provided with suitable face protection, gloves and protective clothing (BS 3316 Part 4, 1987). Regular maintenance of the incineration plant is essential.

Air incinerators

The effluent from biological safety cabinets or chambers where aerosols are generated for investigational purposes must be made safe for discharge to the outside environment. High-efficiency filters are commonly used but methods of heat sterilization have also been studied. Mullican et al (1971) developed an experimental test apparatus for the rapid mixing of air from a hot-air sterilizer with spores of *B. subtilis* subsp. *niger* from an aerosol generator. With this system, the heat-up times were reduced almost to zero so that more accurate data could be obtained on the kill rate of dry heat on aerosolized spores. They found that the spores were destroyed by hot air at 260°C in 0.02 seconds. Calculations based on extrapolation of their findings were in accord with the resistance to dry heat of bacteria on solid surfaces if allowance was made for the heating time of the supporting material.

REFERENCES

ANSI/AAMI ST40 — 1992 Table-top dry heat (heated air) sterilization and sterility assurance in dental and medical facilities. American National Standards Institute, New York

AS 2487 1981 Dry heat sterilizers (hot air type). Standards Association of Australia, Sydney

AS 4187 1994 Code of practice for cleaning, disinfecting and sterilizing reusable medical and surgical instruments and equipment, and maintenance of associated environments in health care facilities. Standards Australia, Homebush, NSW

Barbeito M S, Gremillion G G 1968 Microbiological safety evaluation of an industrial refuse incinerator. Applied Microbiology 16: 291–295

Bennett N MᶜK 1988 Disposal of medical waste. Medical Journal of Australia 149: 400–402

Block S S 1991 Infectious medical wastes: treatment and sanitary disposal. In: Block S S (ed) Disinfection, sterilization, and preservation, 4th edn. Lea & Febiger, Philadelphia, ch 42, p 742

Bond W W, Favero M S 1977 *Bacillus xerothermodurans* sp. nov., a species forming endospores extremely resistant to dry heat. International Journal of Systematic Bacteriology 27: 157–160

Bond W W, Favero M S, Korber M R 1973 *Bacillus* sp. ATCC 27380: a spore with extreme resistance to dry heat. Applied Microbiology 21: 614–616

Bond W W, Favero M S, Petersen N J, Marshall J H 1971 Relative frequency distribution of D_{125C} values for spore isolates from the Mariner-Mars 1969 spacecraft. Applied Microbiology 21: 832–836

British Pharmacopoeia 1993 HMSO, London 2: A197

Brunker T, Fernández B 1972 Effect of flaming cotton-plugged tubes upon the contamination of media during culture transfers. Applied Microbiology 23: 441–443

BS 3316 Part 1 1987 Incinerators. Specification for standard performance requirements for incineration plant for the destruction of hospital waste. British Standards Institution, London

BS 3316 Part 2 1987 Incinerators. Methods of test and calculation for the performance of incineration plant for the destruction of hospital waste. British Standards Institution, London

BS 3316 Part 4 1987 Incinerators. Code of practice for the design, specification, installation and commissioning of incineration plant for the destruction of hospital waste. British Standards Institution, London

Darmady E M, Brock R B 1954 Temperature levels in hot-air ovens. Journal of Clinical Pathology 7: 290–299

Darmady E M, Hughes K E A, Jones J, Tuke W 1958 Sterilisation by conducted heat. Lancet ii: 769–770

Darmady E M, Hughes K E A, Tuke W 1963 Instrument container for dry-heat sterilisation. Lancet ii: 498–499

Douglas C, Burke B, Kessler D L, Cicmanec J F, Bracken R B 1990 Microwave: practical cost-effective method for sterilizing urinary catheters in the home. Urology 35: 219–222

Doyle J E, Ernst R R 1967 Resistance of *Bacillus subtilis* var. *niger* spores occluded in water-insoluble crystals to three sterilization agents. Applied Microbiology 15: 726–730

Doyle J E, Ernst R R 1969 Alcohol flaming — a possible source of contamination in sterility testing. American Journal of Clinical Pathology 51: 407–408

Forrester N, Douglas C W I 1988 Use of the 'Safe air' dental heater for sterilising endodontic reamers. British Dental Journal 165: 290–292

Fox K, Pflug I J 1968 Effect of temperature and gas velocity on the dry-heat destruction rate of bacterial spores. Applied Microbiology 16: 343–348

Gordon R C, Davenport C V 1973 Simple modification to improve usefulness of the Bacti-Cinerator. Applied Microbiology 26: 423

HTM 1994 Health Technical Memorandum 2010 Part 3: Validation and verification. Sterilization. NHS Estates, London

Jeng D K H, Kaczmarek K A, Woodworth A G, Balasky G 1987 Mechanism of microwave sterilization in the dry state. Applied and Environmental Microbiology 53: 2133–2137

Kindle G, Busse A, Kampa D, Meyer-König U, Daschner F D 1996 Killing activity of microwaves in milk. Journal of Hospital Infection 33: 273–278

Latimer J M, Matsen J M 1977 Microwave oven irradiation as a method for bacterial decontamination in a clinical microbiology laboratory. Journal of Clinical Microbiology 6: 340–342

Lindsay R E, Krissinger W A, Fields B F 1986 Microwave vs. conventional oven cooking of chicken: Relationship of internal temperature to surface contamination of *Salmonella typhimurium*. Journal of the American Dietetic Association 86: 373–374

Lund B M, Knox M R, Cole M B 1989 Destruction of *Listeria monocytogenes* during microwave cooking. Lancet i: 218

Mullican C L, Buchanan L M, Hoffman R K 1971 Thermal inactivation of aerosolized *Bacillus subtilis* var. *niger* spores. Applied Microbiology 22: 557–559

NHMRC 1988 National guidelines for the management of clinical and related wastes. National Health and Medical Research Council, Canberra

Perkins J J 1969 Principles and methods of sterilization in health sciences, 2nd edn. Charles C. Thomas, Springfield, ch 12, p 289, 295

Pflug I J 1970 Dry heat destruction rates for micro-organisms on open surfaces, in mated surface areas and encapsulated in solids of spacecraft hardware. Life Sciences and Space Research 8: 131–141

Pflug I J, Holcomb R G 1991 Principles of the thermal destruction of microorganisms. In: Block S S (ed)

Disinfection, sterilization, and preservation, 4th edn. Lea & Febiger, Philadelphia, ch 6, p 85

Pheil C G, Pflug I J, Nicholas R C, Augustin J A L 1967 Effect of various gas atmospheres on destruction of microorganisms in dry heat. Applied Microbiology 15: 120–124

Rohrer M D, Bulard R A 1985 Microwave sterilization. Journal of the American Dental Association 110: 194–198

Rosaspina S, Salvatorelli G, Anzanel D 1994 The bactericidal effect of microwaves on *Mycobacterium bovis* dried on scalpel blades. Journal of Hospital Infection 26: 45–50

Sanborn M R, Wan S K, Bulard R 1982 Microwave sterilization of plastic tissue culture vessels for reuse. Applied and Environmental Microbiology 44: 960–964

Schifftner K 1990 Wet scrubber systems for incinerators. Journal of Healthcare Materiel Management 8(4): 19–25

Simko G J, Devlin J D, Wardle M D 1971 Dry-heat resistance of *Bacillus subtilis* var. *niger* spores on mated surfaces. Applied Microbiology 22: 491–495

Young S K, Graves D C, Rohrer M D, Bulard R A 1985 Microwave sterilization of nitrous oxide nasal hoods contaminated with virus. Oral Surgery 60: 581–585

6. Sterilization by steam at increased pressure

Sterilization by moist heat depends on the use of saturated steam above 100°C, usually at a temperature in the range 121–134°C. Minimum holding times for sterilization are 15 minutes at 121°C, 10 minutes at 126°C and 3 minutes at 134°C (Working Party on Pressure-Steam Sterilisers, 1959). The slightly shorter holding times of 12 minutes at 121°C and 2 minutes at 132°C recommended by Perkins (1969) may be adequate for aqueous liquids if they are cooled slowly. Steam can be heated to temperatures above 100°C only by increasing the pressure above that of a normal atmosphere at sea level.

PROPERTIES AND QUALITY OF STEAM

Saturated steam

Saturated steam is water vapour, free from any other gases, which is in equilibrium with water in liquid phase. On the boundary between the liquid and vapour phases, evaporation and condensation occur at equal rates and the relative humidity of the vapour is at the maximum value of 100 per cent.

The temperature of steam corresponds to that of the boiling water that gives rise to it. The boiling point, which is 100°C at standard atmospheric pressure at sea level, rises as the pressure is increased. When steam is generated within, or piped under pressure into, a closed vessel from which all of the air has been removed, the temperature rises in a fixed relationship to the pressure, as shown in Figure 6.1, where the phase boundary has been drawn by joining separate temperature-pressure combinations. Any point on the line represents saturated steam. The temperature relationships

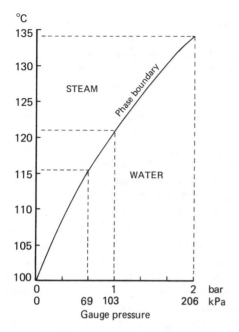

Fig. 6.1 Temperature and pressure relationships in saturated steam.

The biocidal efficiency of saturated steam depends on:

1. Moisture content
2. Heat content
3. Penetration.

Moisture content

Dry saturated steam at the phase boundary has a relative humidity of 100 per cent and a dryness fraction of 1.0, i.e. it is free of moisture carried as droplets in suspension. When the steam condenses on articles to be sterilized, it yields maximum latent heat, as well as moisture, thereby ensuring that the microbial contaminants will be killed rapidly.

Heat content

Steam has a greater heat content than has water at the same temperature, as shown by the figures in Table 6.1.

The sensible heat is the quantity of heat that is required to raise the temperature of water to the boiling point. The latent heat is the additional heat that is absorbed when boiling water is converted to steam at the same temperature (100°C at atmospheric pressure). This heat is converted to energy of motion (kinetic energy) as the water molecules are released from the cohesive forces of the liquid state and acquire the rapid motion that is characteristic of gases. When steam condenses on cooler objects in the sterilizing chamber, the latent heat is released but the sensible heat is retained and the condensate remains at the same temperature. The large amount of latent heat that is released is communicated directly to the surfaces of the load in the sterilizer, heating them rapidly to the temperature selected for sterilization.

that are most often used in steam sterilization are shown by the dotted lines.

On the gauge pressure scale, normal atmospheric pressure is zero; all pressures above atmospheric are positive, while negative values represent degrees of vacuum (e.g. 90 kPa below atmospheric pressure). On the Absolute scale, a complete vacuum is zero and all values are positive. Standard atmospheric pressure at sea level is 103 kPa (equivalent to 760 mmHg) or 1 bar (1000 mbar). Use of the Absolute scale in sterilization technology is limited to extremely low pressures, such as leak tests on prevacuum sterilizers, when the smaller units (Pascals or millibars) may be appropriate.

Table 6.1 Heat content of water and steam

Phase of water	Temperature °C	Heat content (kJ/kg)		
		Sensible heat	Latent heat	Total heat
Liquid	100	419	0	419
Vapour	100	419	2257	2676
Vapour	121	509	2199	2708
Vapour	135	567	2160	2727

Penetration

Penetration of steam through porous paper and cloth wrapping materials to the interior of large textile packs and into partly enclosed cavities of glass or metal equipment is essential for sterilization. Effective penetration depends mainly on removal of air from the chamber and load, but is assisted by the large decrease in volume (e.g. 1600 ml to 1 ml) that accompanies condensation. This is of special importance in the sterilization of textiles.

Quality of steam

Superheated steam

Steam is in a superheated state when the temperature is above that corresponding to the phase boundary at the existing pressure; that is, above the phase boundary line in Figure 6.1. In this condition, the relative humidity is less than 100 per cent and condensation does not occur until the steam is cooled to the phase boundary temperature. Thus, deposition of moisture and release of latent heat are delayed, and the resistance of the bacterial spores is increased (see Ch. 4, Fig. 4.3). The degree of superheat is expressed by the difference between the actual temperature of the steam and the expected phase boundary temperature. If the temperature is 130°C and the pressure is 103 kPa (which corresponds to 121°C in saturated steam), the steam has 9°C superheat. The maximum acceptable degree of superheat in steam sterilization is 5°C. Superheat can result in uneven heating of the load (Smith, 1986). It can also cause failure in sterilization, scorching or cumulative damage of textiles and paper and rapid deterioration of rubber.

The steam in a sterilizer may become superheated from the following causes:

1. Pressure reduction in supply line
2. Dehydration of textiles.

Before steam from the main line enters the sterilizer it passes through a steam separator, where some of the condensate is drained, and finally through a reducing valve which adjusts the pressure to the level required in the chamber. The expansion that occurs when the reduction in

pressure is correct causes evaporation of the remaining water droplets, producing steam which is just dry. However, if the mains steam is too dry when it reaches the reducing valve the reduction is excessive and superheated steam is produced. The problem may be overcome by installing another valve in the supply line, well upstream of the reducing valve fitted to the sterilizer, so that the reduction occurs in two stages. Superheat may occur similarly in prevacuum porous load sterilizers as the full flow of steam expands on entering the evacuated chamber. However, the duration is too short to cause dehydration of the load, especially when steam is introduced in the prevacuum stage of the cycle to assist the removal of air.

A common cause of superheat is dehydration of textile packs prior to sterilization. This may occur if cotton materials are stored in an abnormally dry atmosphere before packing or the packs are placed in a warm, steam-jacketed sterilizer and left for some time before the sterilization cycle commences. If the moisture content of cotton materials is reduced below the normal level of 5 per cent, they will absorb more steam to satisfy their affinity for moisture than is required to heat them to the sterilizing temperature and the excess latent heat liberated raises the temperature of the steam (Henry, 1959). The relationship between dehydration of cotton and superheat is shown in Table 6.2.

Table 6.2 Relation between dehydration and superheating of cotton fabrics (Henry, 1959)

Moisture content of cotton goods (%)	Degree of superheat °C
8	0
5 — normal level (45% RH)	1–2
1	4
0 — completely dehydrated	9

Wet steam

'Wet' steam carries a fog of small droplets of water, usually resulting from condensation in long supply lines that are not adequately insulated. Droplets may be entrained as a result of priming (foaming) in an overfilled boiler and carried forward by high-velocity steam (Joslyn, 1991). Wet steam is undesirable because it soaks porous material, creates a barrier to air removal and delays or prevents drying of textile packs after sterilization. The dryness fraction of steam supplied to sterilizers, expressed as weight of pure saturated steam divided by the weight of steam plus entrained water, should be not less than 0.9–0.95 in the chamber (HTM, 1994). The resolution of problems caused by wet steam depends on correct management of the boiler and adequate insulation of the supply lines. The steam supply to the sterilizer should be tapped from the top of the main line, which should slope downward towards the steam separator and reducing valve adjacent to the sterilizer. The degree of reduction is critical, depending on quality and pressure of the steam supply.

Chemical impurities

The absence of toxic residues is one of the advantages of steam sterilization. However, it has been common practice in the past to add volatile amines (e.g. octadecylamine, cyclohexylamine, morpholine) to the water in the boiler to prevent corrosion. Although traces of these substances in the steam may also reduce corrosion of carbon steel instruments (Holmlund, 1965), their use in boilers that supply steam for sterilization should be generally avoided because the additives may form deposits on the articles that are sterilized and be toxic to patients if they gain access to intravenous solutions or infant feeds. Their presence in tissue culture media is also detrimental to the laboratory culture of viruses (Robbins & Jones, 1971). Other impurities that may be found in steam are phosphates, caustic soda, sulfites (to remove oxygen) and iron salts from rusty steam lines. These may cause staining of instruments and wrappings (Perrotta & Michnikov, 1986). Installation of steam filters may be of assistance for control and prevention of these problems.

Steam and air mixtures

The temperature-pressure relationships of saturated steam shown in Figure 6.1 apply only to pure steam. If air is mixed with steam, it registers as a partial pressure but does not influence the temperature of the steam. If only half of the air in a sterilizing chamber is removed and the pressure is raised to 103 kPa above atmospheric, the steam in the chamber will contain 25 per cent air and the temperature may reach only 112°C instead of 121°C, as expected for pure steam at that pressure (Perkins, 1969). The main effect of air retention is to prolong the time taken for the chamber and load to reach the selected sterilizing temperature. If some residual air is uniformly mixed with the steam when the sterilizing temperature is reached, sterilization efficiency may actually be enhanced (Scruton, 1989a, b). However, if it is concentrated in air pockets within the load, it will interfere with steam penetration and condensation (Smith, 1986). Small amounts of other non-condensable gases (e.g. oxygen, carbon dioxide) entrained from the boiler may cause inconsistencies in tests on porous load sterilizers.

PRESSURE STEAM STERILIZERS

A steam sterilizer is a metal chamber, constructed to withstand the maximum pressure that is required to raise the temperature of steam to the level needed for sterilization. Pressure steam sterilizers of various types are commonly termed 'autoclaves' for historical association and convenient brevity. The term means 'self closing' (Perkins, 1969) and referred originally to a vertical sterilizer with an internally fitted lid which was sealed to the rim of the chamber when steam under pressure was produced internally.

Detailed technical descriptions of the design, construction and controls of modern steam sterilizers are contained in official standards. These documents are prepared for the guidance of sterilizer manufacturers but persons who are responsible for purchasing or operating the sterilizers should also be familiar with them. A brief account of general design and construction will suffice, in this chapter, as an introduction to the special features of sterilizers that are used for processing porous loads, unwrapped instruments and utensils, or aqueous solutions.

General design

Chamber and fittings

The chamber is usually constructed from stainless steel or from mild steel clad with a specified

thickness of stainless steel. Nickel cladding is recommended for bottled fluid sterilizers because it is
more resistant to corrosion. Small chambers may
be cylindrical but larger models are usually rectangular to allow better utilization of the space available for loading. Most are horizontal for the
convenience of front loading but vertical chambers
have some applications in laboratories. The floor
of the chamber slopes downwards to an outlet near
the front of the chamber for discharge of air and/or
condensate. The jacket, which is essential in
porous load sterilizers, is an outer shell that surrounds the wall of the chamber and encloses a
space that can be heated with steam under pressure. The chamber is insulated externally to
prevent heat loss. Internally, a baffle plate is fitted
in front of the steam inlet to distribute the incoming steam and to protect the load from wetting by
condensate. A strainer is fitted over the opening
of the chamber discharge line and ledges or rails
for baskets containing the loads are provided.
Pressure gauges are fitted to the jacket and chamber and a safety valve is set to lift if the pressure
exceeds the maximum for which the chamber is
designed.

Doors

There may be a single door at the front or a door
at each end of the chamber for direct unloading
into the store for sterile supplies. Doors are constructed from material similar to that used in the
chamber and insulated to ensure that parts which
may present a hazard to the operator are maintained at a safe temperature. The door closure is
sealed by a replaceable gasket of heat-resistant material that is fitted to the rim of the chamber.
Hinged doors may be closed manually or mechanically; alternatively, mechanically operated sliding
doors may be used.

Pipework and valves

The steam line adjacent to the sterilizer is fitted
with a steam separator on the high-pressure side
of the reducing valve. If air is removed by
mechanical evacuation, as in prevacuum porous
load sterilizers, air and condensate are removed

separately. The air is evacuated in the prevacuum
stage of the cycle by a water ring-seal pump, steam
ejectors or a combination of both (Knox &
Pickerill, 1964). Condensate is discharged into a
sanitary sewer; backflow in the line is prevented
by a non-return valve and backflow from the
sewer by a mandatory air break and tundish.

All discharge lines for condensate and those
which discharge air and condensate together, as in
conventional downward displacement sterilizers,
slope downwards and are fitted with a balanced
pressure thermostatic steam trap or other suitable
valve. The balanced pressure trap is illustrated in
Figure 6.2. The bellows element contains a small
volume of volatile liquid, which causes it to expand and close the valve when it is surrounded by
saturated steam. An air-steam mixture, which has
a lower temperature than that of pure steam,
brings about contraction of the bellows and the
valve opens to discharge it. The unit should open
automatically in response to a decrease of 1°C in
the temperature of the effluent. Alternative valves
are required for discharge into lines under negative
pressure.

When the sterilization cycle terminates with a
vacuum in the chamber, air must be admitted
through a high-efficiency bacterial filter until atmospheric pressure is restored before the chamber
can be opened. The filter should have a retention
efficiency of 99.997 per cent for particles with a
diameter of 0.3 μm. A non-return valve in the air
intake line prevents wetting of the filter material.
If a prefilter is used, the high-efficiency filter
should have a working life of one year. The air
flow rate into the chamber of a prevacuum porous
load sterilizer should restore it to atmospheric
pressure within 3 minutes.

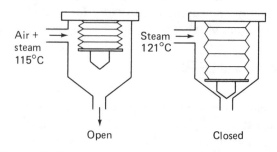

Fig. 6.2 Balanced pressure thermostatic steam trap.

Indicators and controls

Hospital sterilizers are designed to operate an automatic sterilization cycle, which may include the following sequence of stages:

1. Removal of air and heating of the chamber
2. Sterilization of the load
3. Removal of steam, followed by drying of textiles or cooling of liquids
4. Restoration of the chamber to atmospheric pressure.

Each stage is controlled by a timer that is activated by temperature, positive pressure or vacuum, or automatically, under microprocessor control.

The cycle is started by switching on the electric power and opening the steam supply to the unit. The second stage is controlled by a temperature-sensing device in the opening of the chamber drain, where residual air is most likely to accumulate. The temperature in the drain, together with pressure and vacuum readings, is indicated by gauges and recorded on a chart or computer print-out, all located on the instrument panel on the front of the sterilizer casing.

The second stage must be continued, under thermostatic control, until the whole of the load has reached the selected sterilizing temperature and is thereafter maintained at the temperature for a time that is sufficient to kill all the microbial contaminants. At the end of the preset sterilization time, which is the sum of the heat penetration time and a holding time appropriate to the temperature, the steam is exhausted from the chamber. The chamber pressure is reduced slowly to atmospheric for bottled fluids, more rapidly for a load of unwrapped instruments and utensils. Wrapped textiles and equipment (porous loads) are dried by drawing a vacuum for an appropriate time while the chamber is kept hot by the steam jacket.

Indicator lights on the instrument panel show which stage in the cycle has been reached and when the cycle has been completed. If the sterilizer has a door at the opposite end for removal of the sterilized load, appropriate indicators are also located at this end. In the event of failure to achieve the specified sterilizing conditions, the cycle may be terminated prematurely or it may be completed with visual and audible signals. The door remains locked until it is released by an authorized person who can initiate investigation of the fault. Other controls for the operation of the door ensure that the cycle cannot be started until the door or doors have been locked and that they cannot be reopened until the cycle has been completed and the chamber restored to atmospheric pressure. The door of a sterilizer containing bottled fluids should not be released for opening until the temperature has been reduced to 80°C in glass bottles or to 90°C in plastic containers. When the sterilizer has a door at each end, means are provided to ensure that both cannot be open at the same time. A cycle chart that records the number of cycles performed by the sterilizer is useful for maintenance purposes.

Installation and maintenance

The intended location of the sterilizer, whether it is to be built-in or free standing, and the adequacy of steam, water and compressed air supplies should be examined and discussed with the manufacturer before placing an order for purchase. Relevant standards should be consulted.

The engineer who is responsible for preventive maintenance of a steam sterilizer and carrying out minor repairs is usually a member of the hospital staff, who has received the necessary instruction. Some problems may require the advice or assistance of a more highly trained sterilizer engineer who is employed by a regional health authority or by the sterilizer manufacturer (HTM, 1994). Routine engineering tasks which are included in a planned maintenance (PM) program are the checking of the chart records and performance of the operator's daily tasks, observation of an automatic cycle in operation, and inspection of working parts of the sterilizer. The latter includes inspection of the chamber (for signs of corrosion) and the condensate discharge lines (for blockage), the door gasket, door safety interlocks, steam traps, valve seals, drains, air filters, gauges and recorders. The engineer is responsible for the quality and pressure of steam supplied to the sterilizer and ensuring that the pressure settings of steam control valves and safety valves are correct.

Methods of air removal

Steam sterilizers are divided into downward (gravity) displacement or mechanically evacuated (prevacuum) types according to the method that is used for the removal of air in the first stage of the sterilization cycle.

The downward displacement system relies on gravity for the displacement of cool, relatively heavy air by incoming steam. When the steam has filled the upper region of the chamber it moves downwards gradually, displacing the air towards the outlet at the lowest point in the floor of the chamber. Displacement of air from the load occurs more slowly and is critically dependent on methods of packing and loading that ensure minimum resistance to the movement of steam and air.

The downward displacement system is appropriate for sterilization of unwrapped instruments and utensils and for fluids but has now been replaced in porous load sterilizers by mechanical evacuation, using pumps and steam ejectors which reduce the partial pressure of air within the chamber to less than 133 Pa (1.3 mbar) Absolute without the need for a high vacuum (Knox & Pickerill, 1964). When steam is admitted to the evacuated chamber, penetration of the load is almost instantaneous; thus the load heats at the same rate as does the chamber and the heat penetration component of the sterilization time is eliminated. The complete removal of air before the load becomes hot reduces damage to cotton fabric (Henry, 1964) and rubber articles. The overall advantages of prevacuum sterilizers are the certainty of steam penetration into the most difficult loads and reduction of the processing time to 30 minutes or less, compared with 70 minutes or longer in a downward displacement sterilizer.

Particular features of the following types of steam sterilizers and sterilization cycles will now be described: porous load sterilizers (prevacuum type), downward displacement (jacketed) sterilizers, unwrapped instrument and utensil sterilizers, bottled fluid sterilizers and laboratory (general purpose) sterilizers. Further details are given by ANSI (ST8; ST37) and contained in Australian Standards, AS 1410 (1987) for prevacuum type, AS 2192 (1991) for downward displacement (jacketed) type and AS 2182 (1994) for the portable, electrically heated type.

Porous load sterilizers (prevacuum type)

Applications

A porous load comprises surgical linen, instrument sets and any other articles that are wrapped in paper or cloth for sterilization. These materials are also sterilized in reusable, rigid containers with perforated panels covered on the inner surfaces by steam-permeable, high-efficiency bacterial filters.

Mechanically evacuated sterilizers were developed for use in British hospitals after the report of a survey on sterilization practice (Nuffield Provincial Hospitals Trust, 1958) had revealed serious defects in the design and operation of old style, jacketed downward displacement sterilizers. Special attention was given to errors in packing and loading which resulted in failure of steam penetration into packaged materials and equipment.

Special design features

The prototype models were appropriately termed 'high prevacuum' sterilizers (Bowie, 1958) because the chamber was evacuated to 98.8 kPa below atmospheric pressure (corresponding to 2.5 kPa, or 25 mbar Absolute) by means of a water ring-seal pump to remove air from the chamber and load. However, prolonged evacuation (up to 8 minutes) was necessary and it was difficult to prevent air from leaking into the chamber. Furthermore, it was discovered by Harris & Allison (1961), and confirmed by Henry & Scott (1963), that when a test pack was placed in an otherwise empty chamber, thermocouples indicated that sterilizing temperatures were not reached or were not sustained in certain parts of the pack; also, biological indicators gave erratic results. The 'small load effect' was explained by entrainment of residual chamber air (up to 2 per cent of the quantity originally present) by the incoming steam, so that it was concentrated in the solitary pack. When the chamber was filled with packs, the residual air was distributed among the packs so that the amount contained in each was not sufficient to interfere with sterilization.

The problems caused by air leaks and small loads have both been solved by introducing a small amount of steam into the chamber during the evacuation process. A continuous flush of steam, with pumping, was effective in removing all of the air from the chamber. However, a rapid succession of pressure-vacuum pulses, usually combined with steam flushing, improved the efficiency of extracting air from textile packs, without reducing the pressure in the chamber to an extremely low level. Thus, the partial pressure of air in the chamber can be reduced to 67 Pa (0.67 mbar) Absolute (A) without the use of high vacuum (Knox & Pickerill, 1964). The risk of air leaks is also reduced if steam pulsing is performed entirely above atmospheric pressure (Knox & Pickerill, 1967). In the Joslyn process (ANSI, ST46), this is achieved by a series of steam pulses at pressures above atmospheric, alternating with periods of air displacement by steam flushing at atmospheric pressure, thus eliminating the need for negative pressure at any time in the air removal stage of the cycle. The

basic design features of a prevacuum porous load sterilizer are shown in Figure 6.3.

An air detection device is an essential component of a prevacuum sterilizer. In its simplest form, an air detector is a short metal tube, closed at one end, which communicates with the chamber drain and competes with the load for residual air in the chamber (Pickerill et al, 1971). The design of the air detector varies with the brand of sterilizer but the presence of air in the sample can be determined by the temperature recorded by the sensing device in the air detector. If no air is present, the temperature rises to that of saturated steam at the appropriate pressure; but if air is present, then a lower temperature will be reached. The device may also operate by measurement of the pressure that remains after the steam has been condensed by cooling. The sterilizing stage of the process cycle is controlled by the sensing device in

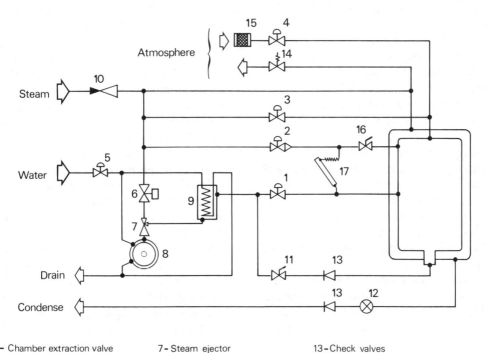

1 – Chamber extraction valve	7 – Steam ejector	13 – Check valves
2 – Steam flushing valve to chamber	8 – Water ring vacuum pump	14 – Safety valve
3 – Main steam valve to chamber	9 – Condenser	15 – Bacteria retentive air filter
4 – Vacuum break valve	10 – Steam pressure reducing valve	16 – Steam flush to chamber isolator cock
5 – Water valve	11 – Chamber discharge setting cock	17 – Air detector
6 – Steam ejector valve	12 – Steam trap to jacket	

Fig. 6.3   Schematic diagram of a prevacuum porous load sterilizer (Courtesy of British Sterilizer Company).

the air detector, which also signals failure to achieve sterilizing conditions if the quantity of non-condensable gas is sufficient to affect steam penetration into the load.

Packing and loading

Double layers of cloth or wrapping paper are generally used as primary packaging for articles undergoing steam sterilization (see Ch. 3). A range of purpose-built, reusable, rigid container systems has been developed for steam sterilization. Guidelines for their selection and use are also available (ANSI, ST33). Regardless of the type of packaging material or container that is used, the overtight packing of textiles must be avoided. Textiles and instruments may be combined in the same pack. In the 'Edinburgh tray' system (Bowie et al, 1963), the instruments are placed in a heavy gauge, heat-retaining aluminium tray; the cloth wrapper is used to line the deep tray and is fastened by cord to the flange. The drapes and surgical dressings required for an operation are laid on top of the instruments and the wrapping material is folded to enclose the contents. The tray itself remains outside the wrappings.

Although linen and metalware can be sterilized in the same load, the latter is a frequent cause of wet packs (Rowe & Kusay, 1961; ANSI ST46). Although the drying process could be extended to the limit imposed by a maximum cycle time of 30 minutes, even this extension might not be sufficient. The problem is caused by deposition of excess condensate on the cool metal surfaces. This tends to coalesce and drain from the site where the latent heat was liberated to another location where heat is not available to revaporize it. If the problem cannot be overcome by adjusting the proportion of textiles and metalware in the load, absorbent material, additional to the normal wrappings, should be placed within packs containing metal instruments or utensils.

The method of loading packs into the sterilizer is not critical, provided that those containing metal are not placed above or in contact with textile packs. The size of packs is limited to 30 × 30 × 50 cm but they may be loaded in more than one layer. It is not necessary, although it may be more convenient, to place the fabric layers vertically.

Sterilization process

The sterilization cycle includes the following sequence of stages:

1. Evacuation of air from the chamber and load, assisted by flushing or pulsing with steam
2. Sterilization of the load for not less than 3 minutes at a minimum temperature of 134°C within a maximum time of 6 minutes for the stage
3. Removal of steam and drying of the load by mechanical evacuation
4. Admission of filtered air to restore atmospheric pressure.

The prevacuum stage may be managed in different ways. A small amount of steam, flushed through the evacuated chamber while pumping continues, is effective in eliminating residual air from the chamber space; however, a considerable amount, sufficient to fail the Bowie-Dick test, remains in the packs (Knox & Pickerill, 1964). This may be removed by a rapid sequence of pressure-vacuum pulses, which reduces the partial pressure of air to a level that is undetectable by the Bowie-Dick test without the need to draw a high vacuum. Two variations of this system are used, one of which is illustrated in Figure 6.4. This represents the system developed by Knox & Pickerill (1967), in which a brief, flush-aided prevacuum is followed by a series of steam pulses in which the pressure remains above atmospheric to avoid the risk of air from the outside atmosphere leaking into the chamber. The other variation, sometimes called the Joslyn process, is one in which the chamber pressure remains at or above atmospheric at all times, eliminating the need for evacuation in the air removal stage. In this system, a short initial steam flush is followed by steam pulses that are separated by short periods of flushing. The time for the stage is 9 minutes. The quantity of steam that is admitted to the chamber in the Knox and Pickerill system is not sufficient to prejudice the validity of the Bowie-Dick test.

The sterilization time of 3 minutes at 134^{+4}_{-0}°C corresponds to the recommended holding time for steam sterilization at that temperature because the heat penetration time has been eliminated by prior removal of air from the load as well as from the

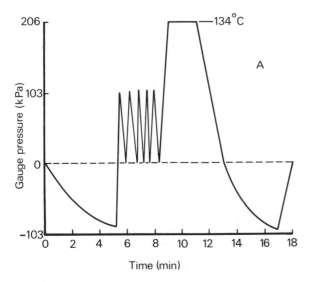

Fig. 6.4 Sterilization cycle in prevacuum porous load sterilizer (Courtesy of D. Mayworm, publisher).

chamber. This also reduces deterioration of fabrics and rubber, which can be sterilized at the high temperature in the absence of oxygen. The minimum exposure time of 3 minutes is standard for routine sterilization of hospital supplies. However, the sterilization of neurosurgical instruments, needles and other material which may be contaminated with the Creutzfeldt-Jakob disease (CJD) agent or other prions which cause human or animal infections, is a notable exception. The standard treatment in the United Kingdom, recommended by Kimberlin et al (1983) and authorized by the Department of Health and Social Security in 1984 (DHSS, 1984), is exposure for 18 minutes at 134°C in a *prevacuum* sterilizer. If the sterilizing stage of the machine is set for 3 minutes at this temperature, the material should be processed in six successive cycles. The recommended treatment in the United States is 1 hour at 132°C in a downward displacement sterilizer (Rosenberg et al, 1986). However, British authorities consider that the use of a downward displacement steam sterilizer is unreliable for inactivation of the CJD agent (Taylor, 1987). In addition, subsequent data indicated that steam sterilization at 132°C for 1 hour is not entirely reliable for the inactivation of the scrapie agent (Ernst & Race, 1993). Even the more efficient

prevacuum steam sterilization process, operating at 134 to 138°C for up to 1 hour, failed to completely inactivate the BSE agent in macerates of bovine brain and scrapie agents in mouse brain (Taylor et al, 1994). However, the macerated samples tested were relatively large in size and probably constituted an unrealistic challenge. Moreover, no evidence of cross-contamination has arisen as a result of the use of 134°C for 18 minutes, as recommended (Taylor et al, 1994).

CJD agent in specimens of formalin-fixed tissue cannot be sterilized by steam processes, as prior fixation of prions in tissue by formalin renders them resistant to subsequent inactivation by autoclaving (Taylor & McBride, 1987; Taylor & McConnell, 1988; Brown et al, 1990). In contrast, although exposure to 1M or 2M sodium hydroxide for 1 hour does not completely inactivate mouse-adapted CJD agent (Tateishi et al, 1988; Tamai et al, 1988), complete inactivation can be obtained by subsequent autoclaving at 121°C for 30 minutes (Taguchi et al, 1991).

The duration of the drying stage may be adjusted to suit the load but the sterilization cycle should be completed within 30 minutes. Failure to dry the packs within this time limit indicates a need to re-examine the methods of packing and loading with respect to the arrangement and proportions of metals and porous material.

Downward displacement jacketed sterilizers

Applications

This type of sterilizer provided the sole method for sterilizing textile packs and wrapped instruments before the development of the more efficient, prevacuum porous load sterilizer. The older type may, however, find use in some circumstances, e.g. where there are financial constraints or a lack of skilled maintenance services. Air removal by downward displacement is less reliable than is air removal by mechanical evacuation. The disadvantages of sterilizing porous loads in a downward displacement steam sterilizer are:

1. Steam penetration of the load is slow
2. The sterilization cycle takes longer
3. Methods of packing and loading are critical
4. Cumulative damage to textiles and rubber occurs.

Special design features

The steam jacket is required to keep the chamber hot between cycles and to assist in the drying of the load under the partial vacuum that is drawn by the venturi steam ejector.

The balanced pressure thermostatic steam trap in the air and condensate discharge line has been described as the 'heart' of the downward displacement sterilizer. It remains open during the air removal stage and re-opens automatically to discharge any air that accumulates during the sterilizing stage. If it malfunctions by sticking in the closed position, or if the line becomes blocked by solids or by an accumulation of condensate because of incorrect installation of the drainline, air will be trapped in the chamber and the sterilizing temperature will not be reached.

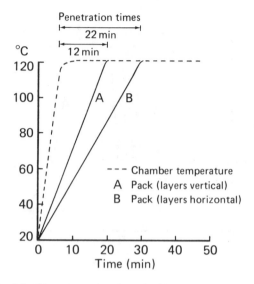

Fig. 6.5 Heat penetration times for identical textile packs in a downward displacement steam sterilizer with parallel layers of fabric positioned (A) vertically and (B) horizontally.

Packing and loading

The critical importance of packing and loading linen packs and wrapped instruments for downward displacement sterilizers and the risks associated with human error led to the development of mechanically evacuated (prevacuum) sterilizers. The packs must be positioned in a downward displacement sterilizer so that air can be freely displaced downwards. Textiles should be packed loosely within cloth and paper wrappings; the layers should be parallel within the pack and vertically oriented in the sterilizer. The large difference between the heat penetration times for similar packs that have been placed vertically and horizontally in a downward displacement sterilizer is shown in Figure 6.5.

Bowls and other empty containers should be placed on edge in the sterilizer; lids, if present, should be separated; if several bowls are packed together, they should be separated by absorbent material. If metalware is sterilized in the same load as textiles, it must be placed so that condensate does not drain on to packs underneath. Instrument sets should be opened and set out on a perforated tray that is lined with absorbent material and placed horizontally in the sterilizer. If rubber sheeting is sterilized, the folded layers must be separated by inserts of porous material. Glass syringes must be disassembled, and the barrel and plunger

placed in the same bag. Tubing and hollow instruments should be wetted internally and drained; tubing should not be tightly coiled. Guidelines on the recommended dimensions (and weights) of textile packs and instrument trays, with illustrations, are available (ANSI, ST8). For textile packs (e.g. the 16-towel test pack), the dimensions are $23 \times 23 \times 15$ cm and weight is 1.5 kg; for instrument trays, dimensions are 50×25 cm and weight 7.2 kg.

Sterilization process

The sterilization cycle consists of the following stages:

1. Gradual displacement of air by incoming steam until the chamber is heated to the selected sterilizing temperature of 121°C
2. Sterilization of the textile packs for the recommended minimum sterilization time of 30 minutes including at least 15 minutes heat penetration time and 15 minutes holding time at 121°C
3. Drying of the load to its original condition by a partial vacuum, assisted by heat from the jacket
4. Restoration of the chamber to atmospheric pressure by admission of filtered air.

The presence of residual air while the load is being heated causes cumulative damage to cotton textiles. Rubber is also damaged by prolonged exposure to the conditions that are used in the sterilization of large textile packs. Mixed loads should therefore be avoided to prevent damage to the smaller or more heat-sensitive articles. The use of a sterilizing temperature above 121°C in a downward displacement porous load sterilizer is not to be recommended because prolongation of the heat penetration time until the load has reached the higher sterilizing temperatures is likely to counterbalance the shorter holding time at the higher temperature and harmful effects may be increased (Perkins, 1969). The drying stage is often the slowest part of the sterilization cycle. Packs that have absorbed surplus condensate from a wet steam supply or by drainage from bowls cannot be dried to the condition that existed before sterilization.

Instrument and utensil 'flash' sterilizers

This type of downward displacement sterilizer is designed to sterilize unwrapped, non-porous articles for immediate use. Although provision may be made for drying instruments and utensils wrapped in a single layer of wrapping material, porous materials cannot be sterilized by this method. Use of these sterilizers in hospitals should be restricted to emergencies, such as unexpected surgery, or dropped instruments (ANSI, ST37; AS 4187, 1994). They should not be used for the routine sterilization of instrument sets. However, they are used for a wider range of articles in medical and dental clinics. These sterilizers must never be used for implantables, suction tubing or cannulae with blind ends (ANSI, ST37; AS 4187, 1994).

Special design features

The horizontal non-jacketed chamber may be cylindrical (e.g. 20 to 25 cm diameter) or rectangular (e.g. 25 by 43 cm) and accommodate 1 to 6 baskets or perforated trays. It is electrically heated and self-contained, with an integral water reservoir above the chamber. An immersion heater generates saturated steam in a covered section on the floor of the chamber or in a well below the floor from

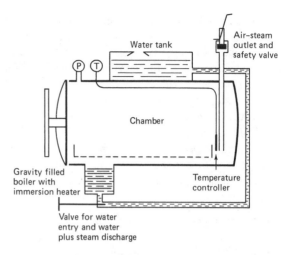

Fig. 6.6 A portable, electrically heated sterilizer, of a manually operated type, for unwrapped instruments and utensils.

water fed by gravity from the reservoir (Fig. 6.6). On completion of the cycle, the steam and the remaining water are returned to the reservoir which acts as a condenser. Automatic controls include pressure and temperature indicators/controllers, stage indicators and timers and a cycle failure indicator (AS 2182, 1994). The heaters must switch off automatically if the water boils dry. If a vacuum is applied in the drying stage, air must be admitted via a HEPA filter.

Loading

The articles for sterilization should be cleaned, decontaminated and inspected (ANSI, ST37). They should be positioned in the baskets or trays so that air can flow out by gravity. If a drying stage is provided, a single wrapper may be applied to individual articles. Hinged instruments should be opened.

Sterilization process

The following stages are carried out under automatic control:

1. Removal of air and heating of the chamber to the sterilizing temperature
2. Sterilization for 3 minutes at 134°C or for 4 minutes at 132°C
3. Restoration of the chamber to atmospheric pressure by rapid exhaustion of steam.

The chamber should be vented and opened immediately because delay increases the wetness of the load and negative pressure in the chamber can cause an inrush of unsterile air. However, if a drying stage is provided, the door remains closed and an independent heater is activated and operates until the load is dry. Aseptic transfer of the sterilized articles must be carefully planned (ANSI, ST37). Ideally, where the sterilizer opens into an operating theatre area, they may be placed directly on an appropriate sterile field.

Fluid sterilizers

Applications

In this context, fluids for sterilization include water and aqueous solutions such as injectable and intravenous solutions and irrigating solutions. Most of these solutions are sterilized commercially; any that are produced in hospitals are processed in the same way and to the same standards that apply to the pharmaceutical industry.

Special design features

The usually non-jacketed sterilizer may be constructed from stainless steel or from mild steel clad with nickel, which is more resistant to corrosion by spilt salt solutions. Sterilizers for use in microbiological laboratories or other places where liquids are sterilized in unsealed containers, which are closed with cotton wool plugs or screw caps, must be programmed for slow exhaustion of steam from the chamber. A rapid spray-cooling system is used when large scale production of sterile water or solutions in hermetically sealed containers is carried out. Although the load can be cooled by means of a cold water spray with a mean droplet size of 80 μm (Wilkinson et al, 1960), cooling with heated condensate, which has been collected in a separate steam-heated tank during sterilization, is more successful. The temperature of the spray is initially close to that of the bottles and is gradually reduced. Compressed air may be admitted to the chamber during cooling to guard against breakage of bottles or bursting of plastic bags. The use of heated condensate for cooling and the filtration of air that is admitted to the chamber after sterilization reduce the possibility of microbial contaminants entering bottles with faulty closures. The sterilization cycle for bottled fluids may be controlled by a temperature sensor in a load simulator, such as a bottle of water or a metal block with similar heating characteristics. The simulator must be cooled or replaced between cycles.

Packing and loading

Glass or plastic bottles, flexible plastic pouches, flasks or test tubes containing water or solutions must be supported on wire shelves, in baskets or other perforated containers from which air can be removed by downward displacement. Wire baskets should be coated with heat-resistant plastic to prevent staining when the liquid is in flexible pouches (Weymes, 1971). The need to use leak-proof containers for discarded cultures of microorganisms will be discussed later.

Sterilization process

There are three stages in a sterilization cycle for fluids:

1. Removal of air and heating of the chamber to the selected sterilizing temperature
2. Sterilization of the liquid, usually at 121°C with a holding time of 15 minutes
3. Cooling the liquid.

It is not necessary for the headspace air to be removed or for steam in the chamber to enter the bottles because steam is produced within the containers when the liquid reaches the sterilizing temperature. Latent heat is released when steam condenses on the wall of the bottles and reaches the contents by conduction. Convection within the liquid assists in the achievement of uniform temperature as heated liquid rises and cooler liquid flows down to replace it. As most of the steam entering a chamber that is filled with a large load of fluids condenses on the containers, air displacement does not commence until the surface temperature of the containers has reached 100°C. The mechanisms of heating are illustrated in Figure 6.7.

Water and heat-stable solutions are sterilized at 121°C; the recommended holding time is 15

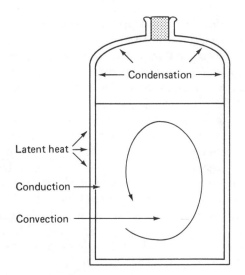

Fig. 6.7 Mechanisms of heat transfer in a bottle of aqueous liquid in a steam sterilizer.

minutes but 12 minutes might be adequate for unsealed containers which must be cooled slowly. A temperature of 115°C and holding time of 30 minutes may be adequate for solutions containing heat-sensitive ingredients but the liquid must be dispensed in small volumes because this temperature-time combination is not equivalent in lethality to 12 minutes at 121°C.

Rapid cooling of fluids in sealed containers is beneficial because it shortens the cycle, minimizing deterioration of heat-labile ingredients and avoiding the danger of breakage or spillage. In sterilizers that are equipped for spray cooling, the cooling time may be reduced from 3 hours to 10 minutes in a small sterilizer and from 22 hours to 17 minutes in a large one (Wilkinson et al, 1960). Rapid cooling prevents the caramelization of sugars in intravenous solutions.

Slow cooling is mandatory for microbiological culture media in unsealed containers because the liquid would become superheated and boil over if the pressure is reduced rapidly. The rate of cooling should be controlled so that the decrease in pressure keeps pace with the falling temperature. The chamber should be vented to atmosphere when it has been restored to atmospheric pressure to avoid the entrance of contaminated air into containers with unfiltered closures, such as screw caps, when a terminal vacuum is released.

Whichever method of cooling is used, the door of the chamber must remain closed until the temperature has fallen to a safe level to prevent explosion or breakage; 80°C is recommended for glass bottles and 90°C for fluids in flexible pouches (HTM, 1994).

Factors influencing sterilization time

The sterilization time for fluids varies widely because the heat penetration time is influenced by the following factors:

1. *Rate of heating of the chamber.* There is little variation in the time required to heat a given volume of liquid from ambient temperature

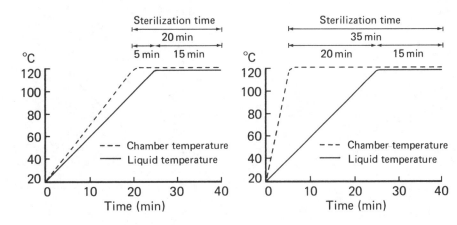

Fig. 6.8 Effect of rate of heating of the sterilizing chamber on the heat penetration time and the sterilization time of bottle fluids.

to 121°C. However the rate at which steam is admitted to the chamber affects the heat penetration time which depends on the heat lag in the liquid when the sterilizing temperature is reached in the chamber. The penetration time, and therefore the sterilization time, is extended when the chamber is heated quickly, as shown in Figure 6.8.

2. *Type of container*. As glass is a poor conductor of heat, a liquid in a thick-walled bottle has a longer heat penetration time than does the same volume in thin-walled flasks or test tubes.

3. *Viscosity of the liquid*. Agar-containing microbiological culture media which have been allowed to solidify before sterilization take 5–10 minutes longer to reach the sterilizing temperature than do media that do not contain agar or are above the setting temperature of 42°C. Particulate matter suspended in a liquid (e.g. cooked meat medium or canned foods) heats slowly and unevenly.

4. *Volume of liquid*. The influence of the size of the container and volume of liquid may be seen by examination of the temperature charts in Figure 6.9.

5. *Trapped air*. The headspace air in vessels containing aqueous fluids does not interfere with sterilization because the upper surfaces of the container are flushed liberally with condensate at the sterilizing temperature. Bottles or bags must be supported in wire baskets or other perforated containers from which air can be removed by downward displacement. The difference in penetration times when a 100 ml bottle containing a microbiological culture medium is placed in an impervious metal container and a wire basket is shown in Figure 6.10.

Perforated containers or wire baskets cannot be used for the collection and sterilization of discarded microbial cultures. Instead, bins or boxes made from metal or polypropylene are used. These containers trap a large amount of air, which results in a prolonged heat penetration time. The air may persist throughout the cycle when the normal downward displacement system is used. The heat penetration time under these conditions is longer for a polypropylene bin than for a metal bin, as shown in Table 6.3. The addition of water to the bin does not result in a dramatic improvement (PHLS Subcommittee, 1981; Lauer et al, 1982), nor does the use of a prevacuum sterilizer (Oates, 1983).

In order to shorten the time required for sterilization of large loads of discarded cultures in hospitals or teaching laboratories, two alternative processes have been designed and successfully tested. Everall et al (1978) described metal containers which were fitted with an inverted funnel, reaching deeply into the bin. The funnels from

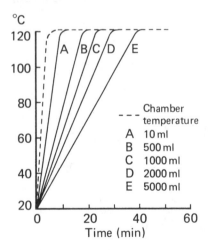

Fig. 6.9 Influence of volume on the heat penetration time of aqueous liquids in a batch sterilization process.

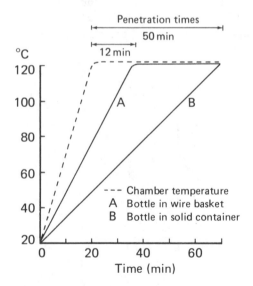

Fig. 6.10 Effect of air trapped in a deep metal container on the heat penetration time of a bottle of aqueous liquid.

Table 6.3 Heat penetration times in containers for discarded cultures[1]

Type of container	Contents	Penetration time (min)
Metal bin	Bijoux bottles (full load)	45–50
Polypropylene bin	Bijoux bottles (full load)	60
Plastic bag	Plastic petri dishes	
	Half-filled	30
	Filled	55–60

[1] Data provided by Gorry J P, Department of Microbiology, University of Melbourne.

four bins were connected to special valves on a branch steam line to the chamber when the discard cycle was used. The efficacy of the method in reducing the heat penetration time to zero was demonstrated; however, the method may be difficult to implement on a large scale. A more practical means of achieving a similar result was described in 1981 by the PHLS Subcommittee on Laboratory Autoclaves. This system, termed full free flowing steam (FFFS), involved the use of a wider bore tube for the chamber drainline and the removal of some unnecessary obstructions. The balanced pressure steam trap was replaced by a valve which was closed manually when the chamber temperature reached 105°C and air removal was complete. The heat penetration time was reduced to 1 minute. With this method, Scruton (1989a) found no difference in penetration times between the metal and plastic bins.

TESTS FOR EFFICIENCY OF STEAM STERILIZERS

The principles have been explained and the methods of testing the mechanical performance of sterilizers and the achievement of sterilizing conditions in the chamber and load have been outlined in Chapter 2. The appropriate tests that are required to qualify each type of steam sterilizer for its intended purpose and to monitor its continued efficiency in routine operation will be described here. Full instructions for performance of the tests are included in Health Technical Memorandum 2010 (HTM, 1994); Steam Sterilization and Sterility Assurance (ANSI, ST46) and Hospital Steam Sterilizers (ANSI, ST8). The recommended frequency of testing varies. Australian recommendations are given in AS 4187 (1994).

Tests for prevacuum porous load sterilizers

Temperature and automatic process control test

In the temperature and automatic process control test, a temperature of 134^{+4}_{-0}°C must be maintained in the chamber for at least 3 minutes in the sterilizing stage. The time for this stage should be no more than 6 minutes and the cycle should be completed within 30 minutes. At the completion of the cycle, the towels in the test pack should be close to the normal air-dry condition.

Leak rate test

The sterilizer controls are switched to an automatic or semi automatic leak test position. A preliminary warming up cycle is required if the test is carried out in the air removal stage but this may be avoided by deferring it to the end of the drying stage. A vacuum is drawn to 50 mbar (5.15 kPa A), the valves are closed and the vacuum source is stopped. After the pressure has stabilized, two readings are taken 10 minutes apart. The result is acceptable if the average leak rate is no more than 1.3 mbar (134 Pa) per minute (HTM, 1994).

Thermocouple test

Thermocouples can be placed at various sites in a sterilizing chamber. One recommended placement for a thermocouple is in a Bowie-Dick test pack while a second is placed in the chamber drain. This test should be carried out with the pack alone in the chamber and, if the result is successful, repeated with a full load of similar packs. The result is successful if the temperatures are within the specified range of 134^{+4}_{-0}°C and the temperature in the pack is the same as that in the chamber drain for the last 2 minutes of the prescribed 3 minute holding time.

Bowie-Dick test

The Bowie-Dick test, which uses a temperature-sensitive indicator in a standard test pack, was designed for convenience in daily performance because complex equipment is required for the thermocouple test. It is a test for satisfactory air removal from the pack in the prevacuum stage of the cycle, and the resulting uniformity of steam penetration. As it does not measure time-at-temperature, it does not confirm that sterilizing conditions have been achieved in the pack.

The test pack contains 24–36 cotton towels of specified quality and size, which are folded to provide 8 thicknesses and stacked horizontally to a height of approximately 250 mm and a density of 150–170 kg/m³. The towels must be washed to remove dressing before they are put into use. The indicator may be a plain sheet of duplicator paper of the same area as the pack, which bears a St Andrew's cross made from specified brands of autoclave tape, or a manufactured sheet of the same size incorporating broken strips of the indicator material. The indicator is placed between towels at the midpoint of the horizontal stack, which is then wrapped in cotton fabric or a sterilizing grade of wrapping paper. The autoclave tape indicator sheets have a 12-month shelf life provided that they are stored under appropriately cool and dry conditions.

The test should be performed at the start of each working day. The pack is placed with layers horizontal, alone in the chamber, at the approximate centre and 100–200 mm above the base. The sterilizing stage of the cycle must not exceed 3.5 minutes at 134°C. Before the test is conducted, a preliminary warming-up cycle (without inclusion of the drying stage) may be required to ensure that a satisfactory cycle is not failed. When the cycle is completed, the pack is opened and the indicator is examined carefully to detect nonuniformity of the colour change. A corner should be compared with the centre of the sheet. Any paler area indicates

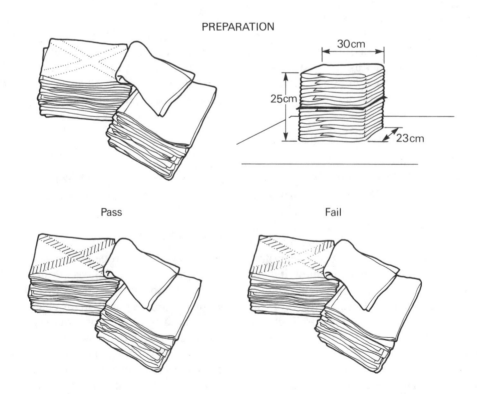

PREPARATION

Pass

Fail

Fig. 6.11 Preparation and interpretation of a Bowie-Dick test (Courtesy of Department of Health, London).

retention of air and that the sterilizer has failed that test. It has been shown that an induced air leak of 1–2 litres per minute will produce a fault signal in the Bowie-Dick test, whereas biological indicators do not yield positive cultures until the leak is increased to 3 litres per minute (Kropp, 1987). The preparation of the pack, insertion of the indicator and examples of pass and fail results are illustrated in Figure 6.11.

The Bowie-Dick test is the principal routine test, in conjunction with the weekly leak test, for monitoring the efficiency of prevacuum sterilizers. Batch variations in the indicator or storage for many years in various climates have been shown not to affect the result of the test (Bowie & Dick 1969; Bowie, 1974) and the quantity of steam used in the preliminary steam flushing or pulsing does not affect the colour of the indicator. The used indicators should be labelled and retained for at least three months as a record. The towels must be unfolded and aired for at least one hour between tests; they should be washed once a week but should not be starched, ironed or calendered. If the test has produced a failed result, the sterilizer must not be used until the fault has been identified and rectified. It cannot be made safe by increasing the sterilizing stage until a uniform colour change is indicated. However, if a subsequent thermocouple test fails to show a temperature difference between the centre of the test pack and the chamber drain, the steam supply should be examined for the presence of noncondensable gases.

Ready-to-use Bowie-Dick type test packs are commercially available. The sensitivity of a number of these packs has been tested by introducing known volumes of air into autoclave chambers containing the packs and comparing the responses to that obtained with the traditional Bowie-Dick test. In these comparisons, the performance of some of the ready-to-use packs was found to be unsatisfactory (Goullet & Hambleton, 1989).

Air detector tests

The function of the air detector is to pass or fail the sterilization cycle according to the amount of air in the chamber. The sensitivity of the air detector must be adjusted, in the first place, to signal a fault if the amount of air in the chamber is sufficient to impair the sterilization process. A variable flow device and an absolute pressure gauge are connected to the chamber to admit measured amounts of air during the prevacuum stage of the sterilization cycle.

For the first stage of the test, a Bowie-Dick test pack with temperature sensors installed is placed in the otherwise empty chamber. A sequence of cycles, covering a range of air leaks, is performed under automatic control until the induced air leak causes the temperature of the pack to be more than 2°C below that in the chamber drain at the commencement of the sterilizing stage. The pressure rise on the absolute pressure gauge, which should not exceed 10 kPa (100 mbar) during the 10 minute test period, is recorded.

The above procedure is repeated with a full load accompanying the test pack and the pressure rise that was determined in the first test. The pressure rise that is required to cause a difference of 2°C between the pack and the chamber drain and to activate the 'fault' signal may be greater than that determined in the first test.

A function test is used to confirm that the air detector is functioning correctly. For this test, the air flow metering device is set as for the small load test. A standard test pack is placed in the chamber at a distance of 100–200 mm above the centre of the chamber base. The test is satisfactory if the operating cycle is aborted and a fault is indicated (HTM, 1994).

Biological and chemical indicators

The status accorded to biological indicators in steam sterilization varies widely from the recommendation that they be used in each cycle to their use as only one component of a qualifying program. Between these limits, their use is recommended either once a day or once a week (ANSI, ST46). Thermocouple tests, which are more reliable, are recommended in the United Kingdom (HTM, 1994). Frequent use (e.g. in every cycle) increases the chance of obtaining false positive cultures which may cause confusion, especially if thermocouple tests do not show any abnormality. Biological indicators intended for use in steam sterilization are prepared from spores of *Bacillus stearothermophilus* as conventional spore papers or self-contained biological indicators.

There are many brands of internal chemical indicators which can be used in conjunction with biological indicators for the advantage of obtaining an immediate indication of a gross error in sterilizing conditions. Integrators which provide a graded response indicating under-or over-exposure are also available.

Downward displacement jacketed sterilizers

The Bowie-Dick test is not applicable to downward displacement sterilizers because the indicator is likely to change colour completely while air is still present in the pack. It is also inappropriate for use in the steam-flush pressure-pulse sterilizers.

Temperature and automatic process control test

Close attention is paid to correspondence of temperature and pressure, clearance of the discharge line and correct functioning of the balanced pressure steam trap in the temperature and automatic process control test.

Thermocouple test

Thermocouple tests are essential to determine the heat penetration time and the temperature reached in the chamber and load. The recommended test pack (ANSI, ST8; ANSI, ST46) is made from 16 freshly laundered, huckaback or surgical towels, each measuring 40×65 cm. Each towel is folded lengthwise into thirds and then once across the middle. The folded towels are piled, with the folds facing in opposite directions, to form a pack measuring $23 \times 23 \times 15$ cm. One, but preferably two, biological indicators and a chemical indicator, if desired, are placed between the seventh and eighth towels. A thermocouple is also placed in the pack at its approximate geometric centre. In positioning the thermocouple, care must be taken to avoid the creation of a passage for steam tracking. The pack is secured with autoclave tape. For the small load test, the pack is placed on the shelf at the front of the chamber, with its layers in a horizontal position. At the conclusion of the test, the time-at-temperature record provided by the thermocouple is read, as are the indicators.

The small load test is repeated in three consecutive cycles. The same test pack is included with full loads for sterilization in the chamber and the full load tests are carried out.

Instrument and utensil 'flash' sterilizers

The temperature and automatic process control test is carried out with a mixed load of instruments and utensils and particular attention to accuracy of timing in the sterilizing stage. A thermocouple test should be performed with two leads in the chamber, one close to the air outlet and one fixed to the surface of an article in the full load. Regular observation of the temperature and pressure gauges is sufficient for routine testing. Biological and chemical indicators are not required in these sterilizers.

Fluid sterilizers

Temperature and automatic process control test

The need for special attention to the correct operation of the balanced pressure steam trap was high-lighted in 1972 when failure to investigate a discrepancy between the temperature and pressure readings, due to a faulty steam trap, was responsible for the death of several patients who received intravenous infusions that were contaminated with Gram-negative bacteria (Clothier, 1972). The control mechanism that prevents opening of the door of the sterilizer until the liquid has cooled to the prescribed temperature (80°C in bottles and 90°C in flexible plastic pouches) must also be checked. Four readings of temperature and pressure should be taken in the sterilizing stage of the temperature and automatic process control test.

Thermocouple test

Thermocouple tests are essential for the determination of the sterilization parameters for a particular liquid, in particular containers, to be sterilized in a particular sterilizer. Penetration times determined in one set of circumstances do not apply in another situation.

A full load of bottles or other containers, which may be a production batch for which a record has been established during commissioning, is used for the test (HTM, 1994). The containers should be filled with 1 litre of fluid and the initial temperatures should not vary by more than 10 per cent. Ten thermocouples are installed in the containers at locations which have been predetermined from heat distribution studies when the chamber was empty and when it was fully loaded. Three thermocouples are placed in containers at the slowest heating sites and three at the fastest heating sites. Three more are placed at the slowest cooling site and one in the chamber drain. The thermocouples must be firmly held in position at 85 per cent of the depth in rigid containers and at the geometric centre of plastic bags.

The result is satisfactory if the fluid in the test containers has been maintained at 121°C for a minimum of 15 minutes and the values for other process variables are within specified limits. Additionally, all temperature sensors must be still in place, the test containers must not have leaked and no more than one container or 1 per cent of the containers (whichever is the greatest) must be broken or burst. The door should remain locked until the temperature in the test containers has fallen to 80°C for bottles or 90°C for flexible containers. When a cooling system is used, the coolant should be tested for particulates and dissolved salts. It should contain no more than 0.01 per cent w/v of these substances.

REFERENCES

ANSI/AAMI ST8 — 1994 Hospital steam sterilizers. American National Standards Institute, New York

ANSI/AAMI ST33 — 1990 Good hospital practice: guidelines for the selection and use of reusable rigid sterilization container systems. American National Standards Institute, New York

ANSI/AAMI ST37 — 1992 Good hospital practice: Flash sterilization — steam sterilization of patient care items for immediate use. American National Standards Institute, New York

ANSI/AAMI ST42 — 1992 Steam sterilization and sterility assurance in office-based, ambulatory-care, medical and dental facilities. American National Standards Institute, New York

ANSI/AAMI ST46 — 1993 Good hospital practice: steam sterilization and sterility assurance. American National Standards Institute, New York

AS 1410 1987 Sterilizers — Steam — Pre-vacuum. Standards Association of Australia, Sydney

AS 2182 1994 Sterilizers — Steam — Portable. Standards Australia, Homebush, NSW

AS 2192 1991 Sterilizers — Steam — Downward displacement. Standards Australia, Sydney

AS 4187 1994 Code of practice for cleaning, disinfecting and sterilizing reusable medical and surgical instruments and equipment, and maintenance of associated environments in health care facilities. Standards Australia, Homebush, NSW

Bowie J H 1958 Requirements for an automatically controlled, high pre-vacuum steriliser. Health Bulletin (Edinburgh) 16: 36–40

Bowie J H 1974 Bowie and Dick test. Lancet i: 1233

Bowie J H, Dick J 1969 Autoclave tape test. British Hospital Journal and Social Service Review 79: 868

Bowie J H, Campbell I D, Gillingham F J, Gordon A R 1963 Hospital sterile supplies: Edinburgh pre-set tray system. British Medical Journal 2: 1322–1327

Brown P, Liberski P P, Wolff A, Gajdusek D C 1990 Resistance of scrapie infectivity to steam autoclaving after formaldehyde fixation and limited survival after ashing at 360°C: practical and theoretical implications. Journal of Infectious Diseases 161: 467–472

Clothier C M (Chairman) 1972 Report of the Committee appointed to inquire into the circumstances, including the production, which led to the use of contaminated infusion fluids in the Devonport Section of Plymouth General Hospital. HMSO, London

DHSS 1984 Management of patients with spongiform encephalopathy [Creutzfeldt-Jakob disease (CJD)]. Department of Health and Social Security circular DA (84)16: 1984

Ernst D R, Race R E 1993 Comparative analysis of scrapie agent inactivation. Journal of Virological Methods 41: 193–202

Everall P H, Morris C A, Yarnell R 1978 Sterilisation in the laboratory autoclave using direct air displacement by steam. Journal of Clinical Pathology 31: 144–147

Goullet D, Hambleton R 1989 Le test de Bowie-Dick: vérifications expérimentales des conditions de virage des systèmes prêts a l'emploi. Revue de l'ADPHSO 14(4): 11–26

Harris H F, Allison V D 1961 Steam sterilisation. Lancet ii: 603–604

Henry P S H 1959 Physical aspects of sterilizing cotton articles by steam. Journal of Applied Bacteriology 22: 159–173

Henry P S H 1964 The effect on cotton of steam sterilization with pre-vacuum. Journal of Applied Bacteriology 27: 413–421

Henry P S H, Scott E 1963 Residual air in the steam sterilization of textiles with pre-vacuum. Journal of Applied Bacteriology 26: 234–245

Holmlund L G 1965 Steam corrosion and steam corrosion inhibition in autoclave sterilization of dental and surgical steel materials. Biotechnology and Bioengineering 7: 177–198

HTM 1994 Health Technical Memorandum 2010 Part 3: Validation and verification. Sterilization. NHS Estates, London

Joslyn L J 1991 Sterilization by heat. In: Block S S (ed) Disinfection, sterilization, and preservation, 4th edn. Lea & Febiger, Philadelphia, ch 29, p 511

Kimberlin R H, Walker C A, Millson G C et al 1983 Disinfection studies with two strains of mouse-passaged scrapie agent. Journal of the Neurological Sciences 59: 355–369

Knox R, Pickerill J K 1964 Efficient air removal from steam sterilisers without the use of high vacuum. Lancet i: 1318–1321

Knox R, Pickerill J K 1967 Steam sterilisation: a pre-sterilising stage combining a flush-aided pre-vacuum with bursts of steam above atmospheric pressure. British Hospital Journal and Social Service Review 77: 2377, 2379–2380, 2382

Kropp D 1987 Air leaks and sterilization effectiveness. Journal of Healthcare Materiel Management 5(6): 65–67

Lauer J L, Battles D R, Vesley D 1982 Decontaminating infectious laboratory waste by autoclaving. Applied and Environmental Microbiology 44: 690–694

Nuffield Provincial Hospitals Trust 1958 Studies of sterile supply arrangements for hospitals. Present sterilizing practice in six hospitals. The Nuffield Provincial Hospitals Trust, London

Oates K, Deverill C E A, Phelps M, Collins B J 1983 Development of a laboratory autoclave system. Journal of Hospital Infection 4: 181–190

Perkins J J 1969 Principles and methods of sterilization in health sciences, 2nd edn. Charles C. Thomas, Springfield, ch 7, p 154; ch 9, p 193

Perrotta K A, Michnikov O 1986 Variations in the quality of steam entering the hospital sterilizer. Journal of Healthcare Materiel Management 4(4): 50–52

PHLS Subcommittee 1981 Public Health Laboratory Service Subcommittee on Laboratory Autoclaves. Specifications for laboratory autoclaves. Journal of Hospital Infection 2: 377–384

Pickerill J K, Perera R, Knox R 1971 Air detection in dressings steam sterilizers. Laboratory Practice 20: 406–413

Robbins J H, Jones G A 1971 Autoclave which sterilises with highly purified steam for tissue-culture laboratories. Lancet ii: 1236–1237

Rosenberg R N, White C L, Brown P et al 1986 Precautions in handling tissues, fluids, and other contaminated materials from patients with documented or suspected Creutzfeldt-Jakob disease. Annals of Neurology 19: 75–77

Rowe T W G, Kusay R 1961 Steam sterilisation. Lancet ii: 604–605

Scruton M W 1989a The effect of air with steam on the temperature of autoclave contents. Journal of Hospital Infection 14: 249–262

Scruton M W 1989b The effect of air on the moist-heat resistance of Bacillus stearothermophilus spores. Journal of Hospital Infection 14: 339–350

Smith R F 1986 Sterile? The ten parameters of steam sterilization. Journal of Healthcare Materiel Management 4(4): 34–36, 38–39

Taguchi F, Tamai Y, Uchida K et al 1991 Proposal for a procedure for complete inactivation of the Creutzfeldt-Jakob disease agent. Archives of Virology 119: 297–301

Tamai Y, Taguchi F, Miura S 1988 Inactivation of Creutzfeldt-Jakob disease agent. Annals of Neurology 24: 466–467

Tateishi J, Tashima T, Kitamoto T 1988 Inactivation of the Creutzfeldt-Jakob disease agent. Annals of Neurology 24: 466

Taylor D M 1987 Autoclaving standards for Creutzfeldt-Jakob disease agent. Annals of Neurology 22: 557–558

Taylor D M, Fraser H, McConnell I et al 1994 Decontamination studies with the agents of bovine spongiform encephalopathy and scrapie. Archives of Virology 139: 313–326

Taylor D M, McBride P A 1987 Autoclaved, formol-fixed scrapie mouse brain is suitable for histopathological examination, but may still be infective. Acta Neuropathologica 74: 194–196

Taylor D M, McConnell I 1988 Autoclaving does not decontaminate formol-fixed scrapie tissues. Lancet i: 1463–1464

Weymes C 1971 Sterilization of water for topical use in plastic bags. British Hospital Journal and Social Service Review 81: 1553, 1555, 1557

Wilkinson G R, Peacock F G, Robins E L 1960 A shorter sterilising cycle for solutions heated in an autoclave. Journal of Pharmacy and Pharmacology 12 (Suppl): 197T–202T

Working Party on Pressure-Steam Sterilisers 1959 Sterilisation by steam under increased pressure. A report to the Medical Research Council. Lancet i: 425–435

7. Sterilization by gaseous chemicals

Modern medical practice has seen the development and production of an increasing amount and variety of medical equipment which cannot withstand sterilization at high temperatures. The equipment may be separated into two categories:

1. Relatively simple devices that are produced and sterilized commercially; they are usually intended to be used once only and then discarded
2. Complex surgical or diagnostic equipment which is reusable and is sterilized on the hospital premises if a suitable process is available.

Phillips & Kaye (1949) reviewed the properties, bactericidal activity and toxicity of ethylene oxide with a view to its future use as a sterilizing agent for heat-sensitive medical equipment, among other materials. The conditions of concentration, temperature, humidity and time required for efficient biocidal action were reported in more detail by Phillips (1949) and Kaye & Phillips (1949). Since that time, ethylene oxide has increased in importance as a sterilizing agent in hospitals and in the large scale industrial production of sterile medical devices. It has been used in a nonflammable mixture with chlorofluorocarbon-12 but this CFC is implicated in depletion of the earth's ozone layer and its use is being phased out.

Commercial producers of sterile devices may choose between ethylene oxide at a temperature within the range 37–55°C and ionizing radiation at ambient temperature by gamma rays or electron beam. The decision is based on the nature of the equipment to be sterilized, the availability of an irradiation facility and the relative costs of installing and operating the two processes. Radiation sterilization is not normally available in hospitals but a choice of low-temperature sterilizing processes is available. Pure (100 per cent) ethylene oxide may be used in a self-contained sterilization system at the temperatures of 37 or 55°C. An alternative low-temperature steam and formaldehyde process is usually operated at 73°C. Some diagnostic instruments and electronic devices might not withstand the higher temperature of the formaldehyde process. The gas plasma systems, which were developed in the 1980s, are other suitable systems for the sterilization of heat-sensitive equipment and materials at temperatures below 55°C.

Gas sterilization should not be used for equipment or materials that withstand steam or dry heat sterilization. The low-temperature processes are slower, more expensive to operate, and may leave toxic residues which necessitate aeration of the sterilized products before they can be released for use. The steam and formaldehyde process, which was developed in the United Kingdom as an alternative to ethylene oxide, is quite distinct from older methods in which formaldehyde vapour is used as a disinfectant in rooms and cabinets where control of concentration, temperature and humidity is usually lacking.

The following explanation of mechanisms of biocidal action applies to ethylene oxide and formaldehyde; thereafter, the processes will be described separately.

BIOCIDAL ACTION OF ALKYLATING AGENTS

Ethylene oxide (C_2H_4O) and formaldehyde (H.CHO) are alkylating agents. Alkylation involves the addition of saturated hydrocarbon groups to reactive amino (NH_2), sulfydryl (SH), hydroxyl (OH) or carboxyl (COOH) groups on protein molecules and to imino (NH) groups in nucleic acid bases.

Typical alkylation reactions with reactive groups on proteins or nucleic acids are:

$$- NH_2 + C_2H_4O \rightarrow - NH(C_2H_4OH)$$
$$- SH + H.CHO \rightarrow - S(H.CHOH)$$
$$> NH + C_2H_4O \rightarrow > N(C_2H_4OH)$$

The biocidal activity of ethylene oxide parallels its alkylating power and depends on an unstable three-membered ring structure, as shown in Table 7.1. Cyclopropane, with a non-reactive ring structure, has neither alkylating power nor biocidal activity. At the other extreme, ethylene imine is so reactive that it is unsuitable for sterilization. The substitution of a hydrogen atom in ethylene oxide by a carbon-containing side chain, as in propylene oxide, reduces activity.

Alkylation of nucleic acids by ethylene oxide has been proposed as the principal mechanism of biocidal action (Gunther, 1980) because these vital cell components control protein synthesis. The ring nitrogen atoms of purine and pyrimidine bases are involved (Bruch, 1973). The principal site of action of ethylene oxide in the DNA of human cells (e.g. lymphocytes) is the N7 position in guanine (Sega & Generoso, 1988). Adducts with histidine, valine and cystine in proteins (e.g. haemoglobin) are also found (Yager, 1987). Formaldehyde has also been found to react with DNA during the replication process, when the double-stranded helix is unwinding (Vologodskii & Frank-Kamenetskii, 1975; Shikama & Miura, 1976).

Table 7.1 Biocidal activity of alkylating agents

Agent	Formula	Biocidal activity
Ethylene imine	H_2C —— CH_2 \ / NH	Very high
Ethylene oxide	H_2C —— CH_2 \ / O	High
Propylene oxide	H_2C —— $CH.CH_3$ \ / O	Moderate
Cyclopropane	H_2C —— CH_2 \ / CH_2	None

Chemical alkylating agents resemble ionizing radiation in their potential for toxicity, mutagenicity and carcinogenicity. They also share with ionizing radiation a broad spectrum of biocidal action, with a less than tenfold difference between the resistance of bacterial spores and the vegetative cells. This contrasts with a very large difference, up to

5 powers of 10, in the heat resistance of bacteria and their spores.

STERILIZATION BY ETHYLENE OXIDE (EO)

Physical and chemical properties of EO

Ethylene oxide, which boils at 10.7°C at atmospheric pressure, is liquefied at an increased pressure in storage cylinders. The pure gas is 1.5 times as heavy as air and usually diffuses downwards if it escapes into the atmosphere. However, upward movement has been demonstrated when small amounts are released, together with warm air, from a sterilizing chamber (Samuels & Corn, 1979; Korpela et al, 1983). Ethylene oxide is highly diffusible, moving through air pockets, wrapping materials (paper, cloth and some plastic films) and dissolving in rubbers, plastics, silicones and oils. The vapour is freely soluble in water, with which it reacts to form ethylene glycol. Reaction with sodium chloride in solutions or solids that have absorbed ethylene oxide yields nonvolatile ethylene chlorohydrin (2-chloroethanol).

Flammability

Ethylene oxide is flammable and highly explosive at all concentrations above 3.6 per cent by volume in air; the explosive force is 50 times as great as would be expected for a purely oxidative reaction. The pure gas may be used below atmospheric pressure in sterilization chambers from which air has been removed by evacuation. Mixtures containing 12 per cent by weight of ethylene oxide (EO) and 88 per cent chlorofluorocarbon-12 (CFC-12) or 10 per cent in carbon dioxide are nonflammable.

The carbon dioxide mixture has the following disadvantages:

1. The high pressure of the mixture requires a more robust chamber to provide for an adequate concentration of ethylene oxide
2. Change in composition as the carbon dioxide is withdrawn from the cylinder leads to a decrease in the amount of ethylene oxide delivered to the chamber and the possibility of a flammable mixture in the cylinder (Ernst & Doyle, 1968)
3. Reaction between carbon dioxide and water vapour in the chamber creates acidity which causes corrosion of the sterilizer and of some materials sterilized
4. The mixture promotes polymerization of ethylene oxide at a rate 10–20 times faster than does the ethylene oxide/CFC-12 mixture (Ernst & Doyle, 1968; Conviser, 1989).

Ethylene oxide is the sole sterilizing agent in the nonflammable gas mixtures; the diluent gases have no biocidal activity. The mixture with fluorocarbon-12 is more expensive than pure ethylene oxide and the carbon dioxide mixture but was widely used in hospital ethylene oxide sterilizers. However, because of environmental considerations rather than economic factors, 100 per cent ethylene oxide is now used.

Polymerization

Ethylene oxide tends to polymerize in storage cylinders, pipelines and sterilizing chambers. Rust, rough metal edges, constrictions in pipes and valves, and the polymer itself act as catalysts. The polymer can also absorb ethylene oxide and could increase the risk of exposure to workers or patients if it is formed within the pores of the materials of some devices (Conviser, 1989). Stainless steel should be used in the construction of sterilizing chambers and storage cylinders. The rate of polymerization is accelerated by a rise in temperature. The products may be solid, semi-solid or liquid and the colour may be white, yellow, green or brown. A white powder is formed in the sterilizing chamber at sites where water accumulates but a yellow liquid, which turns to gum, is formed in pipelines where the temperature and pressure are highest (Ernst & Doyle, 1968). Accumulation can be prevented by the use of high quality liquid ethylene oxide in single-use cartridges which becomes a gas when released into the sterilizing chamber. The empty cartridge is removed, aerated with the load and discarded. This means that there are no large storage tanks or external valves or gas lines between sterilant and chamber to act as sites for polymerization.

Absorption by natural and synthetic materials

Natural rubber absorbs up to 35 000 p.p.m. and synthetic rubbers up to 20 000 p.p.m. ethylene oxide. Polyvinyl chloride (PVC) absorbs as much as 25 000 p.p.m. of the sterilizing gas because ethylene oxide reacts with the phthalate plasticizer. Polyethylene and polypropylene absorb smaller but significant amounts. Paper wrapping material absorbs up to 10 000 p.p.m. and cotton absorbs less than 5000 p.p.m. The figures have been taken from published reports (e.g. Bruch, 1973; McGunnigle et al, 1975) but are subject to wide variation because the amount of ethylene oxide absorbed varies with the concentration and time of exposure and may be affected by the diluent gas. Accurate estimation is difficult because the amounts of ethylene oxide are small and must be extracted quantitatively from the solid material before analysis by gas chromatography (McGunnigle et al, 1975).

Samples of small devices or representative portions of larger devices are selected for the estimation of residual ethylene oxide. In selecting representative, 'worst case' samples for testing, variables affecting the amount of ethylene oxide absorbed should be taken into account. These include size, material composition, packaging, ethylene oxide exposure, water content and conditions of aeration. A method of exhaustive extraction, which is intended to recover all the ethylene oxide in a device, is required if the device is in contact with blood or tissue for more than 30 days. Simulated-use extraction suffices if the contact period is 30 days or less. The maximum dose of ethylene oxide in exposed patients is not to exceed 20 mg in the first 24 hours, 60 mg in 30 days or 2.5 g in a lifetime (ISO 10993.7, 1995).

The headspace method of extraction, in which the absorbed ethylene oxide is volatilized into the headspace of a closed vial by heating, is used for exhaustive extraction. An alternative method is solvent extraction. Quantitation is by analysis of the headspace gas and/or chromatography for the solvent extract. Water, or a physiological solution, is recommended for the simulated-use extraction (ISO 10993.7, 1995). A method in which ethylene chlorohydrin and ethylene glycol can be determined along with ethylene oxide in a single chromatographic analysis has been described (Ball, 1984).

Desorption

The rate at which ethylene oxide desorbs from various materials has been studied extensively to determine when sterilized articles are safe to use. The times required for desorption from packaged articles on open shelves at ambient temperature range from a few hours for those which contain only a small component of absorbing material to about 2 days for articles made from polyethylene and polypropylene and to 1–2 weeks for PVC and some types of rubber. Some silicones are reported to desorb rapidly (White & Bradley, 1973; McGunnigle et al, 1975). As desorption is an exponential process, most of the ethylene oxide is lost quickly but the final stages are very slow. Aeration of sterilized products in ambient conditions is satisfactory in commercial production because sufficient time elapses between sterilization and use. Special aeration cabinets are required in hospitals, where the types of articles that are sterilized by ethylene oxide are often required for use on the following day. The gas is driven out of the material at 50–60°C and flowing air removes it from the cabinet. Aeration times usually range from 2–24 hours but sometimes need to be longer (Gunther, 1974; McGunnigle et al, 1975).

Toxicity

Long-term occupational exposure to low levels, or occasional exposure to higher levels, of ethylene oxide are recognized causes for anxiety about the potential mutagenic, teratogenic or carcinogenic effects of this alkylating agent. The mutagenic effects are detected microscopically by sister chromatid exchanges (SCEs), chromosome breaks and other aberrations in the DNA of human and animal lymphocytes. SCEs are regarded as the most sensitive indicator of exposure to ethylene oxide (Yager et al, 1983). A link between ethylene oxide and human cancers, such as leukaemia, has not been established because statistically significant epidemiological evidence is slow to accumulate and exposure to other chemicals cannot always be ruled out (Nicholls, 1986). Yager

(1987) found that ethylene oxide was strongly mutagenic to rodents but low in carcinogenic and teratogenic activity. Studies in Sweden have accumulated eight cases of cancer in a total number of 733 workers in three factories where medical devices are sterilized by ethylene oxide (Hogstedt et al, 1986). However, none of these cases occurred in one factory where the workers were exposed to ethylene oxide only and their significance was questioned by Divine & Amanollahi (1986). Three other retrospective studies, covering several decades and large numbers of workers (727–2876), have failed to find any evidence of a direct association between exposure to ethylene oxide and the incidence of deaths from cancer (Bommer et al, 1985; Gardner et al, 1989; Greenberg et al, 1990). A single report of spontaneous abortions (Hemminki et al, 1982) remains uncorroborated (Nicholls, 1986). Exposure of patients or workers to ethylene oxide may lead to acute or chronic reactions.

Acute reactions

The immediate effects of inhalation have been likened to the effects of ammonia. They include irritation of the eyes and respiratory tract, headache, nausea, vomiting and dizziness. The condition may result from release of ethylene oxide when the door of a sterilizer is opened without the recommended precautions, leakage from a cylinder valve or the emergency of a major spill. Concentrations below 700 p.p.m. cannot be detected by smell, whereas levels above 1 p.p.m. may be toxic.

Harmful effects may also result from contact of skin and tissues with materials containing absorbed ethylene oxide. Liquid ethylene oxide evaporates too quickly to burn or blister the skin, but sustained contact with clothing, shoes, rubber gloves, anaesthetic face masks, endotracheal tubes and wound dressings which have not been adequately aerated after sterilization may cause dermatitis in hospital patients or staff. In a single episode, 19 patients were seriously burned by surgical drapes and gowns containing 3600–10 800 p.p.m. of residual ethylene oxide; healing took 3–6 weeks in some individuals (Biro et al, 1974). Synthetic materials, sterilized by ethylene oxide and used in cardiopulmonary bypass surgery, have been identified as the cause of severe

toxic shock and some deaths in small children (Stanley et al, 1971). The degree of tissue toxicity depends on the concentration of ethylene oxide in the material and the duration of contact. Reyniers et al (1964) reported that multiple tumours developed on the skin of mice that were in contact with bedding material that had been treated with ethylene oxide, instead of gamma radiation as intended.

An acute, hypersensitivity type reaction has been reported frequently in haemodialysis patients. The severe, sometimes fatal, anaphylactoid reactions usually occur within a few minutes of the start of a dialysis treatment, when the blood returns from the dialyzer to the patient's circulation. The symptoms include dyspnoea, wheezing, urticaria, flushing, headache, hypertension and, less commonly, bronchospasm, cardiac arrest and death. In the United Kingdom, 70 per cent of dialysis centres have experienced cases, with 243 separate reactions in 117 patients over a period of three years (Nicholls, 1986). The incidence is low in peritoneal dialysis, despite the use of tubing that has been sterilized with ethylene oxide (Marshall et al, 1984). However, reactions in the transfusion of haemophiliacs (Vermylen et al, 1988) and in surgery on spina bifida patients (Moneret-Vautrin et al, 1990) are important.

The role of ethylene oxide as the cause of the acute anaphylactoid reactions has been confirmed by the presence of antibodies to ethylene oxide in the patient's blood or tissue. The antibodies are of the IgE type, which is associated with hypersensitivity. Few patients react in the absence of antibodies which are specific to ethylene oxide (Bommer et al, 1985). Regular testing for antibody in haemodialysis patients with anaphylactic symptoms has been recommended (Rumpf et al, 1985). Sensitization is usually initiated during a previous dialysis treatment; when it happens at the first treatment, it is assumed to have occurred during previous diagnostic tests when the patient was in contact with other devices from which residual ethylene oxide had not been successfully removed.

The reactions are associated with new hollow fibre dialyzers which are sterilized with ethylene oxide and intended for single use only. The fibres, which are made from cuprammonium cellulose membrane, are held together at each end by a polyurethane 'potting compound' in which ethylene oxide is retained and from which it can only be removed by thorough rinsing before use (Bommer et al, 1985; Henne et al, 1984). Plate dialyzers, which are made from the same membrane material, do not cause reactions. Symptoms in some patients were reduced dramatically after dialyzers which had not been sterilized by ethylene oxide were used for eight weeks (Bommer et al, 1985). Antibodies to ethylene oxide have not been detected in patients who were treated with dialyzers that had been sterilized by gamma radiation.

Chronic reactions

Cytogenetic effects, such as SCEs, have been demonstrated in the peripheral lymphocytes of workers who have been exposed to low levels of ethylene oxide in hospital sterilizing departments or industrial facilities. Varied opinions have been expressed concerning the significance of the chromosomal aberrations to human health. Chromosome breaks, polyploid and chromatid aberrations were reported by Van Sittert et al (1985) and Clare et al (1985) in workers who had been exposed to ethylene oxide for periods up to 14 years. However, the frequency was not considered to be significant because the levels of ethylene oxide were below detection by air sampling and the subjects could also have been exposed to other chemicals. More serious views were expressed by Sarto et al (1984) and Stolley et al (1984), who found a significantly increased number of SCEs in workers who were categorized as high-exposure groups than in others in the workplace or in community control groups. As the frequency of the aberrations only rarely decreased when exposure to ethylene oxide was reduced or interrupted, Richmond et al (1985) recommended that workers should be under surveillance initially and yearly thereafter.

Less is known about the effects of ethylene oxide on the nervous system. Peripheral neuropathy, with or without CNS symptoms, has been demonstrated by task performance tests in eight workers who were exposed to the levels of ethylene oxide which may occur in hospital sterilizer operations (Estrin et al, 1987). Ohnishi et al (1985; 1986) demonstrated axonal degeneration of myelinated nerve fibres in rats, comparable to mild axonal degeneration in patients with signs of ethylene oxide toxicity.

Ethylene chlorohydrin has less than 15 per cent of the toxicity of ethylene oxide (Gunther, 1974). A report that ethylene chlorohydrin may be present in toxic amounts in PVC if the material has been previously sterilized by gamma radiation (Cunliffe & Wesley, 1967) has been contradicted by subsequent investigations in which no significant amount of ethylene chlorohydrin was detected in irradiated or unirradiated PVC (Bogdansky & Lehn, 1974). However, the amount of chlorides in some pharmaceuticals and foods might result in the production of toxic levels of ethylene chlorohydrin, and ethylene oxide is not used for the sterilization of such materials, with the possible exception of spices or other additives that are used in small quantities (Wesley et al, 1965; Ragelis et al, 1968; Holmgren et al, 1969).

Exposure limits

Standards for exposure by inhalation have been set in the United States by the Occupational Safety and Health Agency (OSHA, 1984) and are widely accepted in other countries. The permissible exposure limit (PEL) of 1 p.p.m. of ethylene oxide in air is calculated as a time-weighted average (TWA). This allows for some variation in concentration during a specified period; this is usually 8 hours, corresponding to the usual work shift. An action level of 0.5 p.p.m./8-h TWA is recommended as the goal to be met in hospital and industrial facilities where ethylene oxide is used. A short-term excursion limit (STEL) of 5 p.p.m., as a 15-min TWA, was defined in an amendment (OSHA, 1988). This represents a lower dose than the 1 p.p.m./8-h TWA as it refers to short-term risks, such as unloading the sterilizer or transferring the load to the aerator (Kruger, 1989).

Susceptibility of microorganisms

All types of microorganisms are susceptible to ethylene oxide if they are exposed to suitable conditions of concentration, temperature and relative humidity for an adequate time. The relatively small difference between the susceptibility of vegetative bacteria and spores is an advantageous feature of the biocidal action of ethylene oxide.

Dadd & Daley (1980) compared the resistance of different bacteria, spores and fungi with that of the spores of *Bacillus subtilis* subsp. *niger* (NCTC 10073), which are commonly used as a biological monitor of ethylene oxide sterilization. The vegetative bacteria, fungi, and the spores produced by *Bacillus stearothermophilus* and *Clostridium sporogenes* constituted a highly sensitive group. Strains of *Bacillus pumilus*, *Clostridium thermosaccharolyticum*, *Bacillus megaterium* and *Bacillus sphaericus* produced spores which were intermediate in resistance between the first group and *B. subtilis* subsp. *niger*. However, some species of *Bacillus* isolated from natural habitats produced spores of higher resistance. The spores of the reference strain of *B. subtilis* subsp. *niger* were only 8 times as resistant as the corresponding vegetative cells of this species. The virus that causes foot-and-mouth disease in domestic animals is susceptible to ethylene oxide (Tessler & Fellowes, 1961). Hoff-Jørgensen & Lund (1972) showed that vaccinia virus, Newcastle disease virus and representative enteroviruses were also susceptible to ethylene oxide treatment despite being tested in the presence of a high concentration of organic matter and allowed to dry before exposure to the gas process.

Factors influencing efficiency of biocidal action

The efficiency of ethylene oxide sterilization depends on achieving an adequate concentration of the chemical vapour at an appropriate temperature and relative humidity. Efficiency may be adversely affected if the microorganisms have previously been desiccated or are occluded within dried organic or crystalline material.

Concentration and temperature

The influences of concentration and temperature are interrelated (Ernst & Shull, 1962). If the concentration is above 440 mg/l, the temperature can vary between 45°C and 60°C without affecting the time required for sterilization. Conversely, when the temperature is above 45°C, an increase in

effective concentration above 440 mg/l has little effect on biocidal action. However, concentrations exceeding 700 mg/l are used in hospital sterilizers to overcome penetration barriers and to allow for absorption by packaging material. If the concentration and relative humidity are constant, the rate of sporicidal action will double for every 10°C rise in temperature (Caputo & Rohn, 1982).

Moisture

Relative humidities below 30 per cent are consistently adverse to the biocidal action of ethylene oxide. Levels ranging from 50–90 per cent, depending on the nature and bulk of the materials to be sterilized, are generally used in hospital and industrial sterilization processes; 70 per cent is recommended for processes which are operated at 55°C. The limiting factor in sterilization efficiency is more likely to be the penetration of moisture than penetration of ethylene oxide gas.

The critical role of moisture was emphasized by Kaye & Phillips (1949). Gilbert et al (1964) found that the optimum relative humidity for biocidal action at ambient temperature was 33 per cent. A similar result has been obtained more recently by Caputo & Rohn (1982) and Dadd et al (1985). At humidity levels below 33 per cent, the death rate curves tailed sharply as a small proportion of spores survived despite increases in time or concentration. Above 33 per cent, the curves were invariably linear but the rate of killing decreased slightly. The resistant spores which survived from the original desiccated population could be restored to sensitivity immediately by wetting or, more slowly, by exposure to a relative humidity above 75 per cent.

These phenomena are subject to different explanations, both of which are probably correct. Gunther (1980) proposed that moisture is necessary for combination of ethylene oxide with reactive groups on the bacterial surface. A surface film of water would promote contact by dissolving ethylene oxide to form a concentrated solution and would also provide a medium for ionization of the reactive groups.

The alternative explanation, proposed by Doyle & Ernst (1967), is that a high moisture level is necessary to dissolve organic or crystalline material which may protect some of the spores. This proposal was based on the observation that only about 1 per cent of desiccated spore populations survive exposure and their sensitivity can be restored rapidly by wetting them. This was confirmed by demonstrating that the difference in the susceptibility of spores of *B. subtilis* subsp. *niger* on impervious and on porous materials disappeared if the spores were thoroughly washed before inoculation on the carriers (Doyle & Ernst, 1968). The higher resistance on impervious material, such as metal foil or plastic, was explained by incrustation with material from the suspending fluid, whereas this was absorbed into the interstices of a porous material such as filter paper, leaving the bacteria in a cleaner condition on the surface and thus more susceptible. The decrease in susceptibility at high humidity which was found by Gilbert et al (1964) does not appear to apply to the higher levels of ethylene oxide concentration and temperature that are used in the hospital sterilization process.

Associated materials

Organic deposits do not confer complete protection on the microorganisms unless the material is very dry. However, occlusion in crystalline material confers complete protection unless the humidity in the sterilizer is high enough to dissolve it (Doyle & Ernst, 1967).

Sterilization by pure (100 per cent) gaseous ethylene oxide

The requirement for an ethylene oxide sterilization process and the availability of trained staff to operate it should be evaluated before a decision is made to install a sterilizer. The quantity of reusable medical, surgical and diagnostic equipment that cannot withstand heat sterilization should be assessed in order to ensure that the capacity of the sterilizing chamber will be fully utilized. If the calculated workload and throughput of a particular hospital are insufficient to justify the cost, the use of an ethylene oxide sterilizing service at a larger hospital or health care institution or the provision of supplies from a commercial source should be considered.

The sterilizer, together with an aeration cabinet, should be installed in a central sterilizing department where the suitability of the process for different types of heat-sensitive equipment can be assessed and the proper preparation and packaging can be supervised. The advice of a microbiologist who has studied the ethylene oxide process should be readily available because regular biological tests are required for qualifying the sterilizer and monitoring it in routine operation. The services of a specially trained engineer are also required.

Applications of ethylene oxide sterilization

Sterilization by ethylene oxide is required for articles that are made partly or entirely from heat-sensitive rubber or synthetic materials or contain electronic components, telescopes and lamps. Most of the articles withstand treatment at 50–60°C but a lower temperature (e.g. 37°C) may be required for some equipment. The manufacturer's advice concerning the sterilization of complex equipment should be sought because components are changed from time to time. The ethylene oxide process is recommended for sterilization of endoscopic instruments; however, it is too slow for the decontamination of an instrument that must be used for successive patients in an operating session.

Ethylene oxide gas sterilization is not applicable to liquids or to articles in impervious packaging material. It is also unsuitable, because of possible toxic effects, for producing sterile diets for infection-susceptible patients or germfree animals. The availability of ethylene oxide sterilization in a hospital does not justify the resterilization of devices which are intended for a single use only. Some types of hospital equipment for which an ethylene oxide process is appropriate are listed in Table 7.2.

Preparation and packaging

Articles to be sterilized by ethylene oxide must be thoroughly cleaned. They should be rinsed with distilled water (not saline), dried at room temperature to avoid excessive dehydration and inspected for cleanliness and absence of water droplets. It may be difficult to check cavities in hollow instruments and it is impossible to verify the cleanliness

Table 7.2 Some articles that may be sterilized by ethylene oxide in hospitals

Types of articles	Examples[1]
Anaesthetic and respiratory therapy equipment	Airways Endotracheal tubes Masks (other rubber items) Mechanical ventilators
Cardiac equipment	Cardiac catheters Heart-lung apparatus Transducers
Devices and materials for implantation	Breast implants Cardiac pacemakers and leads Cardiac valves Orthopaedic prostheses
Diathermy equipment	Tissue implants Cautery pencils Cautery tips Electrical leads
Endoscopic instruments	Arthroscopes Cystoscopes Laparoscopes Resectoscopes
Medical and dental equipment	Equipment for blood cell separation Cryoprobes Dental handpieces (air rotor type) Dermatomes (some types) Drills (battery powered) Electronic equipment Microsurgical accessories Nebulizers Oxygen tents Plastic bath linings Tourniquets Urological stone extractors

[1]Electrical equipment should be checked by an electrician before use

of fine tubes such as cardiac catheters, which should not be reprocessed. The presence of water droplets is not desirable because the free water is able to absorb the gaseous ethylene oxide sterilizing agent. Over-dried packaging material may absorb moisture in the sterilizer thereby depleting the amount that reaches the articles to be sterilized.

Packaging materials recommended for hospital use are similar to those used for steam sterilization because permeability to air, steam and ethylene oxide vapour is essential. Bags made from paper or from paper and transparent plastic film (window pack) are most convenient for small articles but wrapping sheets of crepe paper or cotton fabric may be required for trays containing endoscopes or other large objects. Thin polyethylene film is permeable to ethylene oxide but sealed packages made entirely from the film are impermeable to moisture and are likely to burst under vacuum because air cannot be removed. A porous paper-like material (Tyvek®) made from spun-bonded polyethylene is ideal for ethylene oxide sterilization but its use for hospital packaging may be limited by its high cost. It may be sealed as a breathable patch in a web of transparent plastic.

Pure EO sterilizers

Pure ethylene oxide is the principal form of the sterilant since the implementation of the world-wide ban on chlorofluorocarbon-12 (CFC-12). CFC-12 was formerly used as an inert diluent in a non-flammable gas mixture for hospital use. For economic reasons, pure ethylene oxide was used earlier in industrial sterilizing processes. Flammability is controlled by operating the sterilization cycles at subatmospheric pressure in relatively small chambers from which air has been evacuated. In addition, the humidity level is established before gaseous ethylene oxide is released into the chamber from a unit dose canister.

An ethylene oxide sterilization facility should be accommodated within the hospital sterile supply department (SSD) as a separate section with dedicated packaging and sterilizing rooms (ANSI, ST43; HBN 13.1, 1994), where clean room conditions (BS 5295.1, 1989) and appropriate airflow gradients are established. Access should be restricted to authorized personnel. The suitability of the process for different types of heat-sensitive equipment needs to be checked and proper preparation and packaging supervised. The advice of a microbiologist should be available because regular microbiological tests are required for qualifying the sterilizer and monitoring its performance. The services of a trained engineer are also required.

Design and construction of sterilizers

Relatively small sterilizers fulfil a need for hospital scale operation but multiple units are often used in industrial processes. Chamber sizes of 0.13, 0.14 and 0.22 m³ are available. The following description of this type of sterilizer and the alternative sterilization cycles for which it is designed applies to Sterivac™ sterilizer/aerators.

The chamber is constructed of anodised aluminium, with a stainless steel door. The larger sizes may have a door at each end. A distilled water tank provides steam for humidification of the load. The internal fittings are a cartridge holder and a load basket. Connections to the chamber include a venturi type vacuum pump.

A local exhaust hood is mounted externally above the door of the chamber to draw vapours away from the area when the door is opened by the operator. The exhaust hood is compulsory or optional, depending on local or national regulations. The vents from the sterilizing chamber and exhaust hood may be connected to a common dedicated exhaust system discharging to outside atmosphere or the exhaust gases may be detoxified in an emission control system (Donaldson Abator™) in which a catalyst converts the ethylene oxide to carbon dioxide and water. General room ventilation of 10 air changes per hour is recommended, the intake and outlet being positioned so as to draw vapours away from the operator. Ventilation of the sterilizer/aerator and any separate aeration cabinets should meet OSHA (1984, 1988) standards for protection of the workers.

The large (0.22 m³) sterilizer may be recessed into the wall; smaller sizes are mounted on a table, bench or trolley. Adequate space is required on all sides for service access and a clear space beneath the chamber provides for the circulation of air over the electrical components.

Comprehensive labelling on the front of the sterilizer includes warning of potential hazard, with instructions for immediate first aid and also for operation of the sterilizer. Warnings of toxic, flammable gas and hazardous voltage are placed on the back of the machine for persons who install and service the equipment.

Process indicators and controls

The sterilization process is fully automated, with microprocessor controls, for safe and efficient sterilization. The door interlock system ensures that a cycle cannot be started until the door has been closed and locked and that the door cannot be opened unless ethylene oxide has been completely purged from the chamber. A partly opened (latched) position is provided for use immediately the door has been opened. If the chamber has a door at each end, the cycle can be started only from the loading side. Temperature and vacuum levels are monitored continuously and a printer provides a permanent record of temperature, pressure and time. Indicator lights show the stage of the cycle, including the time of aeration if this is carried out in the sterilizer. Three types of malfunction are detected and signalled automatically:

1. If the malfunction occurs before the cartridge has been punctured, the cycle may be stopped and the load removed
2. If the malfunction occurs during the period of exposure to the gas, the cycle proceeds to completion, signalling a fault with a continuing audible alarm. The door may then be opened as the gas has been removed
3. If the chamber still contains ethylene oxide, the door remains locked and a service call is usually required.

A comprehensive list of causes, remedial measures and emergency procedures is in the operator's manual. Visible spurting or dripping of liquid ethylene oxide from a cartridge constitutes an emergency; a very cold or underweight cartridge indicates leakage.

Sterilization cycles

Automatic settings provide for alternative cycles: a warm cycle at 55°C, requiring 2 hours 45 minutes for completion; and a cool cycle at 37°C, requiring 4 hours 45 minutes. If an exhaust hood is not fitted or not operating, the final air purge is automatically extended by 3 hours before the cycle is completed. Figures 7.1 and 7.2 show a cycle.

The door of the preheated sterilizer is opened to insert a gas canister into the holder and to introduce the baskets containing the load for sterilization. The packs should be well spaced and placed on edge, with the plastic side of one pouch facing the paper side of the next. The door is then closed and it locks when the cycle start switch activates the locking mechanism. An automatic cycle then proceeds through the following stages:

Stage 1. Preconditioning the load (about 45 minutes). A vacuum is drawn to 24 kPa A to remove air and repeated pulses of subatmospheric steam are injected into the chamber. Time is allowed at the peak of each pulse for moisture penetration and also in the vacuum that is re-established before the next pulse. Ten pulses are used in the warm cycle and four in the cool cycle; the vacuum is extended for a further 8 minutes in the cool cycle to provide equivalent time for moisture penetration.

Stage 2. Exposure to sterilizing gas. The gas cartridge is punctured by the difference between the pressure in the final evacuation of the preconditioning stage and the surrounding atmosphere. The ethylene oxide concentration in the chamber is 725 mg/l; the pressure is maintained at about 70 kPa A and the temperature to within 3°C of that selected for the process. The time for the sterilizing stage is 100 minutes for the warm cycle and 220 minutes for the cool cycle.

Stage 3. Gas exhaust and air purge. The chamber is evacuated to about 10 kPa A to exhaust ethylene oxide to outside atmosphere via the dedicated vent line or, preferably, a Donaldson Abator. It is then purged with fresh filtered air for 15 minutes before the door can be opened to the latched position, with the local exhaust hood in operation. After 5 minutes, the door may be fully opened for transfer of the load to a separate aeration cabinet or for retrieval of the biological indicator.

Aeration of the load

Aeration may be carried out in sterilizers with integral aeration, i.e. those models capable of combining sterilization and aeration in the same chamber. Such equipment may also be used as sterilizers only, with aeration carried out in a separate aeration cabinet, especially if the full time recommended for aeration is not available. The temperature is usually 50–60°C, depending on the heat tolerance of the materials, with an airflow rate of four chamber volumes per minute. All air used for aeration must pass through a bacteria-retentive filter of 99.97 per cent efficiency. The heating system should cut out if overheat exceeds 5°C. The aeration time is affected by the following factors:

1. Composition, thickness, design configuration and weight of the device and wrapping material
2. Ethylene oxide concentration, temperature and time of the sterilization process
3. Temperature and the rate and pattern of airflow
4. Size and arrangement of packs in the aerator and the amount of highly absorptive material being aerated
5. Intended use of the device (external or implantable) which influences the permissible limit of residual ethylene oxide.

The recommended time for aeration may vary from a minimum of 2 hours, for articles consisting mainly of metal or glass, to 12 hours or longer. For convenience, the aeration process is commonly operated overnight.

Testing efficiency of sterilization

Two different programs are involved in testing the efficiency of an ethylene oxide sterilization process:

1. Comprehensive validation before commissioning or recommissioning
2. Monitoring of each sterilization cycle in routine operation.

Validation comprises a wide range of tests, including estimation of the bioburden of the product to be sterilized and also of any contaminated raw materials used in its manufacture, as well as the relevant physical tests and the use of biological and chemical indicators. A less extensive range of selected tests is used to monitor routine operation. Recommissioning is recommended annually, or when there are significant changes in the product, packaging method or loading system. The sterilizer should be subject to a preventive maintenance program at specified intervals or when otherwise required. All tests should be carried out by qualified personnel (ISO 11135, 1994; BS:EN 550, 1994; HTM, 1994).

Monitoring sterilization parameters

The parameters of the ethylene oxide sterilization process are: ethylene oxide concentration, relative humidity, temperature and time of exposure.

Thermocouples are used to measure the temperature at selected sites in the chamber and in the load. Direct measurement of the concentration of ethylene oxide gas in routine operation is not feasible. However, the gas concentration may be deduced from the weight of pure ethylene oxide released from the cartridge that is punctured within the evacuated chamber. Because of absorption by the load, the actual concentration would be less. The precise measurement of relative humidity is also a problem because sensors that can measure relative humidity in a chamber containing ethylene oxide are not available. While the optimum relative humidity in a cycle operating at 55°C is close to 60 per cent, a value within the range of 40 to 60 per cent is permitted (BS:EN 550, 1994; HTM, 1994). The relative humidity may be measured directly by a humidity sensor before the ethylene oxide is admitted to the chamber or it may be calculated from the increase in pressure that occurs when steam is admitted for humidification (ANSI, ST24).

Regular calibration of all controlling, indicating and recording equipment is required. The temperatures of the chamber heat cut-out, the chamber wall and the chamber space should also be checked. The chamber space temperature should be within 2°C of the preset gas exposure temperature at the start of the gas exposure stage (HTM, 1994).

Biological indicators

Types, methods of preparation, standardization and use of biological indicators are described in detail in Chapter 2. Spore preparations of *Bacillus subtilis* subsp. *niger* NCTC 10073 (ATCC 9372) provide the principal means of confirming the efficiency of ethylene oxide sterilization because the sterilization parameters cannot all be determined and controlled, especially within the packaged items to be sterilized. The indicators may be in the form of packaged, spore-impregnated papers, self-contained capsules incorporating the recovery medium or inoculated samples of product or simulated product. The incubation temperature for culture of the spores is 37°C (ANSI, ST21).

Each batch of indicators may be calibrated by fractional exposure times in which the severity of

treatment is increased from that which allows the survival of all units tested to complete inactivation. Further treatment is undertaken to obtain the desired sterility assurance level. Validation of the indicators should be carried out at a temperature of not less than 55°C, with a relative humidity of not less than 70 per cent and a concentration of ethylene oxide not less than 800 mg/l (ISO 11138.2, 1994).

The siting of the biological indicators in validation and routine control tests and the number used are governed by the same principles as apply to steam sterilization.

Chemical indicators

Chemical indicators may provide an early indication of gas penetration but they cannot validate the process (HTM, 1994).

Paper strips, which are impregnated with a dye that changes colour from yellow to blue, and adhesive tapes, which develop coloured stripes on exposure to ethylene oxide, are available as external indicators. In common with all external indicators, these serve only to confirm that packages have been exposed to a sterilization process. However, different brands of integrators for ethylene oxide sterilization have been compared to standard type spore papers and found to provide more exacting tests of sterilizing conditions than do biological indicators (Fitzpatrick & Reich, 1986).

In a combined test involving thermocouples, biological indicators and chemical indicators, Line/Pickerill helices are used to provide a severe challenge to gas and heat penetration. In the test, a biological and a chemical indicator are placed in each of twenty helices, which are then wrapped and sealed in paper bags (BS 6257, 1989). Twelve of these units are placed in positions matching those of thermocouples, as used in a previous thermometric test, and the rest are placed at other sites in the chamber or test load. A concordant result from three identical cycles is regarded as providing the minimum time required for the sterilization of the load (HTM, 1994).

Test packs

A challenge test pack and a routine test pack have been devised for use in hospital sterilizers for performance evaluation of the ethylene oxide sterilization process (ANSI, ST41).

The challenge pack is intended for qualifying tests on a new or repaired sterilizer and for ongoing sterility assurance testing. Challenge pack testing should be conducted at least quarterly and after any major changes in procedures. The pack includes cotton materials, which are not normally sterilized by the ethylene oxide process. However, they are used to serve as a challenge to penetration by water vapour and ethylene oxide. The test pack consists of four huckaback towels, each folded to form six thicknesses; an adult size plastic airway and a 22.5 cm length of latex tubing of specified diameter and wall thickness; and two 20 ml plastic syringes. A biological indicator is placed in the barrel of each syringe between, but not touching, the lower end of the plunger and the outlet of the barrel. A needle is not attached and any tip guard must be removed so that the barrel is left open. All components are held at 18–24°C at 35 per cent relative humidity for at least two hours before they are assembled in the test pack. The syringes, tubing and airway are placed between the folded towels at the centre of the horizontal stack, which is then wrapped in two layers of cotton cloth and fastened with adhesive tape. One to five test packs, depending on the size of the chamber, are placed in an otherwise empty sterilizing chamber for the test. Several biological indicators are used in each cycle in qualifying tests until confidence in the efficiency of the ethylene oxide sterilization process has been established.

In the routine test pack, a syringe containing a biological indicator is placed within the fold of a clean surgical towel and enclosed in a wrapper or peel pack of the type that is used in the hospital. As it is desirable to use at least two biological indicators to increase the reliability of the result (see Ch. 2), the test could be performed with two syringes in a single pack or with each of them in two separate packs. The test pack should be accompanied by a full load that is representative of the most challenging type of hospital load. A test is mandatory in every load that contains implantable devices; and, whenever possible, these should not be released for use until the result of the biological test is known (ANSI, ST41). Otherwise, the recommended testing frequency varies from once a day to once a week. If the biological indicators are not removed prior to aeration, the test pack should be aerated with the load. Otherwise, it is aerated with, or without, the load.

Ethylene oxide safety in the workplace

The limits for human exposure to ethylene oxide have already been stated in this chapter but are reiterated here because they define the goals to be achieved and the standards to be met in the cause of worker safety. The permissible exposure limit (PEL) of 1 p.p.m. (8-h TWA) and action level of 0.5 p.p.m. (8-h TWA) correspond to the normal workshift. The short-term excursion limit (STEL) of 5 p.p.m. (15-min TWA) applies to the performance of particular tasks, which may be carried out only once or twice in the workshift. These include installing gas cartridges, opening the door of the sterilizer on completion of the cycle, removing biological indicators from a test pack before it has been aerated, and transferring the load to the aeration cabinet (Yager et al, 1983). The absence of additional, or background exposure, is implied (Kruger, 1989).

Compliance with the PEL standard

A written plan of action must be prepared in all hospitals where the ethylene oxide level in the vicinity of the sterilizer, aeration cabinet or any service facility exceeds 1 p.p.m. When this level has been achieved, further efforts are required to reach the lower action level of 0.5 p.p.m. Essential features of a compliance program are the methods proposed for reducing exposure, a schedule of periodic surveys for leaks and a special plan of action for emergency situations. Attention should be given to identifying the potential sources of exposure for employees. Finally, a detailed schedule for the implementation of the plan must be prepared and a record kept of all measures taken. The plan must be available to employees and their representatives. No further action is required after the 0.5 p.p.m. level has been achieved unless there are changes in the conditions under which it was reached. Nevertheless, it is recommended that the protocol be reviewed annually.

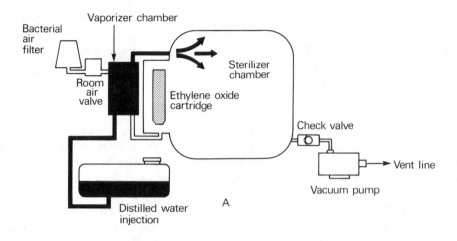

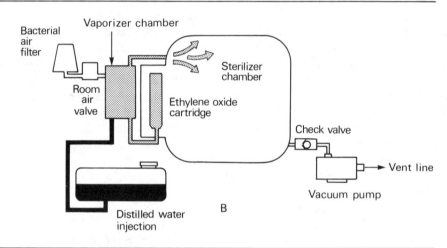

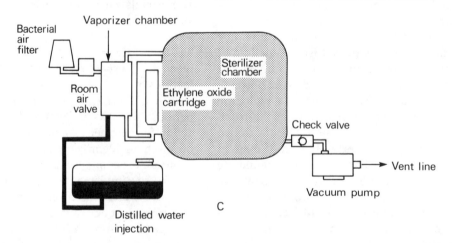

Fig. 7.1 Stages in the operation of a sterilizer using 100% ethylene oxide (A) Humidification (B) Admission of sterilizing gas (C) Sterilization (Courtesy of 3M Company).

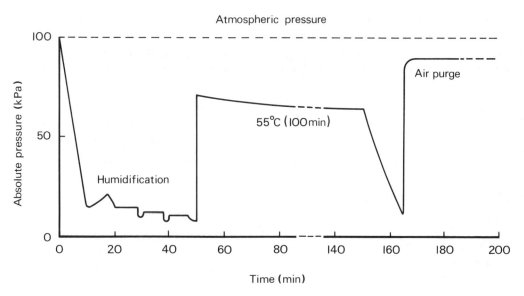

Fig. 7.2 An ethylene oxide sterilization cycle using 100% ethylene oxide at subatmospheric pressure (Courtesy of 3M Company).

A survey which included 1000 US hospitals two years after the standards were introduced showed that 72 per cent had achieved the action level of 0.5 p.p.m. An additional 13 per cent reached 1.0 p.p.m. and the remaining 15 per cent had yet to achieve these levels (Gschwandtner et al, 1986). The main causes of failure were the lack of local exhaust vents over the sterilizer door and aeration cabinet and the absence of a continuing air purge in the exhaust stage of the sterilization cycle. Excess leaks from the gas cylinders or connecting pipelines, and the lack of a leak detection program also contributed. However, in the pure ethylene oxide sterilization process, continuing air purge in the exhaust stage of the cycle occurs for up to 3 hours and the use of gas cartridge units in the sterilizing chamber eliminates the need for large gas cylinders and connecting pipelines.

Control measures

The procedures that are undertaken to comply with the PEL and STEL standards may relate to the design of the workplace; installation of the sterilizer, aerator and gas supply cartridges; engineering surveillance and testing; and safe work practices (Kruger, 1989). The sterilizer and aerator should be installed in a protected alcove within the

sterilizing department, in a separate room (Gourley, 1988) or in a dedicated ethylene oxide unit with packaging, loading and sterilizing areas (ANSI, ST43; HBN 13.1, 1994). Access should be restricted to personnel who operate the process or maintain the equipment. The sterilization cycle should end in an air purge that removes the gases from the chamber and continues automatically until the door is opened. Ventilation of the general area with at least 10 air changes per hour is recommended. In the dedicated ethylene oxide processing unit, the packing, loading, sterilizing, aeration and gas storage areas should be at negative pressure relative to adjacent areas.

One day's supply of gas cartridges (up to a maximum of 12 cartridges) may be stored in the immediate vicinity of the sterilizer, provided that the area is ventilated by, at least, 10 air changes per hour (ANSI, ST43). Additional cartridges should be stored upright in an approved flammable liquid storage cabinet vented to outside atmosphere or in an area suitable for the storage of flammable liquids, with venting to outside atmosphere.

Although the vapours discharged from the sterilizer may be vented directly to outside atmosphere, the use of a catalytic control system, the Donaldson Abator, which was developed for hospital use (Porco, 1988) is recommended. In the Abator, the effluent from the sterilizer and aerator is mixed with preheated air and passed over a dry, granular catalyst before it is vented to atmosphere. In the catalysed chemical reaction, ethylene oxide is oxidized to carbon dioxide and water with the generation of heat. The maximum temperature in the Abator is 138°C and the life of the catalyst is three years. The concentration of ethylene oxide entering the Abator is well below the 3 per cent explosion limit.

If the ethylene oxide is vented directly to atmosphere, the vent lines must be impervious to ethylene oxide and they must not terminate within 7.5 metres of any air intake to the building or near pedestrian traffic inside or outside the building. The sterilizers and aerators must not be used if the ventilation system is not operating.

Attention to work practices is at least as important as are the design features and engineering controls in minimizing or preventing exposure of the staff in sterilizing departments to the risk of ethylene oxide inhalation. Engineers who are responsible for an ethylene oxide sterilization system must be aware of all possible sources of exposure to toxic vapours. They bear the responsibility for regular leak testing as well as for testing the general and local exhaust ventilation and emergency alarms.

Appropriate education of the staff involved in operating the ethylene oxide process is essential. All procedures and work practices must be prominently displayed (HBN 13.1, 1994). Rotation of staff, so that each member serves only part of the workshift, is not permitted as a means of achieving compliance with the OSHA standards.

Tasks which involve known risks of exposure are:

1. Removal and transfer of the load from the sterilizer to the aeration cabinet. The distance should be as short as possible and the load should be pulled, not pushed.
2. Removal of biological indicators from packs before aeration. This is done to assess the efficiency of the sterilization process, independently of the continuing action of residual ethylene oxide on the biological indicators. Protective clothing, including gloves, should be worn.
3. Handling of damaged gas cartridges, which may show signs of leaks or spills by their low

temperature or decrease in weight. They must not be put in the aeration chamber but should be subject to the full sterilization cycle in an otherwise empty chamber.

The use of respiratory protection by sterilizing staff is generally considered unnecessary, unless the engineering and work practices described above are not feasible (Kruger, 1989) or an emergency situation exists.

Emergency situations

The potential for ethylene oxide to cause emergency situations associated with leakage of the liquid or gas from cylinders or other sterilant sources is well recognized and safety measures are clearly defined (ANSI, ST43). However, the risk of catastrophic events has been virtually eliminated by the development of relatively small sterilizers that use pure ethylene oxide at subatmospheric pressure in explosion-proof chambers. Nonetheless, a compulsory written plan must be available; and, in the event of an emergency, it must be implemented immediately (OSHA, 1984). Procedures for routine medical surveillance and emergency treatment of employees must also be available.

The emergency plan requires the installation of automatic, audible and visible alarms (ANSI, ST43) or a public address system. The proper functioning of the alarms requires testing. Escape routes from the source and site of an emergency should be clearly defined. After contact with ethylene oxide, the clothes of the affected person should be taken off and aerated and the person removed to fresh air; or, if necessary, resuscitated with oxygen. Information about the general hospital ventilation systems is required so that the possibility of ethylene oxide reaching other areas of the hospital may be evaluated.

The staff of the sterilizing department and hospital emergency department as well as members of the hospital and community fire services should be familiar with the emergency plan and trained for their roles in its implementation. No untrained or improperly equipped employee should approach the leak source, even to close it down. Supervisors who are responsible for directing the plan and assessing the risk to other hospital areas must be clearly identified. Protective clothing must be stored away from the risk area but immediately accessible.

The main stages of an emergency procedure are as follows (ANSI, ST43):

1. Evacuating and accounting for unprotected personnel
2. Reporting the emergency
3. Entering of the area by protected personnel to evacuate unconscious casualties and then to restore safety by ventilating the facility, washing down with water and disposing of waste in a non-hazardous manner
4. Determining when unprotected workers may safely re-enter the area.

When the emergency plan has been established, a mock drill which involves all participants, but does not cause undue inconvenience in the hospital, should be carried out (Chobin & Engle, 1989).

Monitoring exposure to ethylene oxide

The concentration of ethylene oxide in the workplace can be monitored in two ways:

1. Determination of the concentration in the environment at a particular time, regardless of the presence or absence of staff
2. Estimation of the average concentration to which workers are exposed over a specified time e.g. a workshift.

The ideal monitor should be sensitive to concentrations of ethylene oxide below 1 p.p.m., reliable, easy to use and inexpensive. However, not all of these requirements are generally fulfilled.

Area monitoring. Infrared spectrophotometers, photoionization detectors and gas chromatographs are available. Infrared analyzers are effective in measuring peak levels of ethylene oxide in the atmosphere but are not sensitive enough for monitoring compliance with OSHA standards. Furthermore, frequent maintenance and calibration are necessary to ensure their reliability. These expensive devices are more appropriate to industrial than to hospital use. By contrast, tubes containing specially treated charcoal are portable, inexpensive, sensitive to 0.1 p.p.m. and can be used in hospital facilities. A sample of air is drawn through the tube for a given time and the ethylene oxide is subsequently eluted for analysis by gas chromatography. However, their stability is uncertain.

Personnel monitoring. The monitors must be small enough to be worn by the worker without inconvenience. Charcoal tubes can be clipped to a lapel but a battery powered pump, usually attached to the belt, is also required. These fulfil the requirement for sensitivity but their use has declined with the development of passive diffusion monitors, or badges. Passive monitors operate as follows:

1. A treated charcoal disc absorbs ethylene oxide which is subsequently desorbed and measured by gas chromatography. This may require the return of the disc to the manufacturer (Mullins, 1985; ANSI, ST43).
2. An acid absorbing solution converts ethylene oxide to ethylene glycol which is, in turn, converted to formaldehyde and measured by a colorimetric method in a laboratory (Kring et al, 1984; 1985).
3. Dichromate in silica gel reacts with ethylene oxide to give chromate with a colour change from yellow to green. The silica gel is supported on a plastic strip in the form of a thin layer chromatography (TLC) plate. The exposure is read directly by the length of the green stain in a calibrated gas indicator tube (Gonzalez & Sefton, 1985).

An accuracy of ±13.5 per cent is claimed for each of the dosimeters. This is within the OSHA requirements of ±25 per cent for PEL of 1 p.p.m. (8-h TWA) and ±35 per cent for STEL of 5 p.p.m. (15-min TWA) (Kring et al, 1984).

STERILIZATION BY GAS PLASMA

Plasma is the fourth state of matter, distinguished from solid, liquid and gas. Low-temperature, glow discharge plasma consists of a cloud of reactive ions, electrons and neutral atomic particles, which are produced by the action of a strong electric or magnetic field on a gas precursor (Jacobs, 1989). An example is neon lighting. The visible glow is produced as the reactive species move from states of higher to lower energies. These reactive species are capable of disruptive interactions with the components of microbial cells.

Two plasma sterilization systems are available. In the Sterrad™ system, vapour phase hydrogen peroxide is used as precursor for the generation of plasma by application of a radiofrequency-induced electric field. The vapour phase hydrogen peroxide also exerts biocidal activity during its diffusion phase. In the Abtox™ Plazlyte™ system, two alternating phases are used, both of which are biocidal. The first is vapour phase peracetic acid and the second is the plasma phase; which, in this system, is generated by the action of microwaves on an inert gas mixture of argon, hydrogen and oxygen.

Physical and chemical properties

When the gas precursors of plasma are subjected to radiofrequency energy or microwaves, electrons are removed from atoms and accelerated; molecular species collide and free radicals form. Among the latter are hydroxy and hydroperoxy free radicals. Such free radicals are produced by gamma irradiation of water in the presence of oxygen so are also involved in gamma sterilization. In addition to the various charged particles, ultraviolet radiation is produced with the glow discharge.

Compatibility with natural and synthetic materials

Plasma is not applicable to the sterilization of liquids, oils, powders or biological tissues. In addition, cellulosic-based materials, such as paper, cotton or linen, cannot be used when hydrogen peroxide is the plasma precursor because of their absorption of hydrogen peroxide.

Plasma is applicable to the sterilization of metals, natural rubber, silicone and a range of plastic polymers. Compatible polymers include polyethylene, polypropylene, polystyrene, polyester, polyvinyl chloride and polytetrafluoroethylene (Teflon).

Paper is compatible with the Abtox Plazlyte plasma sterilization system because an inert gas mixture, not hydrogen peroxide, is used for the generation of the plasma in this system. Linen and cotton wraps are approved for use in the longest cycle of this system (cycle III with a 3-hour processing time). However, the data of Alfa (1996) suggest some interference with plasma penetration by linen wrap, as compared to Spunguard™ wrap, in the cycle.

Toxicity and workplace safety

A major advantage of plasma sterilization technologies is the absence of any toxic emissions or residuals. At the end of the sterilization cycle, the reactive elements in plasma combine to form mainly water and oxygen, thereby eliminating the need for aeration. Sterilized articles are safe for immediate patient use.

Aliquots of hydrogen peroxide are safely packaged in a sealed cassette. The cassette incorporates a chemical indicator which changes colour from yellow to red should a leak occur. Once inserted in the sterilizer, the cassette automatically advances through a program, e.g. five cycles of two injection phases. The cycles are conducted under conditions of reduced pressure in the sterilizing chamber.

Strong solutions of hydrogen peroxide and its vapours are potentially irritating to the skin, respiratory tract and the eyes. They may cause serious damage to the eyes. Like ethylene oxide, the PEL for hydrogen peroxide is 1 p.p.m. However, monitoring of the atmosphere in the vicinity of a Sterrad sterilizer has shown that the 8-hour TWA is less than 0.005 p.p.m.

Both the peracetic acid and the inert gas mixture for plasma generation in the Abtox Plazlyte system are supplied in cylinders. Peracetic acid is corrosive in both the liquid and vapour phase. It can damage the skin and eyes and its sharp, pungent odour is irritating to the nose and throat. Operators handling the cylinders are advised to wear heavy-duty, neoprene or rubber gloves as well as eye protection. Since the gas mixture is supplied under high pressure, the cylinders should be handled with care, protected from physical damage and not exposed to heat.

Sterilization cycles that abort because of some failure in compliance with process parameters are programmed to advance to cycle completion. If a power failure occurs, no attempt should be made to open the door of the sterilizing chamber. When power is restored, the sterilization cycle will then proceed to completion.

Susceptibility of microorganisms

The spectrum of antimicrobial activity of plasma-based sterilization systems is broad and includes mycobacteria, sporing bacteria, fungi and viruses.

As required for medical devices, the cycles have been designed to give a sterility assurance level of 10^{-6}. This level has been attained by the plasma-based systems for those microorganisms, such as *B. stearothermophilus*, *B. subtilis* subsp. *niger*, *Deinococcus radiodurans* and the poliomyelitis virus, which are regarded as challenging for other methods of sterilization.

Sporicidal efficacy was validated by the Association of Official Analytical Chemists (Beloian, 1995) test in which penicylinders and sutures are inoculated with *B. subtilis* or *Clostridium sporogenes*, dried, and subjected to the plasma-based sterilization processes. The acceptable end-point for sterility is the complete absence of growth of both spore-formers. This end-point was achieved.

Factors influencing efficiency of biocidal action

Moisture

Although the sterilization cycles were designed to abort in the presence of moisture, recent developments in the system allow for greater tolerance to moisture in loads.

Narrow lumens

Narrow lumens present a challenge to plasma-based sterilization systems. For the Sterrad system, Booster/Adaptors are available for insertion into long, narrow lumened devices. The need for such Booster/Adaptors has been demonstrated by the studies of Alfa (1996). Boosters contain 0.9 ml of 58 per cent hydrogen peroxide to provide a source of extra gas for diffusion along the length of the lumen during the vacuum phase. Adaptors are available in three sizes to fit lumens of 0.1, 0.2 and 0.3 mm diameters. The Booster, which is attached to the insertion end of an endoscope by an Adaptor of appropriate size, is activated just prior to the start of the sterilizing cycle. Only one Booster/Adaptor per endoscope is required.

In general, Booster/Adaptors are used for lumens more than 400 mm and less than 2000 mm in length and from 1 to 3 mm internal diameter. Specifically, for metal reusable devices (e.g. stainless steel and monel metal), the efficacy of the Boosters has been demonstrated for lumens up to 500 mm in length whereas for plastic reusable devices (e.g.

polyethylene, polyvinyl chloride, silicone and Teflon) efficacy has been shown for lengths up to 2000 mm.

Because of possible damage to their material composition, the sterilization of flexible endoscopes by plasma-based systems is not recommended. However, in a hospital-based evaluation of the Abtox Plazlyte system, flexible endoscopes of all sizes and lengths were processed successfully. Negative culture results were obtained for the biological indicators and the various clinical bacterial isolates that were placed in the packaging and portal entries of the endoscopes and no signs of damage were evident (Wilson, 1994).

Organic and inorganic deposits

The presence of serum and salt on articles can seriously compromise the ability of plasma-based sterilization systems to achieve the required sterility assurance level of 10^{-6}. Alfa et al (1996) conducted a comparative study on the low-temperature sterilization processes of gas plasma (Sterrad and Abtox Plazlyte systems), pure ethylene oxide, ethylene oxide/CFC-12 mix and vapour phase hydrogen peroxide. They used carriers inoculated with the species of *Bacillus* which are used as biological indicators and with vegetative bacteria, *Enterococcus faecalis* (ATCC 29212), *Mycobacterium chelonae* (ATCC 19977) and *Pseudomonas aeruginosa* (ATCC 27853). These were tested in the presence and absence of 10 per cent serum and 0.65 per cent salt. All sterilizers tested effected a 6-$\log_{10}$ reduction of all the bacteria tested, except when serum and salt were present. In the presence of these organic and inorganic deposits, only the ethylene oxide/CFC-12 sterilizer generally achieved sterilization. However, none of the sterilizers was capable of effecting a reliable 6-$\log_{10}$ reduction of all bacterial inocula when the carriers were placed in narrow lumens of 125 cm length and 3.2 mm diameter. The investigators commented especially on the unexpectedly high resistance of *E. faecalis* in the presence of serum and salt, even without the additional challenge of placement in a narrow lumen. This species was more resistant than were sporing bacteria to inactivation by the gas plasma systems and vapour-phase hydrogen peroxide. It is speculated that the resistance of *E. faecalis* in the presence of serum and salt may be related to the structure of its bacterial cell wall and its ability to grow in the presence of bile salts. The findings raise concern, particularly in view of the emergence of vancomycin-resistant strains of *E. faecalis* and *E. faecium* as increasingly important nosocomial pathogens. Above all, the findings emphasize the critical importance of meticulous cleaning for the removal of organic and inorganic soil and contamination from articles and equipment in preparation for sterilization. Cleaning assumes even more importance if the devices have narrow lumens.

Gas plasma sterilization in hospitals

Although plasma sterilizers are relatively simple to install, operate and monitor, staff still require specific training in their operation and monitoring and preventive maintenance. Training is usually provided by the sponsor or manufacturer of the system. Critical adjustments and repairs to the sterilizers must be performed only by trained and qualified service personnel.

Applications

The gas plasma-based sterilization technology is applicable to heat- and moisture-sensitive hospital equipment of metal or non-metal construction or composition, including instruments that incorporate complex electronic circuitry. Examples of equipment that may be sterilized by this method include surgical and electrosurgical equipment, defibrillator paddles, fibreoptic cables, camera heads, ophthalmic instruments, dental equipment and respiratory therapy equipment. Qualities of sharpness of cutting edges, flexibility and optical clarity and the electrical and functional integrity of equipment are preserved through repeated cycles of plasma-based sterilization.

Preparation and packaging

All articles require thorough cleaning, in accord with rigid cleaning protocols, as well as drying before processing. They may be wrapped, unwrapped or pouched for sterilization. Hinged instruments and metal containers should be sterilized in the open position.

Packaging materials must permit the free passage of vapours and plasma to all surfaces of the articles. Appropriate wrapping materials for the plasma-based systems are nonwoven polypropylene wraps, such as Kimguard™ or Spunguard™, and Tyvek® (a spun polyolefin wrap) or pouches of Tyvek sealed to Mylar.

Paper wraps and paper/Mylar pouches may be used for the Abtox Plazlyte plasma-based system. Linen and cotton (muslin) wraps have been approved for use in the longest cycle of this system. However, as explained earlier, Alfa (1996) has expressed some reservations about the use of linen wraps because her findings suggest some interference by this material with plasma penetration, even in the long cycle.

Rigid, perforated, gas-compatible trays are supplied as accessories to the systems. Articles for sterilization are loaded into these trays in such a manner as to facilitate the unobstructed circulation of gas sterilants and air, e.g. by placing them vertically and not touching one another. In addition, the loaded trays must not touch the walls of the sterilizing chamber. If indicated, a Booster/Adaptor is inserted into a channel of a lumened device, such as an endoscope.

Gas plasma sterilizers

The sterilizers need to be connected to a power supply for generation of the plasma. This will occur only if the door to the sterilizing chamber is closed and the chamber is at negative pressure. Plasma-based systems of sterilization have error recognition, cycle abortion and error diagnosis and message capabilities.

The original Sterrad 100 sterilizer has been superseded by the Sterrad 100S model and a smaller Sterrad 50 model. The 100 and 100S models have a sterilizing chamber of cylindrical shape with a 100 litre usable volume. The Sterrad 50 sterilizer has a sterilizing chamber of rectangular shape and is of 50 litres in volume. The sterilization cycle for the 100S model has been shortened to 54 minutes for general purpose instruments and equipment and 72 minutes for loads that include endoscopes. Cycle time for the Sterrad 50 plasma gas sterilizer is 43 minutes. The sterilization cycle for the Sterrad 100 model required 75 minutes. A cassette which is placed in the sterilizer holds 10 aliquots of 1.8 ml of a 58 per cent solution of hydrogen peroxide which is sufficient for five separate sterilization cycles in the Sterrad 100S and Sterrad 50 systems since each cycle includes two stages in which hydrogen peroxide is injected, diffused, then used to generate plasma. Cassette advance is automatic and the empty cassettes are finally ejected into an internal collection box which is removed at intervals.

The Abtox Plazlyte sterilizer is equipped with dual chamber technology which permits the generation of the highly reactive, primary plasma in a separate chamber and provides for its subsequent delivery downstream to the sterilizing chamber. The intention is to avoid subjecting the load to an electromagnetic field and to protect it from exposure to the highly reactive, initial components of primary plasma and ultraviolet radiation. In the preceding (first) phase of the Abtox Plazlyte sterilization cycle, a 5 per cent solution of peracetic acid is evaporated into the sterilizing chamber. This phase is alternated with the plasma phase through two, four and six sequential repetitions to give cycles I, II and III of processing times 1, 2 and 3 hours. Cycles I, II and III are designed to cope with increasingly more challenging loads. The sterilizing chamber of the Abtox Plazlyte system is the largest of the gas plasma sterilizers.

On installation of a plasma sterilizer, a program of preventive maintenance is implemented. This provides for servicing at specified intervals e.g. the vacuum pump after every 500 hours of operation.

Sterilization cycles

The original sterilization cycles for the Sterrad 100 sterilizer consisted of phases of vacuum, injection, diffusion and aeration/venting. The shorter cycles of the Sterrad 100S and Sterrad 50 sterilizers consist of the following stages:

Stage 1. Preconditioning stage of vacuum, plasma generation (from air) and venting. It is this stage that permits greater tolerance for the presence of moisture in the loads.

Stage 2. Injection of 1.8 ml of 58 per cent hydrogen peroxide, diffusion and plasma generation.

Stage 3. Injection of 1.8 ml of 58 per cent hydrogen peroxide, diffusion, plasma generation, then venting.

In the Abtox Plazlyte plasma-based sterilization system, successive phases of exposure to vaporised peracetic acid for 20 minutes and to plasma for 10 minutes are preceded and separated by evacuation of the sterilizing chamber. The phases are repeated two, four and six times for the 1-hour, 2-hour and 3-hour cycles. Each cycle is terminated by aeration and venting to atmosphere.

Testing efficiency of sterilization

Process control

The plasma-based sterilization cycles are under automatic, microprocessor control. During operation, the cycle stage and elapsed time are indicated on the front panel of the sterilizer. The sterilizer is also equipped with an audible alarm. All critical parameters of the process are monitored and a printed record for process confirmation and documentation is provided at the conclusion of the cycle. Should a cycle abort, an error message will be displayed on the front panel of the sterilizer and a printout will report or reflect the conditions responsible.

Three different challenge packs simulating hospital loads and similar to those that are used for ethylene oxide sterilization have been devised for testing the three sterilizing cycles of the Abtox Plazlyte system.

Biological and chemical indicators

The single most important criterion for satisfactory performance of a biological indicator is a consistent and reliable log linear dose response to the sterilizing agent. Based largely on this criterion, *B. subtilis* subsp. *niger* (ATCC 9372) was chosen as biological indicator for the Sterrad process and *Bacillus circulans* (ATCC 61) was chosen for the Abtox Plazlyte process. As paper is an inappropriate spore carrier for the Sterrad system, a test pack has been devised with a load of at least 10^6 spores of *B. subtilis* subsp. *niger* (and a chemical indicator) in a Tyvek®/Mylar peel pouch. Paper carriers with at least 10^6 spores of *B. circulans* are used in the Abtox Plazlyte system. The biological indicator for this system is available as either a self-contained unit incorporating an ampoule of culture medium which is crushed to immerse the spore strip or in a packaged configuration from which the spore strip must be removed aseptically for culture.

Appropriate colour changes in the chemical indicators document exposure only to the relevant sterilants and not biocidal efficacy.

STERILIZATION BY VAPOUR PHASE HYDROGEN PEROXIDE

Vapour phase hydrogen peroxide (VPHP) is used for the decontamination of internal surfaces of enclosed spaces, such as flexible film isolators for the performance of sterility testing, or line filling of pharmaceutical products (Rickloff & Graham, 1989; Rickloff & Edwards, 1995). Although potentially corrosive to metals, the low concentrations of VPHP that are effective at ambient temperature (500 to 8000 p.p.m.) minimize the corrosive effects (Rickloff & Edwards, 1995). Hydrogen peroxide is incompatible with cellulosic absorptive materials and it degrades natural rubber and nylon. VPHP is capable of inactivating sporing bacteria, such as *Bacillus stearothermophilus*, *B. subtilis* subsp. *niger* and *C. sporogenes*, as well as fungi and viruses. End products of the action of this oxidant are non-toxic water and oxygen.

The sterilant is produced by vaporizing a 31 per cent solution of hydrogen peroxide into a carrier gas of warm, dry air, which then is delivered into the sealed enclosure. The process has been automated in the VHP®1000 Biodecontamination system (AMSCO). Disposable cartridges of hydrogen peroxide are used to charge the machine and it operates with a slightly positive pressure in the isolator. Any remaining hydrogen peroxide in the exiting air is converted to water and oxygen by passage through a catalyst. An on-board desiccant absorbs moisture and the warm, dry air is charged with fresh sterilant to repeat the cycle. After the requisite time, which depends on the size of the isolator, the flow of warm, dry air serves to aerate and dry the decontaminated surfaces. HEPA filters used in the process are composed of glass fibre, not paper, medium. The VHP 1000 system can also check the integrity of the sealing of the isolator before decontamination by a pressure hold test. Failure to hold the pressure will prevent or abort

the decontamination procedure. The process has been designed to give a sterility assurance level of 10^{-6}. A biological indicator consisting of spores of *B. stearothermophilus* (ATCC 12980) on a non-absorbent fibreglass disc in a Tyvek package is used for validating and monitoring the biocidal efficiency of the process. Adequate distribution of the vapour over the internal surfaces of the isolator can be checked qualitatively by placing strips of a chemical indicator in various positions and observing them for a colour change from light yellow to violet gray (Rickloff & Edwards, 1995).

STERILIZATION BY CHLORINE DIOXIDE

Another powerful oxidizing agent with potential for application to gas sterilization is chlorine dioxide in its gaseous form (Jeng & Woodworth, 1990). Gaseous chlorine dioxide is formed by passing chlorine dioxide through a column of sodium chlorite chips. Prehumidification to 70–75 per cent relative humidity for 30 minutes is necessary for efficient sporicidal activity. Under these conditions, the D value for *B. subtilis* subsp. *niger* ATCC 9372 is 1.6 minutes at a chlorine dioxide concentration of 6–7 mg per litre. Prehumidification by ultrasonic nebulization enhances sporicidal activity even more and reduces the D value to 0.55 minutes. The sterilizing process is conducted at ambient temperature and pressure. The gas penetrates glassine packages, polyvinyl chloride tubes, rigid containers and Tyvek® wrap. Processed plastic materials degas within a few hours. However, fungal spores of *Aspergillus niger* were found to be more resistant to inactivation than were the sporing bacteria tested. It was also noted that extracellular, viscous material could form a protective coating on sporing bacteria. Major advantages of gaseous chlorine dioxide are its lack of mutagenic effects and its low toxicity to humans.

STERILIZATION BY OZONE

Ozone is a rapidly-biocidal, powerful oxidizing agent. Because of its instability, ozone is generated on-site. The humidified gas is fed into an evacuated sterilizing chamber through which it continuously flows at a concentration of 10 to 20 per cent. The sterilizing cycle takes 30 to 60 minutes, including aeration time. Residual ozone is flushed away by the oxygen flow and catalytically converted back to non-toxic oxygen (Karlson, 1989: Stoddart, 1989). However, applications are limited because ozone damages many plastics (except Teflon) and corrodes many metals.

STERILIZATION BY STEAM AND FORMALDEHYDE

The low-temperature steam and formaldehyde process (LTSF) was designed primarily for sterilization or disinfection of cystoscopes and other heat-sensitive instruments (Alder et al, 1966). It is also applicable to a wide variety of equipment that withstands temperatures of 70–75°C but cannot be sterilized by steam above atmospheric pressure. The process requires a specially designed pre-vacuum sterilizer which operates at sub-atmospheric pressure and is quite different from formaldehyde vapour disinfection. Like the ethylene oxide process, the steam and formaldehyde process is too slow for resterilizing equipment that is reused on the same day but the sterilizer can be used for an alternative disinfection process that may be completed within 30 minutes.

Physical and chemical properties

Formaldehyde is not available as a pure gas or liquid. Formalin is an aqueous solution containing 37 per cent w/v formaldehyde, from which the vapour can be released by heating. Formaldehyde polymerizes gradually in the solution, depositing paraformaldehyde as a white powder. It also polymerizes from the vapour state at low temperature and high humidity but this does not occur at the temperature of the LTSF sterilization process. Formaldehyde vapour is nonflammable at the concentration used in this process.

Toxicity

The potential toxicity of formaldehyde is similar to that of ethylene oxide. However, exposure is more readily detected by the odour and irritant effects of the vapour at concentrations below 5 p.p.m. in air. Exposure to 2–5 p.p.m. causes immediate irritation of the respiratory tract and eyes, with the shedding of tears. Skin irritation or allergic contact dermatitis may result from contact with solutions containing formaldehyde. Effects on the respiratory tract and skin have been reviewed by Clark (1983) and Yodaiken (1981).

Earlier retrospective surveys of persons exposed to formaldehyde showed no evidence of a causal association with cancer (Editorial, 1983). However, more recent meta-analysis of multiple studies reveals that, although not linked to lung cancer, substantial formaldehyde exposure is linked to an increased risk of sinonasal and nasopharyngeal cancers (Partanen, 1993).

Absorption by natural and synthetic materials

Relatively high levels of residual formaldehyde have been found in paper and cloth wrappings after treatment by the LTSF process. However, the quantity absorbed by rubber and plastics is reported to be low (Gibson et al, 1968). In view of increased concern about formaldehyde toxicity, further investigation of the quantities absorbed and the rate of desorption are required.

Susceptibility of microorganisms

Formaldehyde has a broad spectrum of biocidal action, similar to that of ethylene oxide. Sporicidal action is slow at room temperature, but is accelerated by combination of the vapour with steam at 70–75°C. Viruses, fungi and tubercle bacilli are susceptible.

Factors influencing efficiency of biocidal action

An increase in the concentration of formaldehyde vapour increases the killing rate if the temperature and relative humidity are constant. The direct effect of an increase in temperature on the killing rate cannot be separated from its other effects of increasing the attainable concentration of formaldehyde vapour, retarding polymerization and decreasing absorption by material associated with the microorganisms, all of which assist the penetration of monomeric formaldehyde to relatively inaccessible sites.

Low-temperature steam and formaldehyde sterilization

Applications

The types of materials and equipment treated by this process are generally similar to those sterilized by ethylene oxide, but the recommended operating temperature of 73°C may be too high for cardiac pacemakers, some pressure transducers and other electronic devices which can be sterilized by ethylene oxide at 37°C. The formaldehyde process should not be used for equipment that withstands conventional steam sterilization. Porous material up to a density of 170 kg/m^3 can be sterilized.

Natural and synthetic rubbers and most plastics are stable to steam and formaldehyde at 70–75°C. Polyethylene, leather, wood and painted surfaces are seriously damaged. The lubricating systems of mechanical ventilators may become contaminated with water but electrical connections can be protected by maintaining slight superheat in the chamber. A list of articles that have been sterilized without adverse effects is given in Table 7.3.

Preparation and packaging

Articles should be clean and dry, as for the other gaseous sterilants. Paper, plain, creped or as bags, and cotton fabric are suitable wrapping materials; polyethylene film and glassine paper are unsuitable, except as an insert in a paper pouch. Cystoscopes may be packed in light cardboard boxes; these should be sterilized in a prevacuum steam sterilizer at 134°C to kill spores and eliminate bituminous material before they are used. Tubing should be loosely packed to avoid retention of air and water droplets, which interfere with steam penetration. Instrument trays or other rigid containers may also be used. Formaldehyde does not diffuse through the wall of plastic tubing. Excessive quantities of porous packaging material may reduce the amounts of steam and formaldehyde reaching the articles to be sterilized.

Design of sterilizers

A low-temperature steam and formaldehyde sterilizer is similar to a prevacuum steam sterilizer, but is operated at negative pressure with

Table 7.3   Some applications of low-temperature steam and formaldehyde sterilization

Types of equipment and materials	Examples
Surgical instruments	Airways Anaesthetic masks, tubing, bags Arthroscopes Cardiac catheters (Teflon, Dacron) Cuffed endotracheal tubes (rubber) Cystoscopes, with leads and lights (including fibre light systems) Laparoscopes
Medical equipment	Blood oxygenators Catheters (gum elastic, latex rubber) Drainage sets Gloves (latex) Humidifiers Hyperbaric equipment parts Mechanical ventilators, with electric motors, switches and heaters Syringes (large polypropylene)
Electrical equipment	Capacitors Defibrillator electrodes Electrode implants for physiological experiments Leads, switches, bakelite plugs and bulbs Motors (water contaminates lubricating system) Potentiometers Transformers

subatmospheric steam at 73°C. The jacket is heated by water under thermostatic control. The floor of the chamber is sloped towards the drain to prevent accumulation of condensate and consequent wetting of the load. Steam and condensate are discharged to an evacuated condenser because the balanced pressure steam traps that are used in steam sterilizers do not operate at negative pressure. Formaldehyde vapour is generated by passing formalin into a steam-heated vaporizer. Air that is admitted to the chamber at the end of the sterilization cycle to remove formaldehyde must pass through a bacterial filter of 99.97 per cent efficiency. Automatic controls include a mechanism to cut out the heating system if the temperature exceeds that selected for the process by more than 2°C.

An exhaust hood should be mounted externally above the door of the LTSF sterilizer. It should be operating just before, during and after the opening of the door (HTM, 1994).

Sterilization cycle

The cycle is carried out below atmospheric pressure. The chamber must be preheated and free drainage of condensate is important because moisture promotes polymerization, leading to failure of the formaldehyde to penetrate into the packs. The cycle may be divided into six stages, as shown by the chart in Figure 7.3 (Alder, 1987).

Stage 1. Air removal. Air is removed by mechanical evacuation; no steam is introduced in this stage. The chamber and contents are dry to prevent polymerization and the only heat source is the chamber wall and the jacket. The jacket should be 4°C above the sterilizing temperature to prevent condensation.

Stage 2. Formaldehyde injection. Three separate amounts of formalin (2 ml per 0.03 m³) are vaporized in a heat exchanger and a period of 3 minutes is allowed after each injection for the pressure to stabilize. Formaldehyde vapour penetrates into tubing and porous material, assisted by vacuum, and sterilization commences in dry conditions.

Stage 3. A larger amount of formalin (8 ml per 0.03 m³) is vaporized and admitted to the chamber. The pressure is allowed to stabilize for 3 minutes before low-temperature steam is introduced slowly to achieve 60–90 per cent relative humidity. This raises the temperature to 73°C and enhances the sterilizing activity of the formaldehyde.

Stage 4. Steam injection is continued for 2 hours to complete sterilization and to commence the removal of formaldehyde via the chamber drain.

Stage 5. Removal of formaldehyde continues by alternating flushes of steam pressure and vacuum.

Stage 6. Filtered air is admitted to the chamber to restore atmospheric pressure.

Aeration

Levels of formaldehyde residues in materials sterilized by the steam and formaldehyde process have not been established. However, it is generally

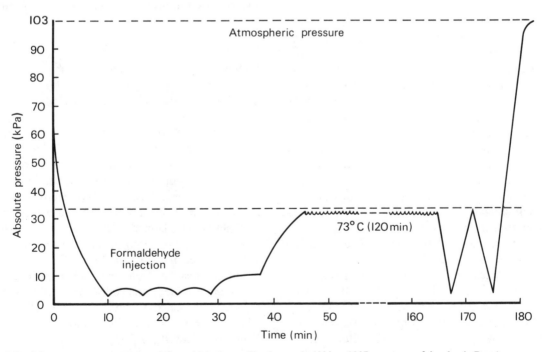

Fig. 7.3 A low-temperature steam and formaldehyde sterilization cycle (Alder, 1987; courtesy of Academic Press).

recommended they receive the same treatment as for ethylene oxide.

Testing efficiency of sterilization

Temperature and automatic process control test

An automatic cycle is performed with an empty chamber and the process variables are observed through each stage or substage. In addition to pressure, temperature, vacuum and stage times, three readings of temperature and pressure should be taken at equal time intervals during the sterilizing stage. The performance is satisfactory if the temperature record is within acceptable levels, the process variables are within limits that have been established during commissioning and no mechanical or other anomalies are observed. The quality of steam may be monitored by the correspondence of temperature and pressure readings; a pressure of 68 kPa below atmospheric pressure corresponds to 73°C.

Thermocouple tests

Thermocouples are used to test the over-temperature cutout mechanism, the temperature of the chamber walls and the penetration of heat into a test pack (HTM, 1994). The over-temperature cutout should come into operation when the temperature reaches 80°C, with the door remaining locked at the end of the cycle. The temperature of the chamber walls (measured by five thermocouples on each side of the chamber) should rise to within 2°C of the process temperature before the automatic cycle can be started. After the first five minutes of the sterilizing stage, the temperature of the wall should be within −5°C and +7°C of the temperature in the chamber drain.

The small load test pack is prepared from the same cotton towels as those that are used in the Bowie-Dick test for prevacuum steam sterilizers. The shape of the pack should be cubic and the volume equivalent to one-fifth of the chamber volume if this is less than 0.15 m^3. One thermocouple is inserted, with care to avoid channelling, into the test pack; a second is placed 50 mm directly above

the pack and a third is located in the chamber drain. The temperatures in the test pack and the free chamber space should be within −2°C and +7°C of the selected process temperature of 73°C. The temperature in the chamber drain should not differ by more than 4°C from that measured in the free chamber space during the sterilizing stage of the cycle. The towels should also be tested for dryness; the gain in weight should not exceed 1 per cent.

Leak monitor test

A small load test pack is placed in the chamber. After evacuation, sufficient air is induced into the chamber by a variable flow device to cause a pressure rise of about 50 mbar over a period of 10 minutes. A fault should be indicated at the end of the cycle.

Formaldehyde concentration

Tests for the concentration of formaldehyde in the air when the sterilizer door is opened should be carried out during commissioning. The estimation of residual formaldehyde in various products is also required in order to determine aeration times.

Biological indicators

Biological indicators which carry 10^6–10^7 spores of *Bacillus stearothermophilus* NCTC 10007 are used in the LTSF process because they are unaffected by steam at 80°C and a lethal effect is indicative of formaldehyde penetration. The biological test is the definitive test for sterilization efficiency and is also used to survey the distribution of formaldehyde throughout the chamber. In the latter test, 27 units, removed from the glassine envelopes and handled aseptically, are attached to a fine thread and placed at planned sites in the free chamber space. Gas penetration is also tested by spore papers placed in two Line/Pickerill helices which are placed near the front and back of the chamber. The helix is a long, fine coiled metal tube, one end of which is sealed to the lid of a small capsule which accommodates the biological indicators (Line & Pickerill, 1973). An alternative device which simulates the shorter, broader metal tube of a cystoscope may also be used, as appropriate, to challenge the efficiency of sterilization (Alder et al, 1971; Gibson, 1977). The seal of the device should be inspected before each test and patency of the lumen checked by purging with air. Biological indicators are used to test for efficiency of sterilization during commissioning, recommissioning, yearly and routine production. At least two biological indicator units should be used in each test because, as explained in Chapter 2, a single unit may yield either a positive or a negative culture if the process is at the borderline of efficiency.

Chemical indicators

Browne Formaldehyde Control Indicator Strips are internal indicators which may be used in conjunction with biological indicators. They do not provide evidence of sterilization but may give prompt warning of inadequate formaldehyde concentration. They may be placed in test or production packs to show that formaldehyde vapour has penetrated in sufficient quantity and for an adequate period of time to turn the colour of the indicator from blue to green. Calibration is carried out in a sterilization cycle operated at 73°C, with introduction of 600 ml of formalin into a 0.6 m³ chamber in a series of 20 pulses. The manufacturer recommends that the controls should be tested in individual sterilizers prior to adoption for routine use.

Browne Formaldehyde Process Detector Spots are available for use as external indication that a process has taken place. These undergo a colour change from blue to yellow.

REFERENCES

Alfa M J 1996 Plasma-based sterilization. The challenge of narrow lumens. Infection Control & Sterilization Technology 2: 19–24
Alfa M J, DeGagne P, Olson N, Puchalski T 1996 Comparison of ion plasma, vaporized hydrogen peroxide, and 100% ethylene oxide sterilizers to the 12/88 ethylene oxide gas sterilizer. Infection Control and Hospital Epidemiology 17: 92–100
ANSI/AAMI ST21 1986 (R1994) Biological indicators for ethylene oxide sterilization processes in health-care facilities. American National Standards Institute, New York
ANSI/AAMI ST24 1992 Automatic, general-purpose ethylene oxide sterilizers and ethylene oxide sterilant sources intended for use in health care facilities. American National Standards Institute, New York
ANSI/AAMI ST41 1992 Good hospital practice: ethylene oxide sterilization and sterility assurance. American National Standards Institute, New York
ANSI/AAMI ST43 1993 Good hospital practice: ethylene oxide gas — ventilation recommendations and safe use. American National Standards Institute, New York
Alder V G 1987 The formaldehyde/low temperature steam sterilizing procedure. Journal of Hospital Infection 9: 194–200
Alder V G, Brown A M, Gillespie W A 1966 Disinfection of heat-sensitive material by low-temperature steam and formaldehyde. Journal of Clinical Pathology 19: 83–89
Alder V G, Gingell J C, Mitchell J P 1971 Disinfection of cystoscopes by subatmospheric steam and steam and formaldehyde at 80°C. British Medical Journal 3: 677–680
Ball N A 1984 Determination of ethylene oxide, ethylene chlorohydrin, and ethylene glycol in aqueous solutions and ethylene oxide residues in associated plastics. Journal of Pharmaceutical Sciences 73: 1305–1307
Beloian A 1995 Disinfectants. In: Cunniff P A (ed) Official methods of analysis of AOAC International, 16th edn. AOAC International, Arlington, vol I, ch 6
Biro L, Fisher A A, Price E 1974 Ethylene oxide burns. A hospital outbreak involving 19 women. Archives of Dermatology 110: 924–925
Bogdansky S, Lehn P J 1974 Effects of γ-irradiation on 2-chloroethanol formation in ethylene oxide-sterilized polyvinyl chloride. Journal of Pharmaceutical Sciences 63: 802–803
Bommer J, Wilhelms O H, Barth H P, Schindele H, Ritz E 1985 Anaphylactoid reactions in dialysis patients: role of ethylene oxide. Lancet ii: 1382–1384
Bruch C W 1973 Sterilization of plastics: toxicity of ethylene oxide residues. In: Phillips G B, Miller W S (eds) Industrial sterilization. Duke University Press, Durham, ch 4, p 49
BS 5295.1 1989 Environmental cleanliness for enclosed spaces Part 1 Specification for clean rooms and clean air devices. British Standards Institution, London
BS 6257 1989 British Standard specification for paper bags for steam sterilization for medical use. British Standards Institution, London
BS:EN 550 1994 Sterilization of medical devices — Validation and routine control of ethylene oxide sterilization. British Standards Institution, London
Caputo R A, Rohn K J 1982 The effects of EtO sterilization variables on BI performance. Medical Device & Diagnostic Industry 4(7): 37–41, 68–69
Chobin N, Engle L 1989 Are you ready for an ethylene oxide spill? Journal of Healthcare Materiel Management 7(3): 56–57, 60
Clare M G, Dean B J, de Jong G, van Sittert N J 1985 Chromosome analysis of lymphocytes from workers at an ethylene oxide plant. Mutation Research 156: 109–116
Clark R P 1983 Formaldehyde in pathology departments. Journal of Clinical Pathology 36: 839–846
Conviser S A 1989 Hospital sterilization using ethylene oxide — what's next? Journal of Healthcare Materiel Management 7(5): 35–36, 38–39, 42
Cunliffe A C, Wesley F 1967 Hazards from plastics sterilized by ethylene oxide. British Medical Journal 2: 575–576
Dadd A H, Daley G M 1980 Resistance of micro-organisms to inactivation by gaseous ethylene oxide. Journal of Applied Bacteriology 49: 89–101

Dadd A H, Town M M, McCormick K E 1985 The influence of water on the resistance of spores to inactivation by gaseous ethylene oxide. Journal of Applied Bacteriology 58: 613–621

Divine B J, Amanollahi K S 1986 Ethylene oxide and cancer. Journal of the American Medical Association 256: 1726–1727

Doyle J E, Ernst R R 1967 Resistance of *Bacillus subtilis* var. *niger* spores occluded in water-insoluble crystals to three sterilization agents. Applied Microbiology 15: 726–730

Doyle J E, Ernst R R 1968 Influence of various pretreatments (carriers, desiccation, and relative cleanliness) on the destruction of *Bacillus subtilis* var. *niger* spores with gaseous ethylene oxide. Journal of Pharmaceutical Sciences 57: 433–436

Editorial 1983 Formaldehyde and cancer. Lancet ii: 26

Ernst R R, Doyle J E 1968 Sterilization with gaseous ethylene oxide: a review of chemical and physical factors. Biotechnology and Bioengineering 10: 1–31

Ernst R R, Shull J J 1962 Ethylene oxide gaseous sterilization 1. Concentration and temperature effects. Applied Microbiology 10: 337–341

Estrin W J, Cavalieri S A, Wald P, Becker C E, Jones J R, Cone J E 1987 Evidence of neurologic dysfunction related to long-term ethylene oxide exposure. Archives of Neurology 44: 1283–1286

Fitzpatrick B G, Reich R R 1986 EtO sterilization monitoring. A performance study. Journal of Healthcare Materiel Management 4(6): 32–35

Gardner M J, Coggon D, Pannett B, Harris E C 1989 Workers exposed to ethylene oxide: a follow up study. British Journal of Industrial Medicine 46: 860–865

Gibson G L 1977 Processing urinary endoscopes in a low-temperature steam and formaldehyde autoclave. Journal of Clinical Pathology 30: 269–274

Gibson G L, Johnston H P, Turkington V E 1968 Residual formaldehyde after low-temperature steam and formaldehyde sterilization. Journal of Clinical Pathology 21: 771–775

Gilbert G L, Gambill V M, Spiner D R, Hoffman R K, Phillips C R 1964 Effect of moisture on ethylene oxide sterilization. Applied Microbiology 12: 496–503

Gonzalez L A, Sefton M V 1985 Laboratory evaluation of stain-length passive dosimeters for monitoring of vinyl chloride and ethylene oxide. American Industrial Hygiene Association Journal 46: 591–598

Gourley R 1988 Safe EtO use: how Utah Valley Hospital controlled EtO in CS. Journal of Healthcare Materiel Management 6(3): 40–41, 43–45

Greenberg H L, Ott M G, Shore R E 1990 Men assigned to ethylene oxide production or other ethylene oxide related chemical manufacturing: a mortality study. British Journal of Industrial Medicine 47: 221–230

Gschwandtner G, Kruger D, Harman P 1986 Compliance with the EtO standard in the United States. Journal of Healthcare Materiel Management 4(6): 38–41

Gunther D A 1974 Safety of ethylene oxide gas residuals Part 2. American Journal of Hospital Pharmacy 31: 684–686

Gunther D A 1980 The chemistry and biology of EtO sterilization. Medical Device & Diagnostic Industry 2(12): 31–35

HBN 13.1 1994 Health Building Note 13 Suppl 1 Ethylene oxide sterilization section. NHS Estates, London

Hemminki K, Mutanen P, Saloniemi I, Niemi M-L, Vainio H 1982 Spontaneous abortions in hospital staff engaged in

sterilising instruments with chemical agents. British Medical Journal 285: 1461–1463

Henne W, Dietrich W, Pelger M, von Sengbusch G 1984 Residual ethylene oxide in hollow-fibre dialyzers. Artificial Organs 8: 306–309

Hoff-Jørgensen R, Lund E 1972 Studies on the inactivation of viruses by ethylene oxide. Acta Veterinaria Scandinavica 13: 520–527

Hogstedt C, Aringer L, Gustavsson A 1986 Epidemiologic support for ethylene oxide as a cancer-causing agent. Journal of the American Medical Association 255: 1575–1578

Holmgren A, Diding N, Samuelsson G 1969 Ethylene oxide treatment of crude drugs Part V. Formation of ethylene chlorohydrin. Acta Pharmaceutica Suecica 6: 33–36

HTM 1994 Health Technical Memorandum 2010 Part 3: Validation and verification. Sterilization. NHS Estates, London

ISO 10993.7 1995 Biological evaluation of medical devices — Part 7: Ethylene oxide sterilization residuals. International Organization for Standardization, Geneva

ISO 11135 1994 Medical devices — Validation and routine control of ethylene oxide sterilization. International Organization for Standardization, Geneva

ISO 11138.2 1994 Sterilization of health care products — Biological indicators — Part 2: Biological indicators for ethylene oxide sterilization. International Organization for Standardization, Geneva

Jacobs P T 1989 Plasma sterilization. Journal of Healthcare Materiel Management 7(5): 49

Jeng D K, Woodworth A G 1990 Chlorine dioxide gas sterilization under square-wave conditions. Applied and Environmental Microbiology 56: 514–519

Karlson E L 1989 Ozone sterilization. Journal of Healthcare Materiel Management 7(5): 43–45

Kaye S, Phillips C R 1949 The sterilizing action of gaseous ethylene oxide IV. The effect of moisture. American Journal of Hygiene 50: 296–306

Korpela D B, McJilton C E, Hawkinson T E 1983 Ethylene oxide dispersion from gas sterilizers. American Industrial Hygiene Association Journal 44: 589–591

Kring E V, Damrell D J, Basilio A N Jr et al 1984 Laboratory validation and field verification of a new passive air monitoring badge for sampling ethylene oxide in air. American Industrial Hygiene Association Journal 45: 697–707

Kring E V, McGibney P D, Thornley G D 1985 Laboratory validation of five commercially available methods for sampling ethylene oxide in air. American Industrial Hygiene Association Journal 46: 620–624

Kruger D A 1989 What is 5 PPM? Understanding and complying with the new EO STEL regulation. Journal of Healthcare Materiel Management 7(2): 34–38, 40–41, 44–45

Line S J, Pickerill J K 1973 Testing a steam-formaldehyde sterilizer for gas penetration efficiency. Journal of Clinical Pathology 26: 716–720

McGunnigle R G, Renner J A, Romano S J, Abodeely R A Jr 1975 Residual ethylene oxide: levels in medical grade tubing and effects on an *in vitro* biologic system. Journal of Biomedical Materials Research 9: 273–283

Marshall C, Shimizu A, Smith E K M, Dolovich J 1984 Ethylene oxide allergy in a dialysis center: prevalence in hemodialysis and peritoneal dialysis populations. Clinical Nephrology 21: 346–349

Moneret-Vautrin D A, Mata E, Gueant J L, Turgeman D, Laxenaire M C 1990 High risk of anaphylactic shock during surgery for spina bifida. Lancet i: 865–866

Mullins H E 1985 Sub-part-per-million diffusional sampling for ethylene oxide with the 3M #3550 ethylene oxide monitor. American Industrial Hygiene Association Journal 46: 625–631

Nicholls A 1986 Ethylene oxide and anaphylaxis during haemodialysis. British Medical Journal 292: 1221–1222

Ohnishi A, Inoue N, Yamamoto T et al 1985 Ethylene oxide induces central-peripheral distal axonal degeneration of the lumbar primary neurones in rats. British Journal of Industrial Medicine 42: 373–379

Ohnishi A, Inoue N, Yamamoto T et al 1986 Ethylene oxide neuropathy in rats. Exposure to 250 ppm. Journal of the Neurological Sciences 74: 215–221

OSHA 1984 Occupational exposure to ethylene oxide, final standard. (29 CFR 1910), June 22. Federal Register 49(122): 25796–25809

OSHA 1988 Occupational exposure to ethylene oxide, final standard (29 CFR 1910), April 6. Federal Register 53(66): 11413–11438

Partanen T 1993 Formaldehyde exposure and respiratory cancer — a meta-analysis of the epidemiologic evidence. Scandinavian Journal of Work and Environmental Health 19: 8–15

Phillips C R 1949 The sterilizing action of gaseous ethylene oxide II. Sterilization of contaminated objects with ethylene oxide and related compounds: time, concentration and temperature relationships. American Journal of Hygiene 50: 280–288

Phillips C R, Kaye S 1949 The sterilizing action of gaseous ethylene oxide I. Review. American Journal of Hygiene 50: 270–279

Porco R D 1988 EtO emission control technology. Journal of Healthcare Materiel Management 6(8): 52, 54

Ragelis E P, Fisher B S, Klimeck B A, Johnson C 1968 Isolation and determination of chlorohydrins in foods fumigated with ethylene oxide or with propylene oxide. Journal of the Association of Official Analytical Chemists 51: 709–715

Reyniers J A, Sacksteder M R, Ashburn L L 1964 Multiple tumors in female germfree inbred albino mice exposed to bedding treated with ethylene oxide. Journal of the National Cancer Institute 32: 1045–1057

Richmond G W, Abrahams R H, Nemenzo J H, Hine C H 1985 An evaluation of possible effects on health following exposure to ethylene oxide. Archives of Environmental Health 40: 20–25

Rickloff J R, Edwards L M 1995 Modern trends in isolator sterilization. In: Wagner C M, Akers J E (eds) Isolator technology. Applications in the pharmaceutical and biotechnology industries. Interpharm Press, Buffalo, ch 7, p 149–172

Rickloff J R, Graham G S 1989 Vapor phase hydrogen peroxide sterilization. Journal of Healthcare Materiel Management 7(5): 45–46, 48

Roberts R B, Rendell-Baker L 1972 Aeration after ethylene oxide sterilisation. Failure of repeated vacuum cycles to influence aeration time after ethylene oxide sterilisation. Anaesthesia 27: 278–282

Rumpf K W, Seubert S, Seubert A et al 1985 Association of ethylene-oxide-induced IgE antibodies with symptoms in dialysis patients. Lancet ii: 1385–1387

Samuels T M, Corn R 1979 Modification of large, built-in, ethylene oxide sterilizers to reduce operator exposure to EO. Hospital Topics 57: 50–55

Sarto F, Cominato I, Pinton A M et al 1984 Cytogenetic damage in workers exposed to ethylene oxide. Mutation Research 138: 185–195

Sega G A, Generoso E E 1988 Measurement of DNA breakage in spermiogenic germ-cell stages of mice exposed to ethylene oxide, using an alkaline elution procedure. Mutation Research 197: 93–99

Shikama K, Miura K-I 1976 Equilibrium studies on the formaldehyde reaction with native DNA. European Journal of Biochemistry 63: 39–46

Stanley P, Bertranou E, Forest F, Langevin L 1971 Toxicity of ethylene oxide sterilization of polyvinyl chloride in open-heart surgery. Journal of Thoracic and Cardiovascular Surgery 61: 309–314

Stoddart G M 1989 Ozone as a sterilizing agent. Journal of Healthcare Materiel Management 7(5): 42–43

Stolley P D, Soper K A, Galloway S M, Nichols W W, Norman S A, Wolman S R 1984 Sister-chromatid exchanges in association with occupational exposure to ethylene oxide. Mutation Research 129: 89–102

Tessler J, Fellowes O N 1961 The effect of gaseous ethylene oxide on dried foot-and-mouth disease virus. American Journal of Veterinary Research 22: 779–782

Van Sittert N J, de Jong G, Clare M G et al 1985 Cytogenetic, immunological, and haematological effects in workers in an ethylene oxide manufacturing plant. British Journal of Industrial Medicine 42: 19–26

Vermylen J, Janssens S, Ceuppens J, Vermylen C 1988 Transfusion reactions in haemophiliac caused by sensitisation to ethylene oxide. Lancet i: 594

Vologodskii A V, Frank-Kamenetskii M D 1975 Theoretical study of DNA unwinding under the action of formaldehyde. Journal of Theoretical Biology 55: 153–166

Wesley F, Rourke B, Darbishire O 1965 The formation of persistent toxic chlorohydrins in foodstuffs by fumigation with ethylene oxide and with propylene oxide. Journal of Food Science 30: 1037–1042

White J D, Bradley T J 1973 Residual ethylene oxide in gas-sterilized, medical-grade silicones. Journal of Pharmaceutical Sciences 62: 1634–1637

Wilson R 1994 Evaluation of the Plazlyte™ sterilization system at The Richmond Hospital, Richmond, B.C. Journal of Healthcare Materiel Management 12(4): 34–40

Yager J W 1987 Effect of concentration-time parameters on sister-chromatid exchanges induced in rabbit lymphocytes by ethylene oxide inhalation. Mutation Research 182: 343–352

Yager J W, Hines C J, Spear R C 1983 Exposure to ethylene oxide at work increases sister chromatid exchanges in human peripheral lymphocytes. Science 219: 1221–1223

Yodaiken R E 1981 The uncertain consequences of formaldehyde toxicity. Journal of the American Medical Association 246: 1677–1678

8. Sterilization by ionizing radiation

Radiation sterilization means treatment by gamma rays, X-rays or accelerated electrons, all of which are ionizing radiations. It excludes ultraviolet light, which is a low energy, non-ionizing radiation with very poor penetrating power.

Ionizing radiations kill all types of microorganisms and usually have enough energy for useful penetration into solids and liquids. They do not heat or wet materials significantly and are widely used for industrial sterilization of heat-sensitive medical and laboratory equipment. Space requirements, safety precautions and cost preclude the installation of large automated sterilization facilities in hospitals and laboratories. However, several small-scale batch-type facilities are now in use. Application of the process to pharmaceuticals, biological products and foods may be limited by the inactivation of some drugs and nutrients and also by development of off-flavours in foods. However, radiation pasteurization of foods, at least up to an average dose of 10 kGy, to extend storage life has been shown to pose no toxicological, carcinogenic or teratogenic hazards. Low-dose irradiation is also useful for reducing the level of microbial contamination of the raw materials used in the manufacture of pharmaceuticals and cosmetics.

A brief review of the properties, mechanisms of biological action and effects of ionizing radiations on microorganisms and materials will precede a description of facilities for radiation sterilization and the main applications of the process.

UNITS AND TERMS

Energy

electron volt (eV): the energy gained by an
   electron moving through a potential difference

of 1 volt. An electron volt corresponds to 1.602×10^{-19} joules (J) and is applicable to electromagnetic and particulate radiation. One mega electron volt (MeV) = 10^6 eV

Power (Output)

joule per second (J/s or Js^{-1}) or watt (W): expresses the power, or output, of a radiation source

Quantity

becquerel (Bq): the quantity of radioactive isotope that undergoes one disintegration per second. The becquerel is the unit in the International System of Units (SI) that replaces the curie (Ci).
1 Bq = 2.7×10^{-11} Ci
1 MCi = 3.7×10^{16} Bq

Absorbed dose

gray (Gy): unit of dose defined as 1 joule of energy absorbed per kilogram of material irradiated. This SI unit replaces the rad (100 ergs/g).
1 Gy = 100 rad
25 kGy = 2.5 Mrad

TYPES OF RADIANT ENERGY

Radiation may be described as energy in motion. It may be non-particulate (electromagnetic) or particulate (accelerated electrons).

Electromagnetic radiation

Electromagnetic radiations travel at the speed of light (3×10^8 m/s). The wavelengths and corresponding quantum energies of each photon in the bands of the electromagnetic spectrum are listed in Table 8.1. The energy of gamma photons from radioactive sources is sufficient to ionize or excite atoms, but is far below the level that could induce radioactivity in the treated material by disrupting the atomic nucleus. Ultraviolet radiation in the range 240–280 nm is biocidal but practical application is limited by its lack of penetrating power to disinfection of air, clear water and clean surfaces which are in the direct path of the radiation. Visible light may damage bacterial nucleic acids but generally has little effect on microorganisms, especially those which are protected by carotenoid pigments (Krinsky, 1976). Infrared radiation is sometimes used as a rapid method of heat transfer in dry heat sterilization processes but its action is limited to heating the exposed surfaces of solid objects. Microwave energy generates heat but the heating is uneven, which limits its application.

Table 8.1   Wavelengths, frequencies and energies of electromagnetic radiations[1]

Type of electromagnetic radiation	Wavelength	Frequency	Energy	
	nm	Hz	eV	J
Gamma	<0.1	>3×10^{18}	>10^4	>2×10^{-15}
X-ray	10^{-4}–1	3×10^{21}–3×10^{17}	10^3–10^7	2×10^{-16}–2×10^{-12}
Ultraviolet				
Extreme	1–20	3×10^{17}–1×10^{16}	60–10^3	10^{-17}–2×10^{-16}
Far	20–200	1×10^{16}–1×10^{15}	6–60	10^{-18}–10^{-17}
Near	200–380	1×10^{15}–8×10^{14}	3–6	5×10^{-19}–10^{-18}
Visible	380–750	8×10^{14}–4×10^{14}	1.5–3	2×10^{-19}–5×10^{-19}
Infrared	750–10^6	4×10^{14}–3×10^{11}	10^{-3}–1.5	2×10^{-22}–2×10^{-19}
Microwave	10^6–3×10^8 (1 mm–300 mm)	3×10^{11}–1×10^9	4×10^{-6}–10^{-3}	7×10^{-25}–2×10^{-19}

[1]Values provided by McKellar B H J, Physics Department, University of Melbourne

Cobalt-60 (^{60}Co) is used as the source of gamma radiation in sterilization facilities. It is prepared by placing the stable ^{59}Co in a nuclear reactor, where it absorbs neutrons to yield radioactive ^{60}Co. The resulting specific activity is 10^{11}–10^{13} Bq/g, depending on the time of irradiation. At each successive disintegration, gamma radiation is emitted at two separate energy levels of 1.333 and 1.173 MeV. The half-life of the isotope is 5.272 years, so that the quantity of radioactivity decreases by approximately 12.3 per cent per annum. Both emissions are suitable for sterilization because they are absorbed by all materials. Penetration depends on the density of the absorbing material; the intensity of the incident radiation falls to about one half after penetrating 12 cm of unit density material. ^{60}Co emits 15 kJ/s (15 kW) per 3.7×10^{16} Bq. Cesium-137 may also be used.

X-rays are similar to gamma radiation but are produced artificially by bombardment of a heavy metal target with an electron or cathode ray beam. The fraction of electron beam energy that is converted to electromagnetic radiation increases steeply with voltage; facilities have been designed to provide the very high doses required for sterilization of medical products or food.

Particulate radiation

Electric current is a flow of electrons. When these are accelerated to very high speeds they gain energy and penetrating power. The energy at which they are produced is restricted, in practice, to 10 MeV as higher energies may induce radioactivity in the treated material. The depth of penetration is 0.33 cm/MeV in unit density material, which is much lower than that for gamma radiation.

MECHANISM OF BIOCIDAL ACTION

The DNA target

All living cells are affected by ionizing radiation in a similar way. The main biological target is deoxyribonucleic acid (DNA), which controls the genetic constitution and reproductive process of the cell. DNA is the most vital cell constituent and it presents a relatively large volume in the microbial cell for absorption of radiation and a large surface for reaction with radiation products. The involvement of DNA as the principal target of lethal action is supported by the following observations (Haynes, 1966; Latarjet, 1972):

1. Frequency of mutations among radiation survivors is above the normal level
2. Replication of DNA, transcription of messenger RNA and synthesis of proteins, which are all controlled by DNA, are more sensitive to irradiation than are other metabolic processes such as respiration (Pollard & Davis, 1970)
3. Artificial incorporation of 5-bromouracil in DNA increases its sensitivity to irradiation but 5-fluorouracil, which is incorporated only in RNA, does not produce this effect (Myers et al, 1977)
4. Oxygen sensitizes bacteria and cell-free DNA to irradiation in a similar way
5. Proteins, such as bacterial toxins (Skulberg, 1965) and enzymes, are relatively insensitive to sterilizing doses of radiation
6. Bacteria that have an efficient mechanism for the repair of DNA damage are highly resistant to irradiation.

The action of radiation on living cells may be considered in three stages, each of extremely short duration:

1. Ionization
2. Radical formation
3. Biochemical changes.

Ionization (10^{-16}–10^{-17} second)

As a gamma photon passes through a material, it interacts with some of the orbital electrons in atoms or molecules. These events are infrequent and randomly distributed along the path. The absorbed energy produces positively charged ions when the electron is ejected from an atom, or unstable excited atoms and molecules. Many of the electrons are ejected at high velocities and produce a great number of additional ions, electrons or excited states. Accelerated electrons from a machine act in the same way as the high-velocity electrons that are produced within the cell; thus the microscopic geometry of events following the passage of gamma or X-ray photons and beams of electrons is the same. Each electron produces denser ionization towards the end of its track through the cell. The linear energy transfer (LET) value is a measure of the absorbed energy per unit length of track and hence of the number of ions and excited species. The atomic nucleus is unaffected by energy levels that are employed for sterilization.

Radical formation (10^{-12}–10^{-14} second)

The ejected electrons finally reach thermal energies of 0.025 eV and may become solvated in polar materials, such as water, giving solvated electrons (e_{aq}^-) or they may react with molecules present in the liquid. Meanwhile, the positive ions and excited atoms or molecules undergo reactions yielding active radicals. The reactive species, such as OH$\cdot$, e_{aq}^- and a few H$\cdot$ atoms, are produced in the intracellular water or the radiation reacts directly with cell constituents that are present in high concentration, producing corresponding ions, excited states and active radicals.

Biochemical changes (10^{-8} second)

The radicals, which are extremely reactive, sometimes react with each other to give the original material, doing little more than heating it up slightly. Alternatively, they may react with cell constituents. In this way DNA, for example, may be affected by the radiolysis of the water. This is known as indirect action. If oxygen is present, it can react with e_{aq}^- and H$\cdot$ producing the perhydroxyl or superoxide radical (HO_2) or with organic radicals giving peroxy species.

Very small amounts of radiant energy can have drastic biological effects, especially in unicellular organisms, but knowledge of the exact nature of the biochemical changes, or lesions, in DNA that are caused by ionizing radiation is far from complete. Two types of DNA damage have been recognized:

1. Breaks in one or both of the DNA strands
2. Lesions in the nitrogenous bases.

One active radical may cause a double-strand break if it is directly produced in the DNA molecule. Indirect action produces single-strand breaks but if the damaged sections on the two strands overlap, the effect would be the same as a double-strand break (Miller, 1970). Death of the cell results from about three double-strand breaks in *Escherichia coli* (Ulmer et al, 1979); 1400 may be required in *Deinococcus radiodurans* (Resnick, 1976). The principal change that has been identified in the nucleic acid bases is the opening and hydration of the 5–6 C = C double bond in the pyrimidine ring structure (Shragge & Hunt, 1974). The stable products of attack on the bond by OH$\cdot$ radicals include monomeric glycols and hydrates along with larger yields of pyrimidine dimers joined by single bonds between any two carbon atoms in the 4–6 position of the two rings (Shragge et al, 1974). The purines are less sensitive, but the main radical formed results in the opening of an N = C double bond at the 2–3 or the 7–8 position (Latarjet, 1972). Direct action may involve the addition of hydrogen atoms to the opened bonds.

Repair of damaged DNA

Some microorganisms have a great capacity for repair of damage to the DNA molecule (Bridges, 1976). *D. radiodurans* and *Deinococcus radiophilus* are more resistant than are bacterial spores (Anderson et al, 1956; Lewis, 1971). Some strains of *Enterococcus faecium* also show an increase above the normal level for non-sporing bacteria (Christensen, 1964). The efficiency of a repair system is often reflected by a large increase in the dose of radiation required for sterilization. The death rate is initially slow and only increases when a dose that inactivates the repair enzymes has been absorbed. Excision repair of damage caused by ionizing radiation involves four main steps which are mediated by enzymes. The enzymes incise the strand near the damaged site (endonuclease), remove or degrade the damaged section (exonuclease), resynthesize the section using the opposite intact strand as a genetic code (DNA polymerase) and, finally, rejoin the break (polynucleotide ligase). Single-strand breaks may be repaired as the open ends are held in place by the opposite strand (Latarjet, 1972; Nair & Pradhan, 1976). Double-strand breaks present greater difficulty and the repair might not be genetically correct. The complex systems which operate to repair damage to DNA that has been caused by irradiation might have evolved to correct naturally occurring errors in replication (Lindahl, 1982). Irradiated microorganisms do not die immediately after a lethal dose has been absorbed. Bacterial motility, respiration and fermentation may continue for several hours and spores may commence germination. Death usually ensues during the first DNA replication and conditions such as low temperature, which delay this process, favour completion of the repair process. Some gaps which remain in the DNA strands after the first replication process has been completed can be repaired by recombination (Bridges, 1976).

STABILITY OF MATERIALS TO IRRADIATION

Many of the materials that are used in the manufacture of medical devices or for their packaging are synthetic polymers. These consist of large molecules and their physical or chemical properties may be adversely affected by small chemical changes. Although most of them are much more stable to irradiation than they are to moist or dry heat, some undergo undesirable changes during or after radiation sterilization (Chapiro, 1974; Plester, 1974; Landfield, 1980). Articles that are intended for a single use only should withstand the highest dose, including local overdose, that will be used in the sterilization process.

Types of radiation-induced changes

Cross-linking between the polymer chains may occur, eventually resulting in a three-dimensional network which changes gums to a rubber-like consistency. Crystalline polymers become hard and brittle, but only at a very high dose. Degradative changes may accompany cross-linking or they may play the predominant role. Polypropylene, nylon and pressure-sensitive adhesives are subject to oxidative degradation. Polyvinyl chloride discolours; polyvinylidene chloride evolves hydrogen chloride and polytetrafluoroethylene (PTFE, or Teflon) evolves hydrogen fluoride. PVC yellows at 25 kGy and Teflon disintegrates to a powder. Glass darkens on irradiation; this may be useful in the preparation of bottles for storing light-sensitive chemicals or pharmaceuticals. Cotton gauze can develop a yellow colour and undergoes a decrease in strength; electron beam radiation does not reduce strength as much as does gamma radiation (Bradbury, 1974).

Factors influencing stability

1. *Physical or chemical structure of the material*: stability is favoured by the presence of a benzene ring in the polymer, especially if it is not part of the chain structure.
2. *Additives*: the presence in the formulation of substances with aromatic ring structures, as in phenolics, improves stability.
3. *Atmosphere during irradiation*: oxygen may enhance radiation-induced degradation. Oxidative deterioration of polypropylene may be reduced by the inclusion of an antioxidant in the formulation but stabilization of Teflon has so far been unsuccessful. PVC may be stabilized by the addition of complexes containing zinc and the problem of the instability of this material has largely been overcome.
4. *Dose rate*: materials such as polypropylene that are subject to oxidative degradation may withstand exposure to a similar dose from an electron accelerator. The very high dose rate of electron beam sterilization does not allow time for diffusion of oxygen into the material to replenish the loss which occurs during irradiation.
5. *Total dose*: as the effects of irradiation are cumulative, materials that are likely to undergo multiple treatments should be tested to dose levels up to or above 1000 kGy.
6. *Post-irradiation storage*: the development of adverse changes following irradiation is attributed to long-lived radicals that persist in materials such as polyethylene, cellulose and Teflon, where they are immobilized in the rigid structure. In rubber-like polymers the radicals are mobile and short-lived.

Levels of stability

Stability is usually rated on the response of the material to a single irradiation in the dose range

25–50 kGy. Teflon is unsuitable for radiation sterilization but fluorinated ethylene copolymers are more resistant. Polyisobutylene is also unsuitable because it is converted to a sticky or oily consistency.

Polyvinyl chloride (PVC) and polypropylene have been modified by the incorporation of stabilizers which overcome the tendencies of PVC to discolour (turn yellow) and polypropylene to embrittle with irradiation. Tygon, a PVC copolymer, is stable to 25–30 kGy. The other materials that are most commonly used — polyethylene (low- and high-density) and polystyrene — present no problems; polystyrene is one of the most stable synthetic materials. Phenolics, epoxy resins and adhesives (e.g. Araldite), polyester resins and mineral oils are also stable to high doses. Silicone rubber is more stable than are other types of rubber; however, silicone oil is stable only at a single-dose level.

SUSCEPTIBILITY OF MICROORGANISMS

Types and species

Microorganisms are much more resistant to ionizing radiation than are higher forms of life. In unicellular organisms the level of resistance is closely related to the volume of the DNA target. The general order of increasing resistance is shown in Table 8.2.

The wide range of doses that may be required for equivalent levels of inactivation reflects variation between genera, species and strains but may also be attributed to variation in the conditions in which irradiation is carried out. Bacterial spores are usually no more than 10 times as resistant as are vegetative bacteria. This is a small difference by comparison with their relative resistances to heat. The DNA in the spore core appears to be protected in vivo because, when extracted from the spore, it is as susceptible to irradiation as is that obtained from vegetative bacteria (Tanooka & Sakakibara, 1968). The mechanism of protection may be similar to that which confers resistance to heat on the constituents of the spore core.

Viruses may be classed as moderately or highly resistant, depending on the DNA volume. D values also vary with the suspending medium of the viruses. A range of 3.9 to 5.3 kGy was found for the D values of 30 viruses of public health significance suspended in Eagle's minimum essential medium (Sullivan et al, 1971). The resistance of the relatively large pox viruses corresponds to that of bacterial spores but the very small viruses that cause poliomyelitis in humans and foot-and-mouth disease in domestic animals are highly resistant. HIV is highly resistant (Conway & Tomford, 1992). Bacterial viruses are extremely resistant. Prions such as those associated with the Creutzfeldt-Jakob

Table 8.2 Sensitivity of microorganisms to ionizing radiation

Group	Microorganisms	Sterilizing dose[1] kGy
Sensitive	Vegetative bacteria (with some exceptions)	0.5–10
Moderately resistant	Moulds and yeasts	4–30
	Enterococcus faecium (suspended in buffer)	10–30
Resistant	Bacterial spores	10–50
	Bacillus pumilus E601	10–30
	Clostridium botulinum (some strains)	30
	Deinobacter spp.	10–40
	E. faecium (dried from serum broth)	10–45
	Most viruses	10–40
Highly resistant	*Moraxella* (some strains)	~50
	Deinococcus radiodurans	55–70
	Bacillus spores (contrived mutants)	35–80
	Foot-and-mouth disease virus, HIV	~50
	Bacterial viruses	wide range (one dose inadequate)

[1]Based on inactivation factor of 10^8 (8D)

disease in man and scrapie in sheep are also highly resistant.

Some exceptions to the general order of resistance among vegetative bacteria, spores and viruses may be seen in Table 8.2. Cultures of Gram-positive cocci which were isolated from dust included strains of *E. faecium* with resistance in the range that is characteristic of bacterial spores (Christensen, 1964). The resistance of *D. radiodurans* (Anderson et al, 1956) and *D. radiophilus* (Lewis, 1971) is equivalent to that of the very small viruses. The micrococci are associated with food sources but the enterococcus is an opportunistic pathogen. These bacteria appear to owe their resistance to the operation of very efficient repair mechanisms and the death rate curves are frequently characterized by a broad shoulder which extends until the absorbed dose is sufficient to inactivate the repair enzymes. Gram-negative bacilli in the genus *Moraxella* may also be highly resistant to irradiation (Welch & Maxcy, 1975). In addition, a radiation-resistant, red-pigmented Gram-negative bacillus, *Deinobacter grandis*, has been isolated from freshwater fish (Oyaizu et al, 1987); and a related *Deinobacter* sp. has been found in irradiated pork (Grant & Patterson, 1989). Some bacterial spores (e.g. *Bacillus sphaericus*, strain C_1A) appear to have increased in resistance by mutation. This might have occurred after repeated exposure to substerilizing doses of radiation; however, this procedure can also result in decreased resistance (Ley et al, 1970).

FACTORS INFLUENCING SUSCEPTIBILITY

Much of the variation in reported D values for organisms of the same or closely related species may be attributable to the influence of the environment before, during or immediately after irradiation. Analysis of the contribution of separate factors, such as oxygen, moisture or temperature, is difficult because the actions are often interdependent.

Oxygen

The resistance of microorganisms is usually increased 2–5 times if anoxic conditions are maintained during and after irradiation. The spores of *Bacillus pumilus* E601, for example, give a D value of 1.75 kGy when irradiated in air and 3.06 kGy in the absence of oxygen (Burt & Ley, 1963a). Potassium permanganate, which is a strong oxidizing agent, can substitute for molecular oxygen; it sensitizes spores to irradiation in anaerobic conditions but does not increase their sensitivity when oxygen is available (Tallentire & Jones, 1973).

Moisture

The influence of moisture on microbial susceptibility is complex because it is interrelated with that of oxygen.

Temperature

Thermoradiation

Radiation sterilization is normally carried out at ambient temperature, although some heat is generated when radiant energy is absorbed by the material treated or extraneous materials, including air, in the environment. Increases of the order of 10°C have been shown to reduce D values by as much as 50 per cent (Pallas & Hamdy, 1976).

The combined effects of radiation and moist or dry heat are potentially useful in the food industry. Kempe (1955) showed that prior irradiation sensitized spores of *Clostridium botulinum* to moist heat; there was no sensitization to irradiation if the order of treatment was reversed. Similar observations apply to *Clostridium perfringens* (Gombas & Gomez, 1978). Synergism is observed under certain conditions when heat and irradiation are applied simultaneously, as in the inactivation of spores of *Bacillus subtilis* subsp. *niger* (Fisher & Pflug, 1977). A synergistic action is one in which the combined effect is greater than the sum of the separate effects. Fisher & Pflug (1977) demonstrated that each agent in the combination must be able to kill spores by itself and that synergism occurs in conditions when they are equally effective as separate sterilizing agents. Synergism has also been demonstrated in certain combinations of dry heat and irradiation (Sivinski et al, 1973). However, Emborg (1974) has expressed doubt about the practicality of combining radiation and heat treatment in the sterilization of medical devices.

Subzero temperature

The effect of irradiation on microorganisms in frozen substrates is important in relation to food. When spores of *C. botulinum* (strain 33A) were irradiated in phosphate buffer and in pork pea broth, there was a sharp increase in resistance when freezing occurred. This was attributed to the reduction of indirect action as the active radicals produced in water were immobilized. A further reduction occurred gradually as the temperature of the phosphate buffer was reduced to −196°C by means of liquid nitrogen. However, reducing the temperature of the pork pea broth below −25°C made no difference; the indirect effects were already nonoperative in this more complex medium at −25°C (Grecz et al, 1967).

Scott et al (1989) described the inactivation of the causative agent of Q fever, *Coxiella burnetii*, by gamma irradiation at a temperature of −79°C. *C. burnetii* shows resistance to disinfection by heat and various chemicals, but its inactivation kinetics are exponential for gamma irradiation at −79°C. A dose of 10 kGy completely inactivated a preparation of *C. burnetii* at a concentration of 10^{11} per ml, without affecting the morphological characteristics of the cells or their antigenicity and ability to elicit an immune response.

Organic substrates

Protection against radiation damage is conferred by dried serum broth (Christensen & Sehested, 1964), grease films (Burt & Ley, 1963a), culture media and other complex substrates (Dyer et al, 1966). The protective effect is reflected by tailing death rate curves.

Chemical agents

Glycerol, thiourea, dimethyl sulfoxide and cysteine protect bacteria against radiation damage, possibly by scavenging free radicals. However other chemicals, including iodoacetamide, iodoacetic acid and potassium iodide, act as sensitizers (Lewis & Kumta, 1975; Nair & Pradhan, 1976). The effect is attributed to the release of free iodine atoms through reaction with hydroxyl radicals (Mullenger et al, 1967) and their incorporation into bacterial cell membranes and interference with repair mechanisms by enzymes associated with the membranes (Shenoy et al, 1968).

The influence of some chemical agents occurs after irradiation, when the treated microorganisms are cultured to detect survivors. The susceptibility of bacterial spores to sodium chloride in the recovery medium increases in proportion to the radiation dose (Roberts et al, 1965).

STERILIZING DOSE

A radiation sterilization process is defined by a single parameter, the minimum absorbed dose. This is the amount of energy absorbed at sites in the load where the lowest dose is received. The time of exposure required to deliver the dose depends on the power, or output, of the radiation source and also on the average density of the material treated. Times range from fractions of a second in electron beam sterilization of small packs to several hours or even days for gamma radiation. Materials of different density, such as scalpel blades and cotton dressings, should not be treated by electron beam irradiation at the same time. Products with different densities can be sterilized simultaneously by gamma radiation if the total weight of material in each container is the same and the irradiation time is based on the high density material.

The dose is maintained at the specified level by adjustment of the conveyor speed as the output of a ^{60}Co source deteriorates. Although economics dictate that a gamma radiation plant should operate 95 per cent of the time, temporary shutdowns are necessary for maintenance, repair or admittance of visitors for educational purposes. The interruptions do not affect the dose to be delivered unless the period is unduly long and the nature of the material permits multiplication of microorganisms that are still viable (Burt & Ley, 1963b; Borick & Fogarty, 1967).

The sterilizing dose must be calculated for the particular goods because it is influenced by the number and resistance of the organisms initially present. The most resistant contaminants are usually bacterial spores but resistant Gram-positive cocci (Christensen, 1964) and yeasts (Ley et al, 1972) have been isolated from medical devices prior to sterilization. A medical device which is moulded at high temperature under hygienic conditions is assumed to have an average total count of 20 microbial contaminants per product unit (Christensen & Kristensen, 1981).

Setting the sterilizing dose

Two alternative methods are recommended for setting the sterilizing dose, i.e. the dose required for a sterility assurance level (SAL) of 10^{-6} (ISO 11137, 1995). One method is based on an estimate of the average bioburden for the product unit. A radiation dose is then read from a table for SAL of 10^{-2}. This dose is applied to 100 product units and the units are tested individually for sterility. If not more than 2 of the 100 units are positive for growth, the table is again consulted for the appropriate sterilizing dose for SAL of 10^{-6}. If more than 2 tests are positive, the use of the other method of dose setting is indicated.

The alternative method is based on information obtained on the natural resistance of the microbial contaminants to small incremental doses of radiation. It uses the results of sterility testing on samples (e.g. 20) of product units that have been subjected to a series of not less than nine exposures to 2 kGy increments of radiation (Davis et al, 1984). From these observations, the dose at which one in 100 units is expected to be unsterile is determined. This corresponds to SAL of 10^{-2}. The dose is then tested experimentally on 100 units, which are irradiated and tested individually for sterility. If the estimated dose for SAL 10^{-2} is verified, the appropriate dose for sterilization (SAL 10^{-6}) is obtained by extrapolation from a computer simulated model.

The conventional sterilizing dose of 25 kGy derives from an assumed initial bioburden of no more than 100 microorganisms per product unit and a D value for *B. pumilus* under anoxic conditions of 3 kGy. Thus, the dose required for SAL 10^{-6} (8D) is 25 kGy. As most articles are irradiated in air, a dose based on a D value under anoxic conditions provides an additional margin of safety. However, use of the currently recommended methods for dose setting provides more flexibility and allows for much lower doses.

INSTALLATIONS FOR RADIATION STERILIZATION

Radiation sterilization is virtually limited to industrial applications because the installations are large, the safety precautions are elaborate and the cost is high. Gamma radiation (^{60}Co) plants are usually more costly than are electron accelerators.

Table 8.3 Performance characteristics of cobalt-60 installations and electron accelerators

Characteristics	Cobalt-60 source	Electron accelerator
Energy	1.333 and 1.173 MeV	Electrostatic 0.2–5 MeV Microwave 2–10 MeV
Penetration (unit density material)	*Ca* 30 cm (depending on source strength)	0.33 cm/MeV
Dose rate	Slow (10 Gy/s)	Fast (10^6–10^{12} Gy/s)
Processing time	Long (several hours)	Short (<1 s)
Size of packs treated	Large (final cartons)	Small (single products or small cartons)
Load conveyors	Horizontal and vertical movements	Horizontal (conveyor belt)
Process controls	Conveyor speed only	Conveyor speed Scan width Beam current, energy Pulse duration and frequency
Safety measures	Source storage tank Chamber construction External indicator/control panel Ozone removal	Machine switched off Shielding to contain X-radiation Ozone removal

The design and construction of ^{60}Co installations and electron accelerators will be described briefly. A comparison of the relevant characteristics is made in Table 8.3.

Cobalt-60 installation

The installation is located within a larger building (Eymery, 1973). It consists of:

1. Irradiation chamber and annexes
2. ^{60}Co, as source of gamma radiation
3. Mechanical load conveyors
4. Process controls and safety systems.

The general layout of an installation designed for sterilization of medical devices is shown in Figure 8.1.

Chamber and annexes

The walls are constructed of reinforced concrete, up to two metres thick. The size of the irradiation chamber is determined by that of the ^{60}Co source and the load conveyors. A storage tank below floor level for the radioactive source is also constructed from concrete, and may be lined with stainless steel; it must be independent of the chamber con-

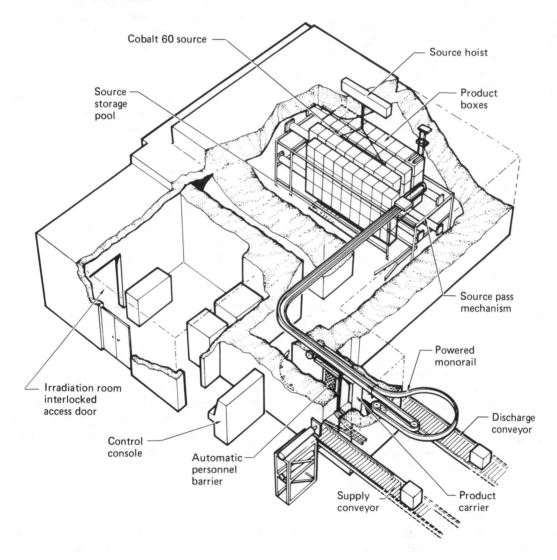

Fig. 8.1 A cobalt-60 installation for radiation sterilization (built by Atomic Energy of Canada Ltd).

struction for protection against earthquake damage. The tank is filled with deionized water to a depth of five metres. Dry storage in a concrete-lined pit, covered with a removable lead plug, may be used for relatively small ^{60}Co sources but is less convenient for adding new elements. The annexes to the chamber include labyrinthine corridors to prevent escape of radiation to the environment during entry and exit of load units. Both chamber and annexes are ventilated to remove ozone and oxides of nitrogen.

Cobalt-60 source

The radioactive isotope is contained in metal tubes, or 'rods'. They arrive at the radiation facility in a lead transport container, which is lowered into the water-filled tank. The depth of five metres allows space for lifting the source elements from the container without emitting more than 10^{-6} Gy at the water surface. They are transferred by means of long-handled tools to a rectangular frame which is suspended by a mechanical hoist. The frame is not filled and rods of different ages are positioned to distribute the dose evenly to the large bulk of material. About once a year new rods are added and the necessary rearrangements are made. Spent rods are removed when all frame positions are filled. Large sources can contain 3.7×10^{16} Bq of ^{60}Co, with a power output of 30 kilowatts or 30 kilojoules per second.

Load conveyors

The first conveyor moves standard size cartons or metal containers through a small entry port, which opens automatically at regular intervals to admit one unit, and conveys them through the approach corridors to the irradiation chamber. Here they are transferred to the irradiation conveyor, which is designed so that the load surrounds the source as completely as possible to minimize dose wastage. The cartons are moved slowly through several positions on both sides of the source until the prescribed minimum dose has been delivered. They are then transferred to another conveyor which moves them through the exit to a storage area, which is physically separated from the place where the cartons awaiting treatment are held.

Controls and safety precautions

The control panel outside the unit includes indicators of the position of the ^{60}Co source (elevated or in storage), the conveyor speed and the water level in the storage tank. The conveyor speed is adjusted periodically to compensate for source deterioration. The source elevator must be completely reliable and should return automatically to the storage position if there is any malfunction in the system. Controls are installed to ensure that the source cannot be raised to the operating position unless the chamber has been locked. Entrance of personnel to the irradiation chamber is possible only when the source is in the storage position and monitors have confirmed that the radiation has fallen to the background level. Radiation monitors should be placed at the entrance to the corridor, inside the chamber, near the air exhaust filter and the water deionizer. Monitors to verify that ozone has been effectively removed by the air-exchange system are also required.

Electron accelerators

In an electron accelerating machine low-energy electrons from the emitting surface of a hot filament are accelerated in a vacuum to high velocity and energy levels and emerge through a thin window. In industrial practice, the limit is set at 10 MeV to obviate any possibility of inducing radioactivity in the irradiated material. There are two types of electron accelerators.

Electrostatic accelerators

This type operates at 0.2–5 MeV. The electrons are accelerated by travelling in an evacuated tube through a high voltage, which may be generated by an insulating core transformer, a 'dynamitron', a Van de Graaff generator or a simple power transformer.

Microwave linear accelerators

These machines operate at 2–10 MeV. Energy is supplied to a pulse of electrons in the accelerating tube by a synchronized travelling microwave field or by a series of standing microwave fields specifically phased and positioned along the path of the electrons. In pulsed systems the dose is delivered almost instantaneously (Haimson, 1974).

Accelerator equipment and operation

Accessory equipment for electron accelerators includes a vacuum pump, water cooling system, operational controls and safety interlock systems. The beam of high-energy electrons is focused and shaped before emerging through a thin metal window. It may be rapidly scanned to and fro across the width of a horizontal conveyor belt, which carries a single layer of small packs. The operating characteristics of an electron accelerator are described by the energy (penetration), power (voltage × current), and efficiency. In pulsed systems allowance must be made for the pulse duration and pulse frequency.

Electrons penetrate effectively 0.33 cm/MeV into material of unit density but sometimes irradiation is carried out from both sides. Dual purpose machines have been designed which can readily be converted to X-ray mode to irradiate bulky packages.

Controls and safety precautions

Unlike a gamma radiation source, the electron beam can be turned off by a switch. Larger accelerators require shielding which is similar to that of a ^{60}Co installation because X-rays are produced when the electrons strike metal parts of the conveyor. Small machines may be locally shielded.

VALIDATION AND CONTROL OF RADIATION STERILIZATION

Commissioning the installation

The following procedures are involved in commissioning a gamma radiation facility:

1. Investigation of the level and distribution of activity of the radioactive source
2. Determination of the dose distribution in a load of suitable density and configuration
3. Determination of the time spent by each product unit in the various positions around the source.

The performance of conveyors and settings of timers must also be checked and recorded.

Auditing the dose

The principles governing determination of the appropriate radiation dose for a particular product and the procedures for dose setting based on the bioburden level or its radiation resistance have been explained in an earlier section. Periodic audits of the sterilization dose are required for the detection of any changes in the bioburden that might necessitate a change in the dose. Dose auditing needs to be performed every 3 months, as a minimum, and after any change that might affect the number and nature of the bioburden. The procedure is to irradiate 100 product units at the dose for SAL 10^{-2} and to test each unit for sterility. From the findings, a decision is made to affirm, augment or re-establish the set dose for SAL 10^{-6}. Similar methods of dose setting and auditing apply to gamma irradiators that use ^{137}Cs and to irradiators that use a beam from an electron or X-ray generator.

Many plastic items and clean materials are sterilized by gamma radiation in the 10 to 20 kGy range. Products and materials which are not required to meet the SAL level for medical sterility may be irradiated to a SAL level of 10^{-3}. Some materials are irradiated to reduce the bioburden only.

Where sterilization doses lower than the conventional 25 kGy for gamma radiation can be validated, their use may help reduce effects such as the loss of material strength or colour change that are induced in some materials by radiation. In addition, lower dosage means financial savings. On the other hand, doses above 25 kGy may sometimes be required.

Measuring the dose

Dosimeters are classified as primary, reference and routine. Primary dosimeters, which are located in national standards laboratories, are the most accurate. They consist of ionization chambers and calorimeters for the measurement of absorbed doses in carbon or metals (BS:EN 552, 1994).

Chemical reference dosimeters are used for gamma radiation and calorimeters for electron beam applications. Examples of the former are ceric-cerous sulfate, ferrous sulfate and dichromate solutions and solid alanine (BS:EN 552, 1994; ISO 11137, 1995). Dosage is usually read in an ultraviolet (UV) spectrophotometer but an electron spin resonance spectrometer is used for alanine (ISO 11137, 1995). Reference dosimeters are used in dose mapping and for checking routine dosimeters (BS:EN 552, 1994).

Routine dosimeters may also be used for dose mapping but their main usage is in routine monitoring. Routine dosimeters consist of strips or pellets of dyed polymethyl methacrylate or clear plastic film which change colour or darken in proportion to the dose of radiation. The degree of darkening of the dyed dosimeters is read by the absorption of visible light of suitable wavelength in a spectrophotometer. Changes in the clear films are read in a UV spectrophotometer. These dosimeters are affected by changes in humidity and temperature; but, provided such effects are taken into account, they are satisfactory for measuring doses up to 40 kGy. However, they need to be calibrated at regular intervals by a calibration system which is traceable to, and consistent with, the primary standard dosimeters (BS: EN 552, 1994; ISO 11137, 1995). Dosimetry records should be kept for all phases of irradiation.

Process indicator discs with various dyes are commercially available. The colour changes include yellow to red, green to brown and other combinations. These discs do not verify a sterilizing dose and they should not be used as the sole means of distinguishing processed from unprocessed products (ISO 11137, 1995).

Biological indicators

If the use of biological indicators is desired, spores of a designated strain of B. pumilus (E601; ATCC 27142) may be used to validate or monitor processes for a dose of 25 kGy. Specified strains of more resistant microorganisms (e.g. E. faecium $A_2 1$, a bacteriophage or spores of a mutant strain of B. sphaericus, $C_1 A$) have been used for doses exceeding 25 kGy (Christensen et al, 1969). Although biological indicators for routine control are usually considered unnecessary (ISO 11137, 1995), the use of resistant test strains of bacteria or spores has been recommended as part of the

procedure of commissioning a new radiation facility (Christensen, 1978).

Product sterility tests

Sterility testing on articles is limited to dose setting procedures or to situations where a gross fault in preparation, packaging or sterilization might have occurred. Soybean casein digest broth, which is incubated at 30 to 32°C for 14 days, is the recommended sterility test medium (ISO 11137, 1995). Controls are required to monitor bacteriostatic or bactericidal activity in the test samples. The packages should be inspected for integrity of the material and the sealing area before a sterility test is carried out.

Product release

The use of biological indicators for process monitoring or of sterility testing of the irradiated product is not recommended for product release (ISO 11137, 1995). Naturally occurring contaminants often include microorganisms that are more radiation resistant than are the spores of B. pumilus (Christensen & Kristensen, 1981). Sterility testing is not feasible as a means of substantiating SALs higher than SAL^{-2}. For example, with SAL^{-6}, a million items would require individual sterility testing. Not only is this impractical but the false positive rate of 0.1 per cent for sterility testing would invalidate the findings (ISO 11137, 1995).

APPLICATIONS OF RADIATION STERILIZATION

The sterilization of medical supplies by gamma radiation from ^{60}Co or high-energy electrons commenced in parallel with the introduction of synthetic materials that do not withstand moist or dry heat sterilization. Radiation sterilization must compete with industrial ethylene oxide sterilization. The high capital costs of gamma installations and electron accelerators can be a deterrent and availability at a convenient location is also important. Some installations are operated independently, accepting goods from different manufacturers and also, on a small scale, from hospitals. Others are installed by large companies to sterilize their own products.

Advantages of radiation sterilization are:

1. The process is operated at ambient temperature
2. The materials are not wetted or significantly heated
3. Packaging materials which act as a complete bacterial barrier may be used and the articles may be packed and sealed into the outer containers
4. The process is continuous and controlled by the time of irradiation (i.e. the speed of the in-cell conveyor).

The principal disadvantage is the possibility of deleterious effects on the articles or packaging material. These may limit or preclude radiation sterilization of some electronic equipment, devices made from unstable plastics and many pharmaceuticals and foods. The low penetrability of electrons limits electron beam sterilization to small volume, low-density products.

Medical equipment

Commercially produced items of equipment for medical use are usually classed as therapeutic devices and covered by regulations similar to those that apply to pharmaceuticals. Most are intended for a single use only; if limited reuse is permissible, directions for resterilization should be specified. Polyethylene, which may be laminated with polyester, nylon, paper or metal foil is the most widely used packaging material. Tyvek®, a spun-bonded polyethylene, may also be used. Other plastics, e.g. PVC, acrylics and polypropylene, have been modified to make them stable.

Reusable heat-sensitive equipment, which has been cleaned and packed in a hospital, may be sent to a gamma radiation facility for sterilization. This is a useful service, provided the necessary prerequisites of physical cleanliness and a low contamination level can be fulfilled, but it involves certain risks. Fine tubes, such as cardiac catheters, should not be reused because internal cleanliness cannot be verified. Knowledge of the stability of the articles and packaging material to repeated irradiation is required and the effect, if any, of irradiation on the function of electronic components. These precautions are the responsibility of the hospital authority, not of the radiation facility.

Some types of articles which may be sterilized by ionizing radiation are presented in Table 8.4. However, they represent only a small fraction of the total and no list would be complete because new heat-sensitive items may be added, while others may be altered in design or construction with the result that they can be sterilized by heat and removed from the list.

Pharmaceutical and biological products

Irradiation is used as a method of sterilizing heat-sensitive organic materials, including anaesthetics, enzymes, therapeutic drugs, antibiotics, hormones and vaccines. Each product must be evaluated in relation to its intended use and the possible risks. Official approval of the process, based on prescribed safety tests for new pharmaceutical products, is required because chemical changes may inactivate drugs or antibiotics, destroy emulsions or produce harmful substances.

Electron beam sterilization at high dose rates, which create anoxic conditions in solutions, may be less damaging to some products than is sterilization by gamma radiation (Diding et al, 1978). Dry solids and oily preparations are generally more stable to irradiation than are aqueous solutions and suspensions. Discoloration does not necessarily indicate loss of antimicrobial or pharmacological activity. Freeze-dried penicillin and streptomycin and some other antibiotics are stable to irradiation. Cortisone and adreno-corticotrophic hormone may be irradiated in solid form but suspensions and solutions are unstable. Irradiation is satisfactory for albumin, iodinated albumin and dry protease enzymes but blood plasma proteins, iodinated albumin in solution, insulin, heparin, thrombin, thyroxine and organometal compounds are very unstable. Sodium alginate and acacia gums are stable in powdered form but lose viscosity if they are irradiated as solutions (Hartman et al, 1975). Tragacanth, which has been irradiated as a powder, gives solutions of reduced viscosity.

The vitamin B complex is stable in dry and injectable forms but the aqueous form of B_6 is not. Vitamin C can be irradiated in dry form, in

Table 8.4 Examples of materials and equipment sterilized by irradiation[1]

Medical, biological and laboratory materials and equipment	Pharmaceuticals and cosmetic materials
Adhesive plasters	Alginate powders
Albumin and iodinated albumin	Anaesthetics
Aortic valves and arterial prostheses	Antibiotics (freeze-dried)
Bandages and dressings	Casein
Blood collecting kits	Creams (e.g. Sunscreen creams)
Bone and cartilage	Cosmetic powders
Bovine serum (frozen)	Detergents and emulsifiers
Catheters and drains	Disinfectants (e.g. alcohol, povidone iodine)
Culture bottles and trays	Eye drops and ointments
Dialyzers	Gelatin capsules
Endotracheal tubes	Gums (e.g. acacia)
Enzymes (freeze-dried)	Herbs and spices
Eye droppers	Lactose (tablet excipient)
Gloves	Lecithin powders
Infusion and transfusion sets	Liposomes
Lancets and scalpels	Microcrystalline cellulose (tablet excipient)
Monoclonal antibodies	Oils (animal, vegetable, mineral)
Needles and syringes	Ointments
Petri dishes	Parabens
Pipettes and pipette tips	Starches (tablet excipient)
Steroids (e.g. dry cortisone)	Talc
Swabs and pads	Vaccines (freeze-dried)
Sutures	Vitamins (dry)
Urine and colostomy bags	Waxes (e.g. beeswax)

[1] Includes data supplied by West G, Steritech, Victoria, Australia

concentrated solutions and in dilute frozen solutions. Vitamin E, calciferol and ergosterol are unstable. Morphine sulfate, ergometrine maleate and procaine hydrochloride are moderately stable when dry, but atropine sulfate cannot be irradiated successfully.

Non-living graft materials, such as blood vessels, freeze-dried bone, cartilage and homograft aortic valves have given satisfactory performance after sterilization by irradiation. Some success has been achieved with vaccines and antisera.

Complex formulations of pharmaceuticals, cosmetics and toiletries, which do not have to be sterile, and some heavily contaminated raw materials, such as starch, talc and pancreatin, may be treated by a dose up to 10 kGy to reduce the number of viable organisms to an acceptable level. Some advances in the irradiation of drugs and antibiotics have been discussed by Diding et al (1978) and Power (1978). Among the chemical disinfectants, isopropyl alcohol, povidone iodine and quaternary ammonium compounds are stable to irradiation (e.g. as skin swabs) but chlorhexidine is inactivated.

Food

The irradiation of plant and animal food products can have beneficial effects in promoting food safety and reducing food losses (WHO, 1994). A dose up to 1 kGy kills insects, pests and parasites; delays the ripening of fresh fruits and inhibits the sprouting of root crops. Doses of radiation in the 1 to 5 kGy range extend the shelf-life of foods by reducing the levels of spoilage microorganisms (WHO, 1994; Pauli & Tarantino, 1995). A dose of 3 kGy destroys *Salmonella* and *Campylobacter* on poultry (WHO, 1994; Pauli & Tarantino, 1995). Less than 1 kGy is also effective against *Escherichia coli* 0157:H7, a causative agent of potentially fatal haemolytic uraemic syndrome, in chicken meat and ground beef (Thayer & Boyd, 1993). This is particularly relevant to the treatment of uncooked meats that are used in fermented sausage products (Robins-Browne, 1995).

Commercial radiation treatment of foods does not induce any radioactivity in the foods. Moreover, no evidence of adverse toxicological effects has been found in numerous feeding experiments on animals (WHO, 1994). Furthermore, although a theoretical possibility, mutant microorganisms of increased pathogenicity have never emerged in practice. Animal studies also indicate the equivalence of irradiated and nonirradiated foods in nutritional quality. Indeed, it has been noted that food processes involving heating often result in greater nutrient losses (WHO, 1994). In general, irradiation of foods results in no hazards for the consumer and can contribute to a safer and more plentiful food supply (WHO, 1994).

Industrial materials

Animal products such as hides, wool or hair for use in carpet manufacture, are sometimes heavily contaminated with anthrax spores and constitute a serious health risk for people who handle them. A dose of 15 kGy would provide a margin of safety for *Bacillus anthracis* (Horne et al, 1959) but would not be effective against the foot-and-mouth disease virus.

REFERENCES

Anderson A W, Nordan H C, Cain R F, Parrish G, Duggan D 1956 Studies on a radio-resistant micrococcus. 1. Isolation, morphology, cultural characteristics, and resistance to gamma radiation. Food Technology 10: 575–578

Borick P M, Fogarty M G 1967 Effects of continuous and interrupted radiation on microorganisms. Applied Microbiology 15: 785–789

Bradbury W C 1974 Physical and chemical effects of ionizing radiation on cellulosic material. In: Gaughran E R L, Goudie A J (eds) Sterilization by ionizing radiation. Multiscience, Montreal, vol I: 387–402

Bridges B A 1976 Survival of bacteria following exposure to ultraviolet and ionizing radiations. In: Gray T R G, Postgate J R (eds) The survival of vegetative microbes. Cambridge University Press, Cambridge, p 183–208

BS:EN 552 1994 Sterilization of medical devices — Validation and routine control of sterilization by irradiation. British Standards Institution, London

Burt M M, Ley F J 1963a Studies on the dose requirement for the radiation sterilization of medical equipment. I. Influence of suspending media. Journal of Applied Bacteriology 26: 484–489

Burt M M, Ley F J 1963b Studies on the dose requirement for the radiation sterilization of medical equipment. II. A comparison between continuous and fractionated doses. Journal of Applied Bacteriology 26: 490–492

Chapiro A 1974 Physical and chemical effects of ionizing radiations on polymeric systems. In: Gaughran E R L, Goudie A J (eds) Sterilization by ionizing radiation. Multiscience, Montreal, vol I: 367–374

Christensen E A 1964 Radiation resistance of enterococci dried in air. Acta Pathologica et Microbiologica Scandinavica 61: 483–486

Christensen E A 1978 The role of microbiology in commissioning a new facility and in routine control. In: Gaughran E R L, Goudie A J (eds) Sterilization by ionizing radiation. Multiscience, Montreal, vol II: 50–64

Christensen E A, Kallings L O, Fystro D 1969 Microbiological control of sterilization procedures and standards for the sterilization of medical equipment. Ugeskrift for Laeger 131: 2123 (Translation p 1–15)

Christensen E A, Kristensen H 1981 Radiation-resistance of micro-organisms from air in clean premises. Acta Pathologica et Microbiologica Scandinavica Section B 89: 293–301

Christensen E A, Sehested K 1964 Radiation resistance of *Streptococcus faecium* and spores of *Bacillus subtilis* dried in various media. Acta Pathologica et Microbiologica Scandinavica 62: 448–458

Conway B, Tomford W W 1992 Radiosensitivity of human immunodeficiency virus type 1. Clinical Infectious Diseases 14: 978–979

Davis K W, Strawderman W E, Whitby J L 1984 The rationale and a computer evaluation of a gamma irradiation sterilization dose determination method for medical devices using a substerilization incremental dose sterility protocol. Journal of Applied Bacteriology 57: 31–50

Diding N, Flink O, Johansson S, Ohlson B, Redmalm G, Öhrner B 1978 Irradiation of drugs with Co-60 and electrons. In: Gaughran E R L, Goudie A J (eds) Sterilization by ionizing radiation. Multiscience, Montreal, vol II: 216–231

Dyer J K, Anderson A W, Dutiyabodhi P 1966 Radiation survival of food pathogens in complex media. Applied Microbiology 14: 92–97

Emborg C 1974 Inactivation of dried bacteria and bacterial spores by means of gamma irradiation at high temperatures. Applied Microbiology 27: 830–833

Eymery R 1973 Design of radiation sterilization facilities. In: Phillips G B, Miller W S (eds) Industrial sterilization: international symposium, Amsterdam, 1972. Duke University Press, Durham, ch 11, p 153

Fisher D A, Pflug I J 1977 Effect of combined heat and radiation on microbial destruction. Applied and Environmental Microbiology 33: 1170–1176

Gombas D E, Gomez R F 1978 Sensitization of *Clostridium perfringens* spores to heat by gamma radiation. Applied and Environmental Microbiology 36: 403–407

Grant I R, Patterson M F 1989 A novel radiation-resistant *Deinobacter* sp. isolated from irradiated pork. Letters in Applied Microbiology 8: 21–24

Grecz N, Upadhyay J, Tang T C 1967 Effect of temperature on radiation resistance of spores of *Clostridium botulinum* 33A. Canadian Journal of Microbiology 13: 287–293

Haimson J 1974 Advances in electron beam linear accelerator technology. In: Gaughran E R L, Goudie A J (eds) Sterilization by ionizing radiation. Multiscience, Montreal, vol I: 71–106

Hartman A W, Nesbitt R U Jr, Smith F M, Nuessle N O 1975 Viscosities of acacia and sodium alginate after sterilization by cobalt-60. Journal of Pharmaceutical Sciences 64: 802–805

Haynes R H 1966 The interpretation of microbial inactivation and recovery phenomena. Radiation Research Supplement 6: 1–29

Horne T, Turner G C, Willis A T 1959 Inactivation of spores of *Bacillus anthracis* by γ-radiation. Nature 183: 475–476

ISO 11137 1995 International Standard Sterilization of health care products — requirements for validation and routine control — radiation sterilization. International Organization for Standardization, Geneva

Kempe L L 1955 Combined effects of heat and radiation in food sterilization. Applied Microbiology 3: 346–352

Krinsky N I 1976 Cellular damage initiated by visible light. In: Gray T R G, Postgate J R (eds) The survival of vegetative microbes. Cambridge University Press, Cambridge, p 209–239

Landfield H 1980 Radiation effects on device and packaging materials. Medical Device & Diagnostic Industry 2 (5): 45–48

Latarjet R 1972 Interaction of radiation energy with nucleic acids. Current Topics in Radiation Research Quarterly 8: 1–38

Lewis N F 1971 Studies on a radio-resistant coccus isolated from Bombay duck (*Harpodon nehereus*). Journal of General Microbiology 66: 29–35

Lewis N, Kumta U 1975 Radiosensitization of *Micrococcus radiophilus*. Radiation Research 62: 159–163

Ley F J, Kennedy T S, Kawashima K, Roberts D, Hobbs B C 1970 The use of gamma radiation for the elimination of *Salmonella* from frozen meat. Journal of Hygiene 68: 293–311

Ley F J, Winsley B, Harbord P, Keall A, Summers T 1972 Radiation sterilization: microbiological findings from subprocess dose treatment of disposable plastic syringes. Journal of Applied Bacteriology 35: 53–61

Lindahl T 1982 DNA repair enzymes. Annual Review of Biochemistry 51: 61–87

Miller D R 1970 Theoretical survival curves for radiation damage in bacteria. Journal of Theoretical Biology 26: 383–398

Mullenger L, Singh B B, Ormerod M G, Dean C J 1967 Chemical study of the radiosensitization of *Micrococcus sodonensis* by iodine compounds. Nature 216: 372–374

Myers D K, Childs J D, Jones A R 1977 Sensitization of bacteriophage T4 to ^{60}Co-γ radiation and to low-energy X radiation by bromouracil. Radiation Research 69: 152–165

Nair C K K, Pradhan D S 1976 Production and rejoining of single-strand breaks in DNA of *Escherichia coli* cells after exposure to gamma-rays in the presence of iodoacetic acid under oxic and anoxic conditions. International Journal of Radiation Biology 29: 235–240

Oyaizu H, Stackebrandt E, Schleifer K H et al 1987 A radiation-resistant, rod-shaped bacterium, *Deinobacter grandis* gen. nov., sp. nov., with peptidoglycan containing ornithine. International Journal of Systematic Bacteriology 37: 62–67

Pallas J E, Hamdy M K 1976 Effects of thermoradiation on bacteria. Applied and Environmental Microbiology 32: 250–256

Pauli G H, Tarantino L M 1995 FDA regulatory aspects of food irradiation. Dairy, Food and Environmental Sanitation 15(9): 558–561

Plester D W 1974 Physical and chemical effects of ionizing radiation on plastic films, laminates and packaging materials. In: Gaughran E R L, Goudie A J (eds) Sterilization by ionizing radiation. Multiscience, Montreal, vol I: 375–386

Pollard E C, Davis S A 1970 The action of ionizing radiation on transcription (and translation) in several strains of *Escherichia coli*. Radiation Research 41: 375–399

Power D M 1978 Physical-chemical changes in irradiated drugs. In: Gaughran, E R L, Goudie A J (eds) Sterilization by ionizing radiation. Multiscience, Montreal, vol II: 237–246

Resnick M A 1976 The repair of double-strand breaks in DNA: a model involving recombination. Journal of Theoretical Biology 59: 97–106

Roberts T A, Ditchett P J, Ingram M 1965 The effect of sodium chloride on radiation resistance and recovery of irradiated anaerobic spores. Journal of Applied Bacteriology 28: 336–348

Robins-Browne R M 1995 Enterohaemorrhagic *Escherichia coli*: an emerging food-borne pathogen with serious consequences. Medical Journal of Australia 162: 511–512

Scott G H, McCaul T F, Williams J C 1989 Inactivation of *Coxiella burnetii* by gamma irradiation. Journal of General Microbiology 135: 3263–3270

Shenoy M A, Singh B B, Gopal-Ayengar A R 1968 Iodine incorporated in cell constituents during sensitization to radiation by iodoacetic acid. Science 160: 999

Shragge P C, Hunt J W 1974 A pulse radiolysis study of the free radical intermediates in the radiolysis of uracil. Radiation Research 60: 233–249

Shragge P C, Varghese A J, Hunt J W, Greenstock C L 1974 Radiolysis of uracil in the absence of oxygen. Radiation Research 60: 250–267

Sivinski H D, Garst D M, Reynolds M C, Trauth C A Jr, Trujillo R E, Whitfield W J 1973 The synergistic inactivation of biological systems by thermoradiation. In: Phillips G B, Miller W S (eds) Industrial sterilization: international symposium, Amsterdam, 1972. Duke University Press, Durham, ch 17, p 305

Skulberg A 1965 The resistance of *Clostridium botulinum* type E toxin to radiation. Journal of Applied Bacteriology 28: 139–141

Sullivan R, Fassolitis A C, Larkin E P, Read R B Jr, Peeler J T 1971 Inactivation of thirty viruses by gamma radiation. Applied Microbiology 22: 61–65

Tallentire A, Jones A B 1973 Radiosensitization of bacterial spores by potassium permanganate. International Journal of Radiation Biology 24: 345–354

Tanooka H, Sakakibara Y 1968 Radioresistant nature of the transforming activity of DNA in bacterial spores. Biochimica et Biophysica Acta 155: 130–142

Thayer D W, Boyd G 1993 Elimination of *Escherichia coli* 0157:H7 in meats by gamma irradiation. Applied and Environmental Microbiology 59: 1030–1034

Ulmer K M, Gomez R F, Sinskey A J 1979 Ionizing radiation damage to the folded chromosome of *Escherichia coli* K-12: repair of double-strand breaks in deoxyribonucleic acid. Journal of Bacteriology 138: 486–491

Welch A B, Maxcy R B 1975 Characterization of radiation-resistant vegetative bacteria in beef. Applied Microbiology 30: 242–250

WHO 1994 Safety and nutritional adequacy of irradiated food. World Health Organization, Geneva

9. Aseptic filtration of liquids and air

Filtration differs from other methods of sterilization as it does not involve killing microorganisms or inhibiting their growth. Living and non-living particles are removed from liquids and gases by passage through fibrous, granular or synthetic membrane filters of appropriate retention efficiency. Fibrous and granular depth filters trap small particles in tortuous channels within the filter bed. Membrane filters act as screen filters; they are traversed by channels which retain particles that are larger than the pore size. The mechanisms by which microorganisms are trapped by depth filters and screen filters are illustrated in Figure 9.1. The filtration of liquids and air will be discussed in separate sections of this chapter.

ASEPTIC FILTRATION OF LIQUIDS

Liquids are filtered for the following purposes:

1. 'Sterile' filtration (removal of microorganisms from heat-sensitive aqueous solutions, organic solvents or oils)
2. Sterility testing of pharmaceutical products and medical devices
3. Collection of bacteria from water samples or other dilute suspensions for enumeration and identification.

TYPES OF FILTERS

Depth filters may be composed of polypropylene, with a wide range of average pore diameters, glass and cellulose fibres. Earthenware, porcelain and sintered glass filters are no longer used for microbial filtration because they are subject to cracking, clog easily and are difficult to clean for

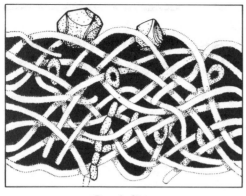

Depth filter

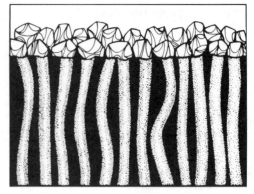

Screen filter

Fig. 9.1 Mechanisms by which microorganisms are trapped in depth and screen filters (Courtesy of Millipore Pty Ltd).

reuse. Ceramic filters are sometimes used for purposes of clarification and purification but will not be discussed in the context of bacterial filtration. Depth filtration is the most economical means of removing the great bulk of particulate burden from a fluid, with membrane filters placed downstream providing highly efficient filtration.

Depth filters

Depth filters are pads containing compacted polypropylene, cellulose or glass fibres. Retention efficiency depends on the nominal pore rating and the selective adsorption of bacteria to the filter material. The pores are much larger than the particles removed but the channels are of uneven diameter and change direction frequently within the filter bed. The maximum pore diameter and retention efficiency of the filter determine the size of particles retained.

Depth filters are available in cartridge format for use. Alternatively, they may be assembled in plate and frame holders for sterilization by steam under pressure at 121°C. Filtration may be carried out under vacuum, with an open funnel, or under positive pressure with a closed funnel. Uniform pressure is important and the pressure differential should not exceed 35–70 kPa because compression of the mat would decrease the flow rate. The liquid which remains in the filter must not be driven or sucked through because the pad will channel or crack, providing

access to the filtrate for microbial contaminants. Filters are discarded or sterilized and reused (×3).

Depth filters may still be used in laboratories for sterilization of heat-sensitive bacteriological culture media or concentrated solutions of heat-sensitive ingredients, such as serum or sugars, before they are added aseptically to an autoclaved solution of the heat-stable components. However, they are not suitable for critical application, where product sterility must be assured. Large multiplate filters, which have been used in the past to produce sterile water in hospitals, are unsuitable for this purpose because the outlet invariably becomes heavily contaminated during use.

Depth filters have a high dirt-holding capacity because they continue to retain particles throughout their depth. However, they have the following disadvantages:

1. A significant volume of the liquid may be lost by retention in the filter pad
2. Components of the liquid (e.g. proteins or enzymes) may be adsorbed, reducing their concentration in the filtrate
3. Filter fibres may be shed into the filtrate
4. Extractables in the filtrate may necessitate rejection of the first portion that passes through the filter or pre-flushing
5. Penetration of microorganisms depends on the time required for filtration and some may eventually pass through, especially if the pressure differentials increase.

Membrane filters

Types of membranes

A variety of polymers are manufactured into membranes for hydrophilic and hydrophobic filters. Hydrophobic membranes will not wet with water. Filter membranes are 125–150 μm in thickness and have regularly spaced pores. The filters are available as discs ranging from 13 to 293 mm in diameter. Hydrophilic filters with hydrophobic rims are used in the sterility testing of liquids containing antimicrobial agents.

Hydrophilic filters for general use are produced from cellulose esters (acetate and nitrate). Polytetrafluoroethylene (PTFE), polyvinyl chloride and polyvinylidene difluoride (PVDF) are used in the manufacture of hydrophobic membranes, although PVDF may be modified to also produce hydrophilic membranes. The low protein binding properties of PVDF is advantageous when used with some liquids.

Membrane filters have a low dirt-handling capacity compared with fibrous depth filters and are easily clogged by particles that are just larger than the pore diameter; however, they have several advantages over the fibrous filters:

1. All particles larger than the pore diameter are retained and bacteria cannot pass through
2. A large open volume (80 per cent of the filter) ensures an adequate flow rate
3. The volume of liquid retained in the membrane is small and can be expelled without breaking sterility
4. The quality of the filtrate is not altered by adsorption of solutes or contamination with foreign material.

Grades of membrane filters

The filters are graded according to the pore size, which is related to their intended use. Prefilters with a pore diameter of 0.8 or 1.2 μm are used to prolong the life of the high-efficiency filters. Two grades of bacterial filters are manufactured; a pore diameter of 0.45 μm is satisfactory for recovering bacteria from liquids but a diameter of 0.22 μm or 0.2 μm is required for producing bacteria-free filtrates. Pore sizes of 0.01–0.02 μm are needed to retain viruses while 0.1 μm is used for the removal of mycoplasmas (Lukaszewicz & Meltzer, 1979).

Cartridges containing filter material provide a large surface area for filtration ('surface filters'). For serial filtration, filter discs of progressively finer pore size may be stacked in a single filter holder.

Membrane filters tend to be blocked by particles just larger than the pore diameter. However, large particles merely form a porous surface mat which assists filtration by retaining smaller particles.

Membrane filter holders

Membrane filters are delicate and must be supported on a porous or perforated disc. Many types of filter holders are available from the firms that manufacture the membranes. The design and efficiency of the holder and provision for collection of the sterile filtrates are as critical to successful filtration as the quality of the membrane itself. Some types of apparatus for use with membranes ranging from 13–293 mm diameter are illustrated in Figure 9.2. The approximate scale of each diagram may be judged from the indicated size of the membrane.

Diagram A in Figure 9.2 represents a filter holder with an open funnel; this model is commonly used for filtration of volumes up to 300 ml. Filtration is operated by suction.

Diagram B shows an assembly with a closed funnel. It may be made from plastic, glass or metal and is designed for sterility testing, when the membrane must be protected from extraneous contamination. The lid is fitted with closed or filtered entry ports for introduction of the liquid, admission of air as the volume of liquid in the reservoir decreases and admission of steam for sterilization. Presterilized filters in small disposable polypropylene chambers have become available for sterility tests. The pooled sample is divided between two or three of these units, as required, by a peristaltic pump. After addition of the appropriate culture media, the units are incubated intact.

Diagram C represents a miniature line filter (Swinny or Swinnex type). It has a Luer-lock fitting on the inlet for connection to a syringe, which holds the liquid and supplies it to the filter under positive pressure exerted by the plunger. This type

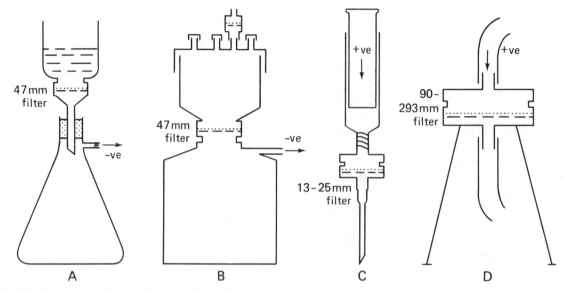

Fig. 9.2 Some types of apparatus for membrane filtration.

of apparatus is designed for small scale filtration of pharmaceuticals, such as intravenous additives, radioactive pharmaceuticals and eye drops in a hospital pharmacy or for similar purposes in a laboratory. Filtration should be carried out in a controlled environment.

Diagram D is a line filter, capable of filtering up to 500 litres if it is fitted with a 293 mm diameter membrane. The inlet of the circular holder is connected to the reservoir of liquid and the exit leads to the receiver. Line filters are used to sterilize relatively large volumes of bacteriological or tissue culture media. They may be operated under positive or negative pressure. Compact polycarbonate units, containing a stack of membrane filters, are now available that can handle volumes of many hundreds of litres, up to 1000 litres. These filter units are disposable but some of the products can be autoclaved up to three times at 121°C for 30 minutes for reuse before disposal. Persons involved in aseptic filtration need to keep abreast of the technological developments in this rapidly advancing field.

THE FILTRATION PROCESS

Sterilization of filters

Membrane filters, such as those that are made from cellulose esters, PTFE or PVDF, are sterilized by steam at 121°C for a holding time of 30 minutes. They can be placed in the holders before sterilization if the funnels are fitted with vented caps to prevent deformation of the membrane by pressure changes during the sterilization cycle. A small amount of distilled water should be added to closed systems to provide steam internally for sterilization. Line filters and cartridge filters can be sterilized in situ by inline steaming to 135°C. Filters that cannot be autoclaved (e.g. hydrophobic) may be sterilized by ethylene oxide or in accordance with the manufacturer's instructions.

Prefilters

Prefilters have the potential to greatly extend the working life of final filters. They serve to retain a large number of the particulates that would otherwise cause premature clogging of the final filters. A type of depth filter is generally used for the purpose.

Because of their composition and structure, depth filters can only be assigned a nominal particle retention rating (Levy & Leahy, 1991). This is determined experimentally by passing through a test fluid with particles of known size distribution and concentration. Polypropylene depth filters have a nominal rating ranging from 0.6 μm to 30 μm. Prefilters of cellulose esters are often used with final filters of 0.45 µm pore diameter, while microfibre glass is used in prefilters for 0.2 µm filters. Alternatively, a membrane filter of 0.8 or 1.2 µm pore diameter can be used. The performance characteristics of the prefilter should be related to those of the final filter. If the latter is a membrane of 0.45 µm pore diameter the prefilter should, ideally, be capable of retaining particles above 5 µm in diameter as this is the size that is most likely to block the bacterial filter. A prefilter that is too coarse will not protect the membrane against the particles which are most likely to clog it whereas, if it is too fine, the prefilter will clog prematurely. In order to ensure an adequate flow rate, the area of the prefilter should be greater than that of the final filter.

Pressure and vacuum filtration

Liquids do not run freely through bacterial filters. Positive pressure must be applied to the reservoir on the upstream side, before passage through the filter, or the receiver must be connected to a vacuum pump on the downstream side, after passage through the filter. Positive pressure filtration requires more elaborate apparatus but has the following advantages over suction:

1. Higher flow rates are possible because pressure differentials greater than one atmosphere can be applied
2. Contamination of the filtrate by air leaks or backflow of water is prevented
3. Protein-containing solutions do not froth in the receiver and volatile solvents do not evaporate
4. The filter assembly can be tested for leaks by a bubble point test before and after use
5. The filtrate can be collected directly in the final containers if the outlet is enclosed in a protective shield or filtration is carried out under clean room conditions.

When filtration is operated by suction, the exit from the receiver should be protected from airborne contamination by a plug of fibrous filter material and a trap should be installed on the vacuum line to prevent backflow of water or oil from the pump. After a sterile filtration has been completed, the membrane is discarded and reusable holders should be cleaned according to the manufacturer's directions.

TESTING EFFICIENCY OF FILTRATION

The efficiency of membrane filters is not affected by thickness, velocity or the pressure differential at which filtration is carried out. Performance may be defined in terms of flow rate (volume filtered in a given time) or throughput (volume filtered before the filter clogs). The flow rate is related to the pore diameter and the total open volume. It varies directly with the pressure differential (provided clogging does not occur) and the effective filtration area, but decreases as the viscosity of the liquid increases. Viscosity can sometimes be reduced by raising the temperature, e.g. to 44°C, as is recommended for filtration of ointments dissolved in isopropyl myristate (United States Pharmacopeia, 1995).

The validation of the process of aseptic filtration is designed to show that the probability of a processed liquid containing a microorganism is 10^{-6} or less.

Integrity tests

The integrity of membrane filters can be tested by measuring the bubble point or the diffusional flow of a gas through a wetted filter. The bubble point, or bubble pressure, is the pressure at which the liquid contained in the channels of the filter is driven out by the test gas. Diffusional flow is the flow of test gas through the wetted filter at pressures below the bubble point. The same technique is used for both tests; diffusional flow measurement is the more sensitive test for filters with surface areas greater than 0.1 m^2.

The testing technique is non-destructive and may be performed on a membrane filter assembly before use, without breaking sterility, then repeated after filtration. This is especially important when radioactive isotopes with a short half-life are sterilized by filtration because they are used before their sterility can be tested. The technique is also used for testing the quality of filter membranes.

Water is the standard test liquid but isopropyl alcohol is used for hydrophobic filters. The test liquid is placed in a vessel on the upstream side and allowed to flow freely to saturate the filter assembly; air pockets are removed by venting. The liquid supply is then disconnected and an upstream connection is made to a test gas. The gas pressure is increased until it is about 80 per cent of the specified bubble point pressure for the filter under test. The liquid displaced on the downstream side is collected into a graduated cylinder and its flow rate is determined in millilitres per minute with the aid of a stop watch. This reflects the rate of diffusion of the test gas through the wetted filter membrane. The result is then compared to a standard rate that has been established for the filter system. An alternative technique is to drain the liquid from the downstream side of the test system and to measure the flow rate of the gas directly through a gas flow meter. Repeated measurements are made and the final calculation should be below specified limits. The gas pressure is then further increased until a sudden increase in the flow rate is observed. This is the bubble point i.e. the pressure at which the marked change in flow rate is observed. It is followed by the appearance of actual gas bubbles in the liquid. The bubble point should be equal to or greater than the recommended value given by the manufacturer for the particular grade of filter. Typically, hydrophilic membranes of 0.45 μm and 0.22 μm average pore diameter have bubble pressures of 220 kPa and 380 kPa with water as test liquid. An automated filter integrity tester has been developed and validated for use (Sechovec, 1989).

Bacterial retention tests

Retention tests are carried out by passing a bacterial suspension containing a known number of cells through the filter. *Serratia marcescens* ATCC 14756 and *Brevundimonas diminuta* ATCC 19146 (0.3 × 1.0 μm) have been recommended (Bowman et al, 1967); the latter provides the most rigorous challenge to a membrane of sterilizing grade. A minimum (relatively high) concentration of 10^7 per cm^2 of filtration area is used. Filtration should be carried out slowly and the entire filtrate should be cultured because the passage of a single cell renders the liquid unsterile.

The size and viability of *B. diminuta* also depends on the composition of the broth medium used for culture and the growth phase of the bacterial culture. *B. diminuta* in the early stationary phase of growth in saline lactose broth medium is recommended (Levy & Leahy, 1991). The filtrate is passed through a secondary 0.22 μm filter which is subsequently transferred to a trypticase soy agar plate and incubated at 30°C for a minimum of 72 hours. A successful test is the retention of all bacteria on the test filter i.e. no bacterial growth on the secondary filter after incubation.

Bacteriological tests do not give an immediate result but are useful for assessing the reliability or reproducibility of particular types of membrane filters or filter holders. The efficiency of a filtration process that has been completed may be tested by passing a bacterial culture through the filter and incubating the filtrate to detect growth.

APPLICATIONS OF MEMBRANE FILTRATION

Membrane filters are more versatile than are depth filters. In addition to the primary purpose of sterile filtration, they can be used in sterility testing and bacteriological studies because the microorganisms are retained on the surface where they may be examined or cultured in situ.

Pharmaceuticals

Heat-sensitive pharmaceuticals, such as ophthalmic solutions, radiopharmaceuticals, irrigating solutions for surgery and peritoneal dialysis, are sterilized commercially by filtration. A bactericide may also be included in the filtered solutions to kill or inhibit the growth of occasional contaminants that might enter during transfer to the final containers, unless the preparation is intended for intravenous administration in volumes greater than 15 ml or for intrathecal injection. If filtration of small volumes of eye drops or additives for intravenous infusions is carried out in hospital pharmacies, the use of a laminar flow cabinet is essential. Products that have been sterilized by filtration are usually subject to more stringent sterility tests than are those sterilized by autoclaving in the final containers.

The sterilization of large volume parenterals by filtration is applied mainly to solutions for total parenteral nutrition. However, intravenous solutions that are sterilized by heat require preliminary filtration through 0.45 μm membranes to remove bacteria, which are pyrogenic even when they are killed, and a variety of other extraneous particles that commonly occur in these products. The particles arise from rubber closures, containers, ingredients of the formulation or precipitation reactions between components (Garvan & Gunner, 1963, 1964; Davis et al, 1970). If the particles are introduced into the blood stream in large numbers, they cause granulomatous lesions in the lungs, brain and other tissues. Subsequent to filtration and sterilization, particles may be introduced into the intravenous solution by additives or by the administration set. In order to overcome this problem, final filters are incorporated at the outlet of the set or close to the cannulation site (Wilmore & Dudrick, 1969; Rapp et al, 1975). A 0.22 μm membrane is required because *P. aeruginosa* and other small Gram-negative bacilli may pass through the 0.45 μm grade (Rusmin et al, 1975; Holmes et al, 1980). The 0.22 μm filters should be replaced every 24 hours to minimize the elution of endotoxin (pyrogens) from the populations of bacteria trapped on their surface (Holmes et al, 1980). Inline filtration has also been recommended as an additional measure that can be taken to prevent peritonitis in continuous ambulatory peritoneal dialysis (Spencer, 1988).

Biological materials

Serum for addition to culture media for propagation of bacteria and viruses can be sterilized only by filtration, and this applies also to antisera and many other blood products. Serum and other materials that have a high content of lipids and colloids may require serial filtration in which the liquid is passed through a depth type prefilter or a membrane of 1.2 μm pore size and then through a 0.22 μm membrane filter. The membranes may be mounted as a stack in the same holder. Alternatively, a fabricated filter of graded density may be used in which the filter material of the outer section has a larger pore size that that of the inner section. The fabricated filtering devices of pleated or stacked configuration provide a much greater membrane surface area with higher volume deliveries and flow rates. Ultrafilters, ranging in pore size from 0.01 to 0.001 μm, are used in tangential-flow devices for filtration with retention of viruses and proteins (Eudailey, 1983). Virus vaccines can be passed through 0.45 μm cellulose triacetate filters to remove bacterial contaminants and tissue culture debris without significant adsorption of virus to the filter membrane (Cliver, 1968), or through PVDF filters.

Microbiological culture media

Most bacteriological culture media are heat-stable to varying degrees but some heat-sensitive ingredients, such as sugars and serum, are sterilized separately and added aseptically to the sterilized solution of heat-stable components. Tissue culture media, which are used for propagation of viruses, are sterilized by filtration; fetal calf serum may be prefiltered and added to the medium before the final filtration.

Industrial applications

Filtration plays a prominent part in the commercial production of antibiotics for parenteral or oral administration. After purification, the concentrated solution is filtered and then distributed aseptically into the final containers, in which it may be freeze-dried. Some heat-sensitive industrial fermentation media may be sterilized in large quantities by filtration. Membrane filters of 0.45–1.2 μm are used to remove yeast cells in the clarification of beer and wines. Ultrafilters and tangential-flow devices also have application in harvesting and concentrating the protein end-products of biotechnology.

Sterility tests

The important role of membrane filtration in sterility tests on commercially produced pharmaceutical products and medical devices has been discussed in Chapter 2. Membranes of 0.45 μm pore size and 47 mm diameter, with a hydrophobic edge, are used for tests on antibiotics and also on injections that contain a chemical preservative.

Residues left on the filter after the liquid has passed through are removed or inactivated by washing with an appropriate diluent and the membrane is cultured for detection of bacteria or fungi. Oil-based pharmaceuticals, such as ointments, are dissolved in isopropyl myristate (United States Pharmacopeia, 1995) and the membrane is washed with a diluent containing a surface active agent to remove oil residues before the membrane is cultured. Membrane filtration has also made it practicable to perform sterility tests on relatively large samples of intravenous infusions.

Bacteriological investigations

This special application of membrane filters is not relevant to sterilization except that it is used to determine numbers and types of microbial contaminants that have been rinsed from solid objects. The main use of the filters is in the analysis of bacterial populations in water samples. An interesting development' in membrane design followed reports that coliform counts varied with the type or brand of membrane used (Presswood & Brown, 1973; Schaeffer et al, 1974). Examination of various membranes showed that they varied with respect to the size of the pore openings; larger openings allowed the bacteria to be immersed in liquid medium during filtration and subsequent incubation of the membrane, eliminating the adverse effect of drying on their viability. The correlation between recovery of faecal coliforms and the number of large openings on the filter surface has been confirmed by scanning electron microscopy (Standridge, 1976), and membranes are now manufactured with enlarged pores of $0.7 \mu m$ average pore diameter for such bacterial counts.

ASEPTIC FILTRATION OF AIR

The human respiratory tract acts as a filter which effectively prevents bacteria-carrying particles greater than $5 \mu m$ in diameter from reaching the alveoli of the lung. This is achieved by the tortuous course of the air stream through the bronchi and bronchioles, where the particles are trapped on the moist mucous lining. However, smaller droplet nuclei ($\leq 5 \mu m$) which arise when droplets

of respiratory tract secretions dry in air, can penetrate this natural filtration mechanism. The surgeon's mask is also an air filter, intended to prevent outward or inward passage of droplets carrying potentially harmful bacteria or viruses. The high-efficiency particulate air filters (HEPA filters) that are now used to provide ultraclean air for medical and industrial purposes are in a different category because they have a retention efficiency of at least 99.97 per cent for airborne particles $0.3 \mu m$ or more in diameter.

Ultraclean air is required in hospital areas where patients undergo surgery or are being nursed in protective isolation, and in industrial premises where sterile pharmaceuticals or medical devices are produced. The supply of sterile air to cultures of bacteria or fungi that are used for production of antibiotics, enzymes or organic acids is a particularly exacting task, as is the aseptic assembly of presterilized components for life-detection space capsules. The following types of filters are used for the various purposes:

1. Fibrous depth filters
2. Granular depth filters
3. Fibrous (paper) sheet filters
4. Membrane filters.

FIBROUS DEPTH FILTERS

Plugs of non-absorbent cotton wool are used in microbiological laboratories to exclude microbial contaminants from culture media in test tubes or flasks. They are adequate for this purpose if they remain clean and dry but cotton wool is relatively inefficient as a filter because it has little mechanical strength and tends to channel during steam sterilization or to break down during use. Finely spun glass fibres, resin-treated natural wool or mineral slag wool are used to make depth filters for industrial fermentation processes. The glass fibres are made by heating borosilicate glass in a high-velocity air stream; they are circular in cross section and of uniform diameter in the range 0.06–6 μm. About 70 per cent of the fibres in mineral slag wool are also less than 6 μm in diameter but a small proportion of much coarser fibres adds strength to the filter.

The fibrous material is packed into tubes or

larger containers, where it is held under pressure from both ends. Cartridge depth filters may be preformed slabs containing mixed fibres which are bonded together by resin. All types of filters must be packed and assembled so that air cannot pass between the medium and container wall. Large and small depth filters are usually sterilized by steam at 135°C and an exposure time of 30 minutes is recommended.

Mechanisms of filtration

The interspaces in fibrous filters are larger than the particles that the filter retains but contact between the particles and the fibres results in adsorption or mechanical trapping as the air flows through uneven channels, which change direction continually along their path through the filter bed. Fibrous filters are generally more efficient in removing bacteria from gases than from liquids because the microorganisms can leave the air stream more easily. The mechanisms of arrest that operate in a particular filter depend on the size, mass, electrostatic charge and velocity of the particles. The following mechanisms are recognized in fibrous depth filters:

1. Interception (direct impact)
2. Inertial impaction
3. Diffusion and gravitational settling (sedimentation)
4. Electrostatic precipitation.

Mechanisms 1–3 are illustrated in Figure 9.3.

Interception

Light particles have little momentum and tend to follow the course of the air stream around the fibres but direct interception may occur. The chance of colliding with a fibre increases with particle size, and is also favoured by fine fibres. This mechanism of capture may occur at low or high velocities, but the magnitude of its contribution to filtration is uncertain.

Inertial impaction

Heavy particles tend to continue in a straight path, colliding with a fibre instead of following the air stream around it. This mechanism of impingement is favoured by high velocity and a matrix of fine fibres which causes abrupt changes in the gaseous flow path. The chance of impaction also increases with the density and size of the particles. Inertial impaction is the principal mechanism of arrest in high-velocity filters; it does not operate at velocities below 30 cm/s.

Diffusion and gravitational settling

Particles less than 0.3 µm in diameter, such as bacteriophage, are too small for direct interception and too light to be collected by inertial impaction. However, if the velocity is very low, they may diffuse out of the air stream by random Brownian movement. This increases the length of their path through the filter and promotes contact with the fibres, to which they adhere. Diffusion is the principal mechanism of retention in low-velocity filters (less than 30 cm/s). Very small particles (less than 0.3 µm) can be removed only by low-velocity filters. Thermal convection and gravitational settling may also participate under these conditions. Electrostatic precipitation may also be involved.

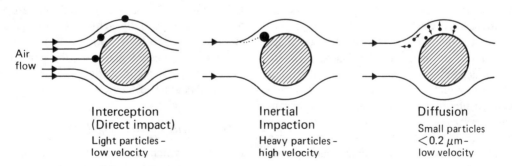

Fig. 9.3 Mechanisms by which airborne particles may be trapped in fibrous depth filters.
Note: Shaded areas represent fibres in cross section.

Electrostatic precipitation

Particles may be retained by the attraction of opposite charges on the filter material and the microbial cells. Electrostatic precipitation is important in resin-treated wool filters, where the charge on the resin coating is opposite to that on the wool. The impregnation of wool with resin increases filtration efficiency from 50 per cent to 99.99 per cent. Electrostatic attraction is independent of air velocity and particle size.

Factors influencing efficiency

Fibrous filters are never 100 per cent efficient because they do not act as mechanical sieves. The level of efficiency is expressed as per cent retention or per cent penetration of the airborne particles. Efficiency is governed by the following factors:

1. Air velocity
2. Filter thickness
3. Fibre diameter and packing density
4. Number and size of particles.

Air velocity

Linear velocity per second is equal to the volume of air per second divided by the area of the filter. If velocity is increased from a very low level, the efficiency of retention for particles of a given size decreases at first to a minimum, which is reached at about 30 cm per second. Beyond this point, efficiency increases with velocity, as shown in Figure 9.4 (curve A). The changing effect of velocity is associated with a difference in the mechanism of retention (Humphrey, 1960). At low velocity, efficiency depends mainly on diffusion, but this mechanism becomes less effective as the velocity increases. Above 30 cm/s, inertial impaction starts to operate, especially for particles exceeding 1 μm in diameter. This mechanism increases in efficiency with the velocity, until a point is reached at which channelling occurs through displacement of fibres or the trapped microorganisms are released by vibration. Submicron particles, such as bacteriophage and viruses, can be removed only by the mechanisms that operate in low-velocity filters, as shown in Figure 9.4 (curve B).

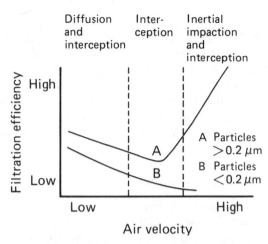

Fig. 9.4 Influence of air velocity on filtration efficiency and mechanisms of interception of microorganisms by fibrous depth filters.

Filter thickness

The proportion of particles retained at different depths in a fibrous filter bed approximates to a logarithmic relationship so that most are trapped in the proximal layers and the number decreases sharply as the depth of the filter is traversed. A penetration constant (k) may be derived from the following formula:

$$\ln \frac{N}{N_o} = -kX$$

where N_o is the number of particles entering the filter, N is the number that penetrate to a given depth, and X is the depth at which the count was determined. The filtration efficiency is frequently expressed in terms of X_{90}, the depth of filter required for the retention of 90 per cent of the number of particles entering the filter (Humphrey, 1960). Glass fibre and slag wool filters operating below 15 cm/s usually achieve 99.99 per cent retention at a depth of 76 mm. When two depth filters are connected in series, the combined efficiency for particles of a given size is the product of their separate efficiencies.

Fibre diameter and packing density

Fine fibres which are densely packed provide minimum pore size with maximum surface for adsorption of particles. Ideally, the fibre diameter should be less than that of the smallest particles to be filtered, but in practice a range of 1–6 μm is satisfactory in glass fibre and slag wool filters. If the packing is too dense, the resistance to air flow is excessive and the fibrous structure may be damaged; if it is too loose, channelling may occur. A suitable packing density is 190–400 kg/m^3. Bonding resins may be used to maintain porosity and to prevent shifting of the filter material during sterilization. The efficiency of a filter is lost if it becomes wet.

Number and size of particles

The bacterial content of filtered air is directly related to the number of microorganisms initially present. Thus the chance of producing sterile air is greatly increased if the air intake is sited high above ground level and prefilters are used.

Single bacteria range from 0.3 μm to about 1 μm in diameter (cocci) or width (bacilli). Bacterial viruses and the large animal viruses are 100–250 nm, but most viruses are 20–100 nm. However, as airborne microorganisms are usually associated with dried residues of non-living material, the particles are larger than the actual size of the microorganisms they contain. Particle size influences filtration efficiency through its effect on the mechanism of retention. The most difficult size to remove is 0.3 μm; larger and smaller particles are both removed with greater efficiency.

Design of fibrous depth filters

The depth of a filter depends on the degree of reduction of the microbial contaminants that is required. This may be calculated from an estimate of the number of bacteria-carrying particles in the incoming air, the volume of air that will pass the filter in a given time, and the maximum acceptable chance of a viable microorganism penetrating the filter. For example, if the initial contamination level of the air is 175 viable particles/m^3 and 14 m^3 of air per minute will pass the filter during a 3 day cycle, the total number entering the filter is 10^7. If the maximum acceptable chance of penetration is 10^{-3}, a reduction factor of 10^{10} is required. Other design parameters, such as optimum diameter, air velocity and pressure drop involve complex calculations because these factors are interrelated.

Low-velocity filters

These operate at 5–12 cm/s. They have a low pressure drop and are large in cross section to give adequate flow rates. They are moderately efficient and relatively insensitive to changes in velocity that occur during operation; a decrease in velocity increases their efficiency. This is the only type of filter that is capable of removing particles less than 0.3 μm in diameter efficiently.

High-velocity filters

These operate above 0.6 m/s. They are more compact than are low-velocity filters and are cheaper to install but they are more costly to operate because they have much greater resistance to air flow and a large pressure drop is required to achieve adequate flow rates. If the air velocity decreases below 0.6 m/s during operation, the efficiency may fall below the level for which the filter has been designed.

GRANULAR CARBON FILTERS

Filters packed with granular carbon of particle size 1–2 μm and mesh range 10–60 are frequently used to provide sterile air for industrial fermentations (Cherry et al, 1963). They are large, low-velocity filters with a pressure drop of 6.9–34.5 kPa. The factors governing their efficiency have not been fully investigated but, as for fibrous filters, they depend on the depth of the filter bed and the initial contamination level of the air. As carbon filters work best under dry conditions, the air should be delivered at a temperature above the dew point to prevent condensation. The carbon may spontaneously ignite if air is passed through the filter while it is still hot after steam sterilization.

FIBROUS (PAPER) SHEET FILTERS

High-efficiency particulate air (HEPA) filters with a low resistance to air flow and a large surface area are required to provide air with an extremely low bacterial count to industrial premises where sterile pharmaceuticals are manufactured, operating rooms and protective isolation facilities in hospitals, and aseptic work areas in microbiological laboratories. Ultraclean environments ('clean rooms') were developed initially for aseptic assembly of presterilized spacecraft components. The highest clean room standard was designated Class 100. The number of airborne particles of 0.5 μm or more should not exceed 3.5/l. Particles over 5 μm diameter should not be detected. The role of air filtration in meeting the standard is limited to removal of bacteria-carrying particles from fresh or recirculated air that is introduced into the room. A conventional or a unidirectional ('laminar') flow system must be established to remove microorganisms that arise from equipment or persons, or work activity within the room, away from the sensitive area and ultimately to the exhaust system.

The HEPA filters that are used for these purposes are large paper sheets, made from glass or cellulose fibres and ranging from less than 1 μm to 5 μm in diameter. They may be used separately or in combination. Esparto grass from South America is a source of long cellulose fibres. Continuous glass fibre may be formed into sheets of graduated density, with relatively loose packing at the inlet surface to prevent clogging and denser packing towards the outlet side to provide mechanical strength and filtration efficiency. The very large fibrous sheets that are required to give adequate velocities and flow rates are pleated around suitable supporting material and are sealed at all edges in a frame to form a compact filter unit. The integrity of the filter depends on absence of pinholes in the paper and perfect edge sealing. Single units are installed in air ducts or, in 'laminar' flow systems, they form a bank of parallel units occupying the whole area of a ceiling or wall.

Efficiency of HEPA filters

HEPA filters have efficiencies ranging from 99.97 to 99.997 per cent retention for particles averaging 0.3 μm in size. Larger and smaller particles may be retained with 100 times greater efficiency. Filtration efficiency may be reduced below the rated level by increased air velocity, neutralization of electrostatic charges on the particles, or relative

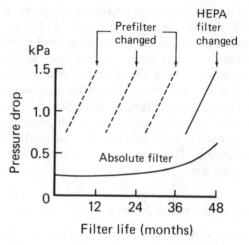

Fig. 9.5 The role of prefilters in extending the working life of a high-efficiency (HEPA) filter.

humidities over 95 per cent (Harstad & Filler, 1969).

HEPA filters have a working life up to 3–4 years if they are used in conjunction with prefilters with a lower pressure drop. The prefilters remove large particles and some of the smaller ones and are relatively inexpensive. The prefilter should be changed several times before the final filter is replaced (Fig. 9.5). Indications for replacement of the HEPA filter are:

1. An inadequate flow rate, which is not remedied by changing the prefilter
2. A pressure drop that exceeds the capacity of the blower fans
3. A leak that cannot be sealed.

Disinfection of used filters

HEPA filters installed in the exhaust systems of rooms or safety cabinets where pathogenic microorganisms have been dispersed should be disinfected in situ, or removed by a person wearing protective clothing and then incinerated or autoclaved. Disinfection in situ may be accomplished by heating elements in the exhaust duct if the filter is fireproof. However, this method has restricted applications. Disinfection by formaldehyde vapour is recommended. Formalin (37–40 per cent w/v formaldehyde) should be vaporized in the duct for 30 minutes at a temperature of at least

24°C, and adequate humidity must be provided by introduction of steam or water spray. The relative humidity should be between 70 and 90 per cent.

MEMBRANE FILTERS

The general properties of membrane filters and the role of hydrophilic membranes in the filtration of liquids have already been described. With air/gas filtration through hydrophobic membranes, electrostatic forces are generated which significantly increase the efficiency of filtration as both electrostatic and mechanical mechanisms of retention operate. Thus, a membrane of 0.8 μm pore diameter can retain particles down to a diameter of 0.5 μm, while the hydrophobic 0.2 μm air/gas membrane is rated to remove particles down to 0.05 μm diameter. These sterilizing membrane filters are commonly used in the supply lines for air and gases and in the vents of culture vessels and tanks for sterile production and manufacturing in the biotechnology and pharmaceutical industries.

TESTS FOR EFFICIENCY OF AIR FILTERS

Filters are tested by determining the per cent penetration of high-density aerosols with a known particle size distribution. Standard tests are based on chemical dusts with a high proportion of 0.3 μm particles, as this size is most difficult to filter. Bacteriological tests are unnecessary if a filter passes the more rigorous chemical tests, but may be used to compare different types of filters for efficiency in removing bacteria or viruses, or for a check on reproducibility of performance in a particular type or brand of filter.

Installations for testing

The various test methods are similar in principle, regardless of the type of filter or aerosol used. For tests with chemical dusts, the filter is installed in a duct which should be of adequate size and length upstream and downstream of the filter to allow the aerosol to be dried and mixed uniformly and to permit the withdrawal of samples for analysis. In bacteriological tests, the filter to be tested may be installed in a line filter holder; the bacterial aerosol

is passed into a mixing chamber before it enters the line to the test filter.

Chemical aerosols

Chemical dusts consisting of sodium chloride or dioctyl phthalate are commonly used. A fluorometric method, in which aerosolized rhodamine B was used as the fluorescent dye, has also been described (Sullivan et al, 1967). In the sodium chloride flame test (BS 3928, 1969), dried particles of 0.02 -2 μm diameter (median 0.6 μm) are generated from a 2 per cent solution of sodium chloride by the evaporation of water from an atomized spray of droplets. The sodium content of the filtered and unfiltered air is measured by the intensity of colour produced in a hydrogen flame photometer. The mean particle size of 'hot' dioctyl phthalate (DOP) is 0.3 μm. The amounts in upstream and downstream samples are measured photoelectrically and the lower limit of detection is 0.001 per cent penetration. If the penetration is less than 0.003 per cent, then the filter has an efficiency of more than 99.997 per cent. The chemical tests provide an immediate result. The 'cold' DOP smoke test is used to detect pinholes or imperfect seals in the filter face of laminar flow installations (Gross, 1978).

Microbial aerosols

Aerosols containing bacteria or bacterial viruses (bacteriophage) are considered to be more sensitive than chemical tests for critical evaluation or comparison of filters with an efficiency rating near 100 per cent. *B. subtilis* subsp. *niger* spores (approximately 1 μm in cross-section diameter) may be generated as predominantly single- or two-celled particles by a DeVilbis nebulizer. An advantage of spores over vegetative bacteria is that they do not tend to die in the test air stream. Aerosols of bacteriophage T_1 (Harstad & Filler, 1969) and a more stable actinophage (Roelants et al, 1968) have been used to evaluate the variables and determine the efficiency of virus retention by air filters. In a less orthodox method, susceptible chickens were used as an indicator of the in-use effectiveness of filters in removing Marek's disease virus, an avian pathogen, from the effluent air of an enclosure containing infected birds (Burmester & Witter, 1972).

APPLICATIONS OF AIR FILTRATION

Protective environments

High-efficiency air filters made from cellulose or glass fibres have a wide range of applications in hospitals, microbiological laboratories and industrial processes, as shown in Table 9.1.

Operating theatres are always supplied with filtered air but the benefit of replacing conventional plenum ventilation with a laminar flow system is difficult to evaluate because it must be assessed by the incidence of infections, rather than by its effect on the number of airborne contaminants. When a laminar flow enclosure is installed in an operating theatre, it is usually for orthopaedic surgery, which incurs a high risk of infection because the operation field is usually large and the time is prolonged. Laminar flow units in which the filters are located in a panel behind the head of the bed or in an overhead canopy are used for individual leukaemia patients.

Table 9.1   Applications of high-efficiency air filters

Locations	Applications
Hospitals	Ventilation of operating theatres and protective isolation facilities
	Decontamination of inspired or expired air in mechanical ventilators and suction apparatus
	Filtration of compressed gases (e.g. O_2) administered to patients
	Filtration of air admitted to steam or gas sterilizers
Microbiological laboratories	Ventilation of safety cabinets and 'sterile' rooms
	Decontamination of exhaust air from cabinets or rooms where aerosols of pathogenic microorganisms have been generated
	Decontamination of effluent air from aerated bacterial or fungal cultures
Industrial premises	Ventilation of rooms or enclosures for aseptic filling of liquids sterilized by filtration
	Ventilation of rooms for sterility testing
	Ventilation of rooms for assembly of micro-electronic equipment

Mechanical ventilators

Mechanical ventilators are used in anaesthesiology and, over longer periods, by patients requiring respiratory therapy in intensive care. Installation of bacterial filters in the inspiratory and expiratory limbs of the breathing circuits of anaesthetic apparatus and respiratory therapy equipment is intended to protect the patient from infection, to decrease the need for frequent disinfection of the complex apparatus and to prevent the discharge of pathogenic bacteria from the patient's respiratory tract into the circuit of the ventilator and the ward environment.

The filters must be small, cheap, disposable or autoclavable and of low air resistance. They should not absorb anaesthetic gases, and residual ethylene oxide must be removed if it has been used to sterilize the circuit (Bryan-Brown, 1972). Glass fibre filters can fulfil these requirements. The inspiratory side of the breathing circuit poses no problems if the filter precedes the humidifier. However, effective filtration of exhaled gases is difficult because moisture increases the resistance of the filter and may block it completely. A wet filter can support growth of Gram-negative bacteria, such as *P. aeruginosa*, which are potentially pathogenic to debilitated patients. Backflow of condensate from tubes beyond the filter may also be responsible for contamination of the circuit and wetting of the filter (Martin & Ulrich, 1969). Methods recommended for retaining filter efficiency in the high humidity of the expiratory limbs of circuits include the use of hydrophobic filters (Lumley et al, 1976; Eudailey, 1983) and the provision of an electrically heated mantle to maintain the filter at 56–76°C during use (Pyle et al, 1969; Holdcroft et al, 1974). The application of disposable fibreglass filters has also been described by Dyer et al (1970) and Shiotani et al (1971).

Suction apparatus

Filtration is necessary to prevent dissemination of bacteria, directly to the room air or through the vacuum system, from bottles that trap mucus and purulent secretions from the respiratory tracts of tracheostomy patients and premature infants. The liquid in the trap should contain an antifoam agent. Disinfectants are not recommended because they tend to promote frothing. A bacterial line filter, made from two layers of fibreglass paper supported by perforated aluminium plates sealed in an aluminium holder has been described (Marshall, 1964). It is placed between the collecting bottle and the vacuum source. Constant performance over a period of four months was reported, but the filter is useless if it becomes wet.

Compressed gases

Compressed gases are drawn from cylinders at high pressure, and low-resistance filters are therefore unnecessary. The Linde filter, designed for the removal of bacteria from clinical oxygen, consists of a tubular brass case, 10.5 cm long and 2.8 cm diameter, divided into five compartments by mesh copper screens which are supported by perforated Teflon discs (Mortensen & Hill, 1964). The compartments are packed with Pyrex glass wool to a density of 0.3 g/cm^3 and the ends are closed with caps adapted to fit standard oxygen connectors. Small, disposable, inline filter units containing single gas permeable, hydrophobic membranes are used in pressure lines with access to the blood stream, as in dialysis (Eudailey, 1983).

Similar filter units, but with multiple membranes, are used in anaesthesia. Although these filters cannot be used with conventional humidifiers, a type incorporating a heat-moisture exchange function is able to replace the humidifier. The units are presterilized by ethylene oxide or gamma radiation.

Laboratory effluents

Filters fitted to the exhaust ducts of safety cabinets which are used for containment of harmful microorganisms must be designed to cope with the maximum air flow rate and the expected contamination level. The filtration of effluents from aerated cultures of pathogenic microorganisms is complicated by their high moisture content. An ingeniously designed filter overcomes this problem by trapping the microorganisms in a heat-resistant mineral fibre filter pad, which is maintained at 200°C by a thermostatically controlled heating element in an adjacent compartment (Cameron & Favelle, 1967).

REFERENCES

Bowman F W, Calhoun M P, White M 1967 Microbiological methods for quality control of membrane filters. Journal of Pharmaceutical Sciences 56: 222–225
Bryan-Brown C W 1972 Bacterial filters. International Anesthesiology Clinics 10(2): 147–156
BS 3928 1969 Method for sodium flame test for air filters (other than for air supply to I.C. engines and compressors). British Standards Institution, London
Burmester B R, Witter R L 1972 Efficiency of commercial air filters against Marek's disease virus. Applied Microbiology 23: 505–508
Cameron J, Favelle H K 1967 An effluent-air filter. Journal of Applied Bacteriology 30: 261–263
Cherry G B, Kemp S D, Parker A 1963 The sterilization of air. Progress in Industrial Microbiology 4: 35–60
Cliver D O 1968 Virus interactions with membrane filters. Biotechnology and Bioengineering 10: 877–889
Davis N M, Turco S, Sively E 1970 A study of particulate matter in I.V. infusion fluids. American Journal of Hospital Pharmacy 27: 822–826
Dyer E D, Maxwell J G, Peterson D E, Mitchell C R 1970 Disposable fiberglass filter to counter bacterial contamination of intermittent positive pressure breathing equipment. Anesthesia and Analgesia 49: 140–147
Eudailey W A 1983 Membrane filters and membrane-filtration processes for health care. American Journal of Hospital Pharmacy 40: 1921–1923
Garvan J M, Gunner B W 1963 Intravenous fluids: 'A solution containing such particles must not be used'. Medical Journal of Australia 2: 140–145
Garvan J M, Gunner B W 1964 The harmful effects of particles in intravenous fluids. Medical Journal of Australia 2: 1–6
Gross R I 1978 Testing of laminar flow equipment. Journal of the Parenteral Drug Association 32: 174–181
Harstad J B, Filler M E 1969 Evaluation of air filters with submicron viral aerosols and bacterial aerosols. American Industrial Hygiene Association Journal 30: 280–290
Holdcroft A, Lumley J, Gaya H, Adams D, Darlow H M 1974 Respiratory filters in clinical practice. Lancet ii: 25–26
Holmes C J, Kundsin R B, Ausman R K, Walter C W 1980 Potential hazards associated with microbial contamination of in-line filters during intravenous therapy. Journal of Clinical Microbiology 12: 725–731
Humphrey A E 1960 Air sterilization. Advances in Applied Microbiology 2: 301–311
Levy R V, Leahy T J 1991 Sterilization filtration. In: Block S S (ed) Disinfection, sterilization, and preservation, 4th edn. Lea & Febiger, Philadelphia, ch 30, p 527
Lukaszewicz R C, Meltzer T H 1979 Filter validation symposium. 1. A cooperative address to current filter problems. Journal of the Parenteral Drug Association 33: 246–249
Lumley J, Holdcroft A, Gaya H, Darlow H M, Adams D J 1976 Expiratory bacterial filters. Lancet ii: 22–23
Marshall M 1964 Bacterial filter for suction apparatus. Lancet ii: 21
Martin J T, Ulrich J A 1969 A bacterial filter for an anesthetic circuit. Anesthesia and Analgesia 48: 944–946
Mortensen J D, Hill G 1964 Clinical and bacteriologic evaluation of a new filter designed specifically for

bacteriologic decontamination of oxygen used clinically. Diseases of the Chest 45: 508–514

Presswood W G, Brown L R 1973 Comparison of Gelman and Millipore membrane filters for enumerating fecal coliform bacteria. Applied Microbiology 26: 332–336

Pyle P, Darlow M, Firman J E 1969 A heated ultra-high-efficiency filter for mechanical ventilators. Lancet i: 136–137

Rapp R, Bivins B, Schroeder H, DeLuca P P 1975 Evaluation of a prototype air-venting inline intravenous filter set. American Journal of Hospital Pharmacy 32: 1253–1259

Roelants P, Boon B, Lhoest W 1968 Evaluation of a commercial air filter for removal of viruses from the air. Applied Microbiology 16: 1465–1467

Rusmin S, Althauser M B, DeLuca P P 1975 Consequences of microbial contamination during extended intravenous therapy using inline filters. American Journal of Hospital Pharmacy 32: 373–377

Schaeffer D J, Long M C, Janardan K G 1974 Statistical analysis of the recovery of coliform organisms on Gelman and Millipore membrane filters. Applied Microbiology 28: 605–607

Sechovec K S 1989 Validation of an automated filter integrity tester for use in bubble point testing. Journal of Parenteral Science and Technology 43: 23–26

Shiotani G M, Nicholes P, Ballinger C M, Shaw L 1971 Prevention of contamination of the circle system and ventilators with a new disposable filter. Anesthesia and Analgesia 50: 844–854

Spencer R C 1988 Infections in continuous ambulatory peritoneal dialysis. Journal of Medical Microbiology 27: 1–9

Standridge J H 1976 Comparison of surface pore morphology of two brands of membrane filters. Applied and Environmental Microbiology 31: 316–319

Sullivan J F, Songer J R, Mathis R G 1967 Fluorometric method for determining the efficiency of spun-glass air filtration media. Applied Microbiology 15: 191–196

United States Pharmacopeia 1995 23rd rev. United States Pharmacopeial Convention Inc, Rockville, p 1689

Wilmore D W, Dudrick S J 1969 An in-line filter for intravenous solutions. Archives of Surgery 99: 462–463

10. Chemical disinfectants

This chapter contains concise descriptions of the properties and main applications of chemical disinfectants that are commonly used as solutions in water or alcohol for disinfection of equipment, surfaces and intact skin or mucous membranes. General discussion of mechanisms of biocidal action, microbial susceptibility and factors influencing efficiency in use will be found in Chapter 11, together with the evaluation of disinfectants and the consequences of incorrect use. Disinfection of living tissues is the subject of Chapter 12.

ALCOHOLS

General properties

Ethyl ($CH_3.CH_2OH$), isopropyl ($CH_3.CHOH.CH_3$) and n-propyl ($CH_3.CH_2.CH_2OH$) alcohols are all colourless liquids, which boil at approximately 80°C. They evaporate at room temperature, leaving no residue. The low surface tension of alcohol-water mixtures confers wetting ability and they penetrate well into crevices of the human skin or inanimate objects. These alcohols are miscible with water. They are flammable at the concentrations that are recommended for disinfection.

Microbial susceptibility

Gram-positive bacteria	highly susceptible
Gram-negative bacteria	highly susceptible
Acid-fast bacteria	susceptible (suspensions)
Bacterial spores	resistant
Lipophilic viruses	susceptible (suspensions)
Hydrophilic viruses	variable

Formulation

Water must be added to alcohols to obtain the maximum rate of biocidal action, which depends on protein denaturation. Recommended concentrations of alcohol range from 60–80 per cent but the method of preparing the solutions (by weight or volume) is rarely stated. Price (1939) recommended 70 per cent ethyl alcohol by weight for skin disinfection. In 1945, Archer recommended 80 per cent by volume which is approximately 70 per cent by weight. The same recommendation is made in this book as it ensures that the concentration of alcohol will be neither too high nor too low for effective bactericidal action. The optimum concentration for disinfection varies with the moisture content of the bacteria and their environment. Isopropyl alcohol is generally regarded as being equally effective at slightly lower concentrations (e.g. 60–70 per cent v/v).

Factors influencing efficiency

Alcohols coagulate or precipitate proteins in serum, pus, sputum and other biological materials. This action may protect microorganisms from effective contact with the alcohol. The concentration of alcohol diminishes as it evaporates and the action may be bacteriostatic at concentrations below 50 per cent. There is no residual action after the alcohol has completely evaporated.

Adverse effects

Alcohols are irritant and toxic to tissue cells and are generally unsuitable for application to mucous membranes. Skin conditioners, such as glycerol or resins, must be added to alcohol-based skin disinfectants if they are applied frequently to the hands because dryness, roughness or cracking of the skin may result from the removal of lipids.

Rubber swells and plastics may be hardened by frequent or prolonged contact with alcohol; contact times should be limited to 10 minutes. The lens cement of optical equipment, such as endoscopic instruments, is weakened by disinfection with alcoholic solutions.

Applications

Alcohols, which are non-selective bactericides, are used in situations where continuing action is not required and the lack of solid residues is an advantage. They have an important role in skin disinfection, either as the sole bactericide or in combination with chlorhexidine or povidone iodine (see Ch. 12).

Ethyl alcohol (80 per cent v/v) is used to disinfect the surface of glass ampoules containing local anaesthetics, cleaned surfaces of hospital trolleys, dental bracket tables and cleaned laboratory benches. However, 70 per cent v/v ethyl alcohol is incapable of inactivating cell-free, dried HIV within 10 minutes and is therefore unsuitable for the inactivation of HIV on surfaces (Hanson et al, 1989). It has also been shown to be ineffective against *Mycobacterium tuberculosis* in the presence of sputum or when dried on surfaces; the antimycobacterial activity is restricted to *M. tuberculosis* in suspensions (Best et al, 1990). Precautions are required to prevent accidental ignition.

ALDEHYDES

General properties

Formaldehyde (H.CHO) and glutaraldehyde (CHO.CH$_2$.CH$_2$.CH$_2$.CHO) are available as aqueous solutions which have a characteristic pungent odour. Formaldehyde polymerizes to form a white deposit (paraformaldehyde) in the concentrated stock solution (formalin) and on articles after prolonged immersion in diluted solutions. Polymerization of glutaraldehyde occurs more slowly but is accelerated when the acid stock solution is rendered alkaline to activate it for use as a disinfectant (Stonehill et al, 1963). Russell (1994) has reviewed the antimicrobial activity, mechanism of action and uses of glutaraldehyde.

Microbial susceptibility

Gram-positive bacteria	highly susceptible
Gram-negative bacteria	highly susceptible
Acid-fast bacteria	moderately susceptible

Bacterial spores	susceptible (slow killing, species variation)
Lipophilic viruses	susceptible
Hydrophilic viruses	moderately susceptible
Fungi	fungistatic or fungicidal

Formulation

Formalin is an aqueous solution containing 37–40 per cent w/v formaldehyde. It may be diluted with water or alcohol to the concentration required for use. If alcohol is used, its final concentration should be 70–80 per cent v/v.

Glutaraldehyde is sold as a 2 per cent w/v aqueous solution, to be used undiluted as a broad spectrum disinfectant or sterilant for heat-sensitive instruments. The acid stock solution (pH 4) is accompanied by a liquid or powdered activator which must be added to adjust it to pH 7.5–8.5 before use. The whole of the contents (usually 2–5 litres) must be activated when the container is opened for use. A working life of 14–28 days is usually specified, but care must be taken to avoid the introduction of organic material or excess water by uncleaned or wet instruments. If only part of the activated solution is required for a single use, the used portion should be discarded.

Ready-to-use formulations of glycol-complexed glutaraldehyde are available in 1 and 2 per cent w/v concentrations. These solutions are of reduced odour and irritancy and do not require an activator. They are stable for two years, with a reuse life of 28 days.

Factors influencing efficiency

Formaldehyde is active at acid or alkaline pH. Alkalinized glutaraldehyde slowly decreases in activity as polymerization occurs. Glutaraldehyde reacts with proteins in nutrient broth, with the production of a reddish colouration and a loss of activity at low concentrations. However, most reports indicate that deposits of proteinaceous material on the articles to be disinfected do not present a significant barrier to penetration.

Adverse effects

Formaldehyde

Formaldehyde vapour is extremely irritant to the eyes and the respiratory tract at low concentrations (2–5 p.p.m.) which can also be detected by smell. Skin irritation and allergic dermatitis may result from contact with solutions containing formaldehyde. Effects on the respiratory tract and skin have been reviewed by Yodaiken (1981) and Clark (1983).

An unusual case of formaldehyde toxicity involved haemolysis in a patient undergoing haemodialysis. The source of formaldehyde was traced to the filters in a newly installed water filtration system (Orringer & Mattern, 1976). Its significance lies in the fact that formalin is widely used as a disinfectant for haemodialysis equipment.

Formaldehyde has recently become a focus of attention as an occupational and community health hazard. Occupations that involve exposure to formaldehyde vapour include pathology and the manufacture of ion-exchange resins, organic chemicals, brake linings and urea-formaldehyde insulating material. Occupants of private homes and other premises that contain urea-formaldehyde insulation are also exposed to significant concentrations of the vapour (Dally et al, 1981).

As an alkylating agent, formaldehyde is potentially carcinogenic and squamous cell carcinomas have been produced experimentally in rats (Yodaiken, 1981). A potent carcinogen, bis-(chloromethyl) ether, is produced if formaldehyde reacts with any source of free chlorine, including chlorine disinfectants (Drew et al, 1975). Care must be taken to avoid contact between these two chemicals, e.g. in histopathology laboratories and mortuaries. The data from more than 30 epidemiological studies on formaldehyde exposure and respiratory cancers have been subjected to meta-analysis (Blair et al, 1990; Partanen, 1993). The aggregated evidence does not indicate a risk of lung cancer from exposure to formaldehyde. However, it does reveal an increased risk and an exposure-response gradient for sinonasal and nasopharyngeal cancers. Simple precautions for handling formaldehyde in pathology laboratories are given by Clark (1983).

Glutaraldehyde

Contact dermatitis in nurses who removed instruments from a solution of glutaraldehyde was reported by Sanderson & Cronin (1968). A variety of adverse reactions has now been recognized (Burge, 1989). These include eye irritation, nose and throat symptoms, nausea, headache and rashes (Norbäck, 1988; Jachuck et al, 1989). The rashes were attributed to direct irritation because patch tests were negative and the severity increased with the extent of exposure. However, some cases of contact dermatitis have been associated with positive patch tests (Maibach, 1975). Asthmatic reactions have also been reported (Benson, 1984). The problem of adverse reactions may be exacerbated in warm, tropical climates, where high ambient temperatures can promote the vaporization of the volatile glutaraldehyde (Mwaniki & Guthua, 1992).

Recommended safety precautions include the wearing of impervious gloves and aprons when handling instruments which have been immersed in a solution containing glutaraldehyde. For respiratory protection, containers should be covered and, when they are opened, appropriate ventilation (e.g. local exhaust) should be provided. Automatic washer/disinfectors for endoscopic instruments are available.

Applications

The use of aldehydes as disinfectants is limited to situations in which biocidal action against bacterial spores, viruses, acid-fast bacilli or fungi is required. They provide an alternative to strong chlorine disinfectants when these are likely to damage instruments or other equipment. The sporicidal action of glutaraldehyde is superior to that of formaldehyde but it may be less effective against acid-fast bacteria than is formaldehyde (Bergan & Lystad, 1971; Collins, 1986). A wide range of viruses is susceptible, including both lipophilic and non-enveloped types (Klein &

Deforest, 1963; Saitanu & Lund, 1975). Hanson et al (1989) showed that 2 per cent alkaline glutaraldehyde inactivated cell-associated HIV and cell-free HIV in the presence of dried serum within 2 minutes. However, a 1 per cent concentration was ineffective even after immersion for 15 minutes. Fungi may be inhibited or killed.

Disinfection of heat-sensitive instruments

Heat-sensitive endoscopic instruments should be sterilized by the ethylene oxide, gas plasma or the low-temperature steam and formaldehyde process. However, the necessary time will not usually be available if the instruments are required for repeated use on the same day. In that situation, the endoscopes should be disassembled after use, thoroughly cleaned, subjected to high-level disinfection in 2 per cent w/v glutaraldehyde and repeatedly rinsed entirely, or at least finally, in sterile water. Alternatively, they may be sterilized by processing through the Steris system. Details of these processes are given in Chapter 14.

Decontamination of soiled instruments

All blood-stained instruments are potentially contaminated with hepatitis viruses or HIV. They can usually be cleaned safely by trained staff wearing protective clothing but glutaraldehyde is a suitable disinfectant if heat treatment is not practicable.

Disinfection in microbiological laboratories

Provided that the extraction fans remove the fumes, glutaraldehyde may be used to disinfect biological safety cabinets after work involving hazardous microorganisms. Formaldehyde vapour, generated within the cabinet, is recommended for disinfection before replacement of exhaust filters. The aldehydes are also effective in decontaminating incubators, cold rooms or benches which have

Cl—〈benzene ring〉—NH.C.NH.C.NH. (CH₂)₆.NH.C.NH.C.NH—〈benzene ring〉—Cl

$$Cl-C_6H_4-NH.C.NH.C.NH.(CH_2)_6.NH.C.NH.C.NH-C_6H_4-Cl$$

with NH groups above and below the carbon centres.

Chlorhexidine

become contaminated with fungi or bacterial spores. Solutions are more effective than vapours; in either case, safety precautions are required.

CHLORHEXIDINE

General properties

Chlorhexidine is a cationic biguanide, with the formula on the previous page.

The potential of chlorhexidine as a bactericide was discovered during a survey to find new anti-malarial agents related to proguanil (Davies et al, 1954). It is a basic substance, forming salts with inorganic and organic acids. The digluconate (usually referred to as chlorhexidine gluconate) is soluble in water and is available as a 20 per cent w/v aqueous concentrate which may be diluted with water or alcohol. Aqueous solutions of chlorhexidine are moderately surface active. They are colourless and odourless but have a bitter, unpleasant taste.

Microbial susceptibility

Gram-positive bacteria	highly susceptible
Gram-negative bacteria	moderately susceptible
Acid-fast bacteria	resistant
Bacterial spores	resistant
Lipophilic viruses	susceptible
Hydrophilic viruses	resistant

Formulation

Aqueous and alcoholic solutions of chlorhexidine, ranging in strength from 0.02–4 per cent w/v, can be prepared from the stock solution containing 20 per cent w/v chlorhexidine gluconate. Distilled water should be used because anions in tap water, such as chloride and sulphate, can precipitate the bactericide. The problem of precipitation may also be encountered when colouring agents are added by the user to identify the concentration or to distinguish between aqueous and alcoholic solutions. When it is necessary to adjust the tonicity of a chlorhexidine solution for application to injured tissue, sodium acetate must be used instead of sodium chloride.

Ethyl alcohol, or a mixture of ethyl and isopropyl alcohols to a total concentration in the range 60–80 per cent v/v, is used to prepare solutions for skin disinfection of hands and operation sites. Several chlorhexidine formulations are available commercially. Alcoholic solutions usually contain 0.5 per cent chlorhexidine, with or without glycerol or resins as skin conditioners. A bactericidal skin cleanser contains 4 per cent chlorhexidine, providing 1 per cent in available form (Lowbury & Lilly, 1973). Obstetric lubricant creams contain 1 per cent of the active agent. Mouth rinses for use in the control of dental plaque are complex formulations containing ingredients to mask the unpleasant taste.

Aqueous solutions containing different concentrations of chlorhexidine, or of a 1:10 mixture of chlorhexidine and cetrimide, are sterilized commercially, in appropriate volumes for the intended use. This overcomes the problem of survival and growth of Gram-negative bacteria which may be introduced by contaminated distilled water or dirty containers when dilutions are prepared in the hospital. This precaution applies particularly to 0.02–0.05 per cent w/v aqueous solutions of chlorhexidine which are used for urinary catheterization and bladder irrigation. The solutions are stable to autoclaving at 115–121°C at pH 5–6 but chlorhexidine is extensively inactivated if heated in poor quality glass bottles that release alkali. A small amount of p-chloroaniline is produced during heat sterilization of aqueous chlorhexidine but the quantity in a dilute solution is unlikely to present a hazard (Goodall et al, 1968). Chlorhexidine is inactivated by gamma radiation but can be sterilized by filtration if the first 10 ml of filtrate is discarded to allow for adsorption by the membrane.

Factors influencing efficiency

Chlorhexidine is active in the pH range 5.5–8; the optimum is usually on the alkaline side because this promotes the availability of anionic groups on the bacterial surface to react with the cationic chlorhexidine. The free base precipitates above pH 8. Soaps and other anionic detergents react with chlorhexidine and inactivate it. Although some nonionic detergents are compatible, nonionic polysorbate 80 (Tween 80) is actually used as an inactivator in bactericidal tests.

Adverse effects

Chlorhexidine is remarkably free from toxicity and its potential for skin irritation and sensitization is very low (Rosenberg et al, 1976). Acute oral toxicity is also low because chlorhexidine is poorly absorbed from the alimentary tract. Animal tests for chronic toxicity resulted in decreased consumption of the unpalatable drinking water, but the effects of long-term consumption are not serious, and are usually reversible. No adverse effects on reproduction and no brain changes of the type associated with hexachlorophene have been detected. Specific problems associated with the use of chlorhexidine are discussed in Chapter 12.

Applications

Chlorhexidine is used mainly as a skin disinfectant in a variety of applications, which are the subject of Chapter 12. It combines the immediate action of iodine compounds with a residual and cumulative action. Dilute aqueous solutions or creams may be applied to mucous membranes or contaminated wounds.

Chlorhexidine also finds applications in urology, e.g. as a urethral antiseptic and lubricant; in obstetrics and gynaecology, e.g. for disinfection of the perineum and vagina; and in oral disease and dentistry, where it has multiple uses. These include a major role in the control of plaque and caries, maintenance of oral hygiene in immunocompromised persons, treatment of mouth ulcers and pre- and post-operative infection control (Denton, 1991).

CHLORINE COMPOUNDS

General properties

The broad spectrum biocidal activity of chlorine (Cl_2) and a variety of organic and inorganic chlorine-releasing compounds is mediated by hypochlorous acid (HOCl), which is formed in aqueous solutions at pH 5–8. Hypochlorite ions (OCl^-), which predominate in strongly alkaline solutions, are virtually devoid of activity. Chlorine dioxide (ClO_2), which does not depend on production of HOCl for its biocidal action, is included in the section on strong oxidizing agents.

All chlorine compounds are oxidizing agents and the end products of their reaction with microorganisms and associated organic material are inactive chlorides (e.g. sodium chloride). The following types of chlorine compounds are most commonly used as disinfectants:

Sodium hypochlorite, NaOCl
Calcium hypochlorite (chloride of lime), $Ca(OCl)_2$
Lithium hypochlorite, LiOCl
Chlorinated trisodium phosphate (sodium hypochlorite in water of crystallization of the strongly alkaline phosphate)
Chlorinated isocyanurates, e.g. sodium dichloroisocyanurate (NaDCC, or SDIC):

Microbial susceptibility

Gram-positive bacteria	highly susceptible
Gram-negative bacteria	highly susceptible
Acid-fast bacteria	moderately susceptible
Bacterial spores	susceptible (optimum pH 7.6)
Lipophilic viruses	susceptible
Hydrophilic viruses	susceptible (high concentration)
Amoebic cysts, algae	susceptible
Fungi	moderately susceptible

| Prions | moderately susceptible (high concentration) |

Formulation

Sodium hypochlorite is available only as aqueous solutions, which are usually prepared by adding chlorine to caustic soda:

$$Cl_2 + 2NaOH \rightarrow NaOCl + NaCl + H_2O$$

Commercial sodium hypochlorite usually contains 12–14 per cent available chlorine when manufactured. When preparing dilutions, allowance should be made for deterioration of the stock solution: for example a 14 per cent solution may be reduced to 10 per cent or less in about 4 weeks. An electrolytically prepared solution containing 1 per cent available chlorine, used mainly for disinfection of infants' feeding bottles when diluted, is more stable.

The strongly alkaline solution is diluted with water to concentrations, ranging from 200 parts per million (p.p.m.) to 5000–20 000 p.p.m. (0.5–2.0 per cent), as required for its various uses. However, sporicidal action is greatly accelerated by buffering the solution to pH 7.6 (Death & Coates, 1979). Calcium and lithium hypochlorites are white solids.

Chlorinated trisodium phosphate and the various chlorinated isocyanurates are marketed as powders; the organic compounds usually contain compatible detergents. They vary in water solubility and it is important to ensure that the solid is completely dissolved before the solution is used. It may be difficult or impossible to prepare concentrated solutions (above 1000 p.p.m.) from some powdered forms.

Concentrations of chlorine-based disinfectants refer to available chlorine, which is a measure of oxidizing power. Available chorine is equivalent to the amount of elemental chlorine (Cl_2) that is required to produce a molecule of sodium hypochlorite (NaOCl). It is therefore double the amount that is actually contained in the hypochlorite molecule because one of the chlorine atoms is included in the inactive sodium chloride. The available chlorine content of a powder is expressed as per cent w/w and that of a concentrated solution as per cent w/v or parts per million (p.p.m.), depending on the strength. One per cent corresponds to 10 000 p.p.m. When a powdered disinfectant contains mixed active and inactive solids, the manufacturer's directions regarding the weight of powder to be dissolved in a stated volume of water must be followed.

Available chlorine content is determined in the laboratory by titration. A solution of sodium arsenite and an external potassium iodide-starch indicator are used. Titration is continued until a drop of the mixture does not give a blue colour with the indicator. A standard 0.141M sodium arsenite solution is convenient for use as 1 ml corresponds to 0.005 g available chlorine. From this relationship, the concentration of available chlorine in a known volume of chlorine-based disinfectant can be calculated. If a 5 ml sample is titrated, then the titration volume in millilitres gives the chlorine concentration directly in grams per litre (Ayliffe et al, 1993).

Factors influencing efficiency

Concentration and pH

The effects of concentration and pH are interrelated and the latter may be more important; for example, 100 p.p.m. at pH 7.6 kills spores of *Bacillus subtilis* as rapidly as does 1000 p.p.m. at pH 9. The alkalinity of sodium hypochlorite stock solutions favours stability during storage but the pH must be in the range 6–8 for effective biocidal action. The solution decomposes at pH 4, evolving chlorine. The dilution factor (e.g. from 10 per cent available chlorine to 1000 p.p.m.) may be sufficient to achieve the optimum range of pH but buffering to pH 7.6 is required for rapid and reliable sporicidal action of dilute solutions (Death & Coates, 1979).

The influence of temperature has practical significance because hypochlorite solutions may be used for hot cleaning and sanitization in the food and dairying industries. An increase of 10°C halves the time required for sporicidal action.

Organic material

Chlorine disinfectants react readily with all types of organic matter, including blood, faeces and tissues. Nitrogenous components are converted to organic chloramines (N-chloro compounds), which retain some activity; however, these are eventually destroyed by oxidative reactions if sufficient chlorine is available. The concentration of available chlorine that is used for disinfection should be high enough to provide an effective residual of the active agent after the chlorine demand of the organic material associated with the microorganisms has been satisfied.

Hard water

The calcium and magnesium ions in hard water do not inactivate chlorine disinfectants but ferrous or manganous cations and nitrite or sulfide anions reduce active hypochlorous acid to inactive chloride. Small amounts of potassium bromide may potentiate the action of hypochlorite (Shere et al, 1962). However, this effect is less obvious at the high concentrations of available chlorine that are used for disinfection in hospitals.

Adverse effects

Strong hypochlorite solutions have a penetrating and irritant odour due to release of gaseous chlorine. They bleach and damage the texture of fabrics and corrode many metals; silver and aluminium are most susceptible but stainless steel instruments and utensils are damaged by the high concentrations that are required for general disinfection in hospitals. Food cans withstand 10 p.p.m. available chlorine in the cooling water but the usual concentration used is about 5 p.p.m.

Chlorine disinfectants are approved for use in the catering, food and dairying industries because the relatively weak solutions (150–200 p.p.m.) that are used as sanitizers produce no toxic residues. Chlorine in swimming pools may cause eye irritation. Chlorinated trisodium phosphate, which is strongly alkaline, is unsuitable for manual cleaning of hospital equipment or in dairying applications because it is too irritant to the skin.

Applications

Chlorine disinfectants have a wide range of uses, from the treatment of water supplies to inactivation of hepatitis B virus and HIV in blood.

Disinfection of water

Chlorine is used for the disinfection of public water supplies, swimming pools and water used for cooling canned foods or washing fresh foods such as fish or poultry (Table 10.1). Sewage may also be treated with chlorine but reliance must be placed on the production of chloramines as the high chlorine demand of the organic materials cannot, in practice, be satisfied. Residual free chlorine in water supplies and swimming pools should be about 0.6 p.p.m. and should fall to 0.3 p.p.m. by the time the water reaches the consumer. Levels of 5–10 p.p.m. are required for ice-water mixtures used in the food industry. Tablets of halazone or other N-chloro compounds may be used for disinfection of suspect drinking water by individual consumers.

Table 10.1　Water disinfection with chlorine for public health and industrial purposes

Application	Available chlorine concentration (p.p.m.)
Public water supplies	0.5 (holding time 1–2 h)
New water mains	20 (2 h)
Swimming pools	0.6, dropping to not less than 0.3, continuous treatment
Industrial process water Can cooling	4–5 (free chlorine must be present)
Poultry processing	10–20 (200 for 10 min for ice-water)
Abattoirs	10 (free residual)
Sea water (fish and trawlers)	40
Washing salads, fruit, raw meat, fish	100 (soak 10–15 min and rinse well)
Fish and shellfish from polluted water	200–6000
Potable water for aircraft	10 (30 min, then dechlorinate)
Drinking water (small scale or individual)	20–30 (15 min)
Algal control	0.2–2.0
Slime control (paper industry, power station cooling water)	Example: 3–5, for 15–20 min every 3 h
Soft drinks industry	Virtual sterility required; super chlorination and dechlorination

Sanitization

Chlorine disinfectants are widely used in the dairying, food production and catering industries because they do not leave toxic residues. The recommended concentration for use on precleaned equipment and work surfaces is 150–200 p.p.m. If detergent-sanitizers are used on uncleaned equipment or surfaces, a higher concentration may be required to allow for inactivation by organic matter. Infant feeding bottles may be disinfected by the use of a 1:80 dilution of a purified 1 per cent w/v stock solution (i.e. 125 p.p.m.) after they have been thoroughly cleaned.

General disinfection

Sodium hypochlorite, at an available chlorine concentration of 10 000 p.p.m. (Bloomfield et al, 1990) is suitable for decontaminating blood that has been splashed or spilled on equipment or floors. For tissue that may contain the Creutzfeldt-Jakob prion, 20 000 p.p.m. is recommended. If the articles (e.g. instruments) or material cannot withstand the high concentration, alkaline glutaraldehyde may be used for inactivating hepatitis B virus and HIV in blood and serum. Solutions containing 500 p.p.m. available chlorine are suitable for general disinfection of environment and equipment in hospitals. A concentration of 2500 p.p.m. may be used in laboratory discard jars in bacteriological laboratories but 5000 p.p.m. is required in virus laboratories unless the discarded material or equipment is to be autoclaved. A lower concentration may provide temporary safety if the contaminated equipment is autoclaved in the container before it is emptied.

HEXACHLOROPHENE

General properties

Hexachlorophene is a bisphenol, in which two chlorinated phenol molecules are linked by a methylene bridging group as shown in the formula in the next column. The white solid has low solubility in water but is more soluble at alkaline pH. It forms emulsions with soap and detergents.

Microbial susceptibility

Gram-positive bacteria	susceptible (killed slowly)
Other microorganisms	resistant

Formulation

Hexachlorophene is used as a 3 per cent w/w skin cleansing emulsion, formulated with non-alkaline detergents. It is also incorporated in dusting powder and bar soaps.

Factors influencing efficiency

Hexachlorophene maintains its activity against pathogenic staphylococci in the presence of soap and alkaline or neutral detergents. The initial action on the skin bacteria is slow but adsorption of hexachlorophene to the skin can provide the sustained and cumulative action that is required for surgical hand disinfection.

Adverse effects

Accidental ingestion of a hexachlorophene emulsion has caused death in adults and children on several occasions (Wear et al, 1962; Lustig, 1963). The use of hexachlorophene as a skin disinfectant or antiseptic can cause an oedematous condition in the white matter of the brain, which may result in convulsions and even death in premature infants and sometimes in adults (see Ch. 12).

Applications

Hexachlorophene usage has declined because of the seriousness of its adverse effects. Nonetheless, a recent WHO publication (Ayliffe, 1996) lists hexachlorophene, among other skin disinfectants, for the treatment of skin sites (e.g. perineum, buttocks) that are colonized by methicillin-resistant *Staphylococcus aureus* in healthy carriers.

IODOPHORS

General properties

Iodophors are organic complexes containing iodine trapped within the micelles of a surface active agent. The amount of free iodine in a concentrated solution is low but it is released from the micelles as the solution is diluted (Berkelman et al, 1982). The organic carrier may be polyvinylpyrrolidone (PVP), another nonionic surface active compound or a cationic detergent. Povidone-iodine (PVP-I) is a brown, water-soluble powder containing approximately 10 per cent w/w iodine. Iodophors are also soluble in ethyl and isopropyl alcohols. Iodine-based disinfectants are stable in acid solutions but decompose, releasing iodine vapour, if heated above 40°C.

Microbial susceptibility

Gram-positive bacteria	highly susceptible
Gram-negative bacteria	highly susceptible
Acid-fast bacteria	susceptible
Bacterial spores	may be susceptible
Protozoan cysts	susceptible
Lipophilic viruses	susceptible
Hydrophilic viruses	susceptible
Fungi (yeasts)	susceptible

Formulation

Povidone-iodine may be used as an aqueous or alcoholic solution. A povidone-iodine antiseptic solution contains 1 per cent w/v available iodine in water or alcohol base, and a surgical scrub, incorporating added detergents, contains 0.75 per cent. Low-foaming products, strongly acidified with phosphoric acid, are used in the dairy industry.

Factors influencing efficiency

The optimum pH is in the neutral and acid range. The influence of temperature on activity is irrelevant because decomposition occurs above 40°C, with evolution of iodine vapour. Soft or hard water may be used to prepare solutions for use as surface disinfectants or sanitizers. Iodine reacts more slowly than chlorine with organic matter because it is a weaker oxidizing agent; this property may outweigh its slower biocidal action.

Adverse effects

In their principal use as skin disinfectants, iodophors have several advantages over the solutions of free iodine which they have replaced. The incidence and severity of hypersensitivity reactions is greatly reduced and stains on clothing or dressings can be removed by washing. However, caution should be exercised in their application to sensitive tissues. Wlodkowski et al (1975) reported that povidone-iodine can cause changes of genetic significance in DNA and Ahrenholz et al (1979) found that human neutrophil function was depressed as a result of application to the peritoneal cavity.

Applications

Povidone-iodine preparations have an important place as an alternative to chlorhexidine for skin disinfection, especially in situations where its equally rapid action and broader spectrum of bactericidal and sporicidal activity are required. However, povidone-iodine lacks the persistent action of chlorhexidine and the colour may discourage its use for hand washing. It is used as a teat dip for prevention of mastitis in dairy cows.

Iodophors may be used to disinfect clinical thermometers used by tuberculous patients; the thermometers should be rinsed after 10 minutes immersion and stored dry. Iodophors may be used as an alternative to chlorine compounds for disinfection of clean equipment or room surfaces in hospitals and for utensils and work surfaces in the food production, catering and dairying industries, although chlorine disinfectants are more widely used. The recommended concentrations of available iodine are 50–150 p.p.m. The presence of iodine can be detected by colour to the lower limit of its bactericidal activity. A strongly acid iodophor is used to prevent or remove milkstone from milking machines and other dairy equipment.

PHENOLS

General properties

Phenol ('carbolic acid') is the parent compound of the substituted phenols which are used to formulate phenolic disinfectants. The substituents may be alkyl groups (methyl, ethyl), halogen atoms (Cl, Br, F) or aromatic ring structures (phenyl, benzyl). All of the compounds retain the alcohol (OH) group of the parent phenol, which is no longer used as a disinfectant because of its irritant nature and lower activity. The formulae of some substituted phenols that are commonly used to formulate the disinfectants are shown below.

Alkylphenols are obtained by collecting coal tar distillate in three fractions with increasing boiling points. Cresols predominate in the first, xylenols in the second, and high-boiling tar acids in the third fraction. Bactericidal activity generally increases and skin irritancy decreases as the boiling point rises. The crude phenols are usually dark brown. Halogenated phenols, which may also contain alkyl or aromatic substituents, are prepared synthetically and are white solids which are insoluble in water. They are generally more active than phenols containing alkyl groups only.

Microbial susceptibility

Gram-positive bacteria	highly susceptible
Gram-negative bacteria	highly susceptible
Acid-fast bacteria	susceptible
Bacterial spores	resistant
Lipophilic viruses	susceptible
Hydrophilic viruses	resistant

Formulation

Most formulations contain mixed phenols, the types and proportions being selected to yield

o-cresol

m-cresol

m-xylenol

p-chlor-m-xylenol

di-chlor-m-xylenol

o-phenylphenol

o-benzyl-p-chlorophenol

products with a desired spectrum of activity. The coal tar phenols act non-selectively against Gram-positive and Gram-negative bacteria but the chloroxylenols are deficient in activity against Gram-negative organisms, especially *Pseudomonas*, *Proteus* and *Klebsiella*. Activity in this area has been greatly improved by the inclusion of aromatic phenols, such as *o*-phenylphenol and *o*-benzyl-*p*-chlorophenol. The formulae are usually trade secrets and only the total phenol content is specified. Some products now on the market are more active against the Gram-negative rods than they are against Gram-positive cocci.

Phenolic disinfectants are formulated with surface active agents or emulsifiers because the active ingredients are insoluble in water. 'Clear soluble fluids' contain natural soaps or synthetic anionic detergents. The relative concentrations of phenols and surfactant are critical because the phenols must escape from their location within molecular aggregates (micelles) of the carrier to the aqueous phase, where they exert their bactericidal action. Clear soluble fluids can be made from crude or refined coal tar phenols, chloroxylenols or complex mixtures of synthetic phenols.

'Black fluids' and 'white fluids' are crude coal tar disinfectants. The former are clear liquids in concentrated form but produce emulsions on dilution. White fluids are prepared as emulsions. Hydrocarbons are used to stabilize the emulsions. Phenolic disinfectants are diluted by volume for use as the exact composition of the concentrated product is usually not known.

Factors influencing efficiency

Phenols have relatively high concentration coefficients and a small reduction in the concentration causes a large increase in the killing time. They are most active at neutral or slightly acid pH because the unionized molecule is the active form but the influence of pH is complex; alkalinity generally reduces activity but the phenates that are formed are more soluble. The emulsifier may also affect the outcome (O'Connor & Rubino, 1991). The activity of chloroxylenols against Gram-negative bacilli is low but it may be increased by formulation with ethylenediamine tetraacetic acid (Russell & Furr, 1977).

Organic matter has little effect on the activity of coal tar disinfectants. The synthetic phenols are affected to a lesser degree than are the chlorine compounds, chlorhexidine and quaternary ammonium disinfectants. Oils and fats reduce activity by extracting the phenols from the aqueous solution.

Natural soaps and anionic detergents are compatible with phenols, subject to being formulated in the correct proportions. Nonionic detergents, such as polysorbate 80 (Tween 80) reduce activity and cationic detergents (quaternary ammonium compounds) are incompatible. Hard water is unsuitable for preparing dilutions; formulae that contain soap are affected more than are those that contain synthetic detergents.

Adverse effects

All phenolic disinfectants are poisonous if swallowed (Joubert et al, 1978). Crude coal tar disinfectants, such as lysol, cause chemical burns if the concentrated solution comes in contact with the skin. Synthetic formulations are less irritant. The odour of coal tar disinfectants is objectionable and is no longer associated in the mind of the user with efficiency. However, its place has been taken by the perfume of added pine oils, which do not contribute significantly to the bactericidal activity. Phenols may stain wool, cotton and synthetic fabrics; cause damage to copper, nickel and zinc; and impart a taint to foods.

Applications

The phenols are general purpose disinfectants for use on inanimate objects and surfaces where bactericidal action in the presence of organic soils is required. They are also effective against lipophilic viruses. Best et al (1990) showed that 5 per cent w/v phenol effectively destroyed *M. tuberculosis* in suspension and carrier tests, with and without sputum as organic load, within 1 minute of contact. Accuracy in diluting phenolics is important because small errors may result in significant changes in disinfectant activity.

Hospital uses

Clear soluble synthetic phenolics are suitable for disinfection of used instruments if this is necessary and heat treatment is not available. They may be used for disinfecting floors, walls, furniture and fittings in high risk areas such as operating theatres, delivery rooms, nurseries, intensive care wards and dialysis or renal transplant units. They are also appropriate for dealing with spillage of biological material other than blood. If sinks, slop-hoppers or wash basins are suspected of being a source of bacteria causing hospital-acquired infection, a strong phenolic may be poured into the waste pipe and left overnight (Maurer, 1985).

Laboratory uses

Phenolic disinfectants are appropriate for routine disinfection in laboratory animal units and of benches that have been contaminated with non-sporing bacteria. They may be used, as an alternative to chlorine compounds, in discard jars in bacteriology, but not in virology, laboratories (Maurer, 1985).

General hygiene

Relatively cheap coal tar disinfectants may be used in unoccupied premises or outdoor situations.

QUATERNARY AMMONIUM COMPOUNDS (QACs)

General properties

The quaternary ammonium compounds are cationic (positively charged) surface active disinfectants. Both characteristics contribute to their bactericidal activity by promoting uptake of the molecules by the microorganisms. The complex cations form salts with chloride or bromide; the associated anions play no part in the antimicrobial action. The active cations may be regarded as derivatives of an ammonium ion (NH_4^+), in which the four hydrogen atoms have been replaced by organic groups. At least one of these groups is a long hydrocarbon chain derived from fatty acids in vegetable oils. The water-repellant chain causes the molecules to concentrate as an oriented layer at the surface of the solution and at all interfaces with colloidal protein, suspended particles and solid surfaces. The charged nitrogen-containing

group has a high affinity for water and prevents the QAC from separating out of the aqueous solution. There are many types of quaternary ammonium compounds; the formulae of cetrimide and benzalkonium chloride are shown.

The QACs are non-crystalline solids, soluble in water and alcohols. The solutions are slightly alkaline, colourless and, with the exception of pyridine-based compounds, odourless. They are stable to heat and radiation sterilization.

Microbial susceptibility

Gram-positive bacteria	highly susceptible
Gram-negative bacteria	moderately susceptible
Acid-fast bacteria	resistant
Bacterial spores	resistant
Lipophilic viruses	susceptible
Hydrophilic viruses	resistant (except HBV)

Formulation

QAC disinfectants are sold as concentrated solutions (10–50 per cent w/v) containing one or more active agents or as a mixture containing other compatible disinfectants, e.g. the biguanide chlorhexidine. These are used to prepare dilute solutions in water or 80 per cent v/v ethyl alcohol. Detergent-sanitizers are formulated with compatible nonionic detergents. Many of these can be regarded only as expensive cleaning agents, but some meet the standard of hospital grade disinfectants. Each product must be evaluated by microbiological tests, regardless of the QAC content.

Factors influencing efficiency

Types of microorganisms

The quaternary ammonium compounds have a narrower antimicrobial spectrum than the synthetic phenols and chlorhexidine. They are very active against Gram-positive cocci but may be less active against Gram-negative bacteria. In the first report of inactivation of hepatitis B virus by low-level disinfectants, Prince et al (1993) showed that two QACs destroyed viral infectivity within 10 minutes. The end points, which correlated, were

$$\left[C_{16}H_{33} \underset{\underset{CH_3}{|}}{\overset{\overset{CH_3}{|}}{N}} CH_3 \right]^{+} \quad Br^{-}$$

Cetrimide

$$\left[C_8H_{17}\text{--}C_{18}H_{37} \underset{\underset{CH_3}{|}}{\overset{\overset{CH_3}{|}}{N}} CH_2\text{--}\bigcirc \right]^{+} \quad Cl^{-}$$

Benzalkonium chloride

read by both the Morphological Alteration and Disintegration Test and chimpanzee infectivity.

Concentration and pH

The concentration coefficients of QACs are low, so that halving the concentration approximately doubles the time for a specified level of inactivation. The optimum pH is on the alkaline side (9–10); values below 7 are unfavourable.

Organic and synthetic materials

The proteins in blood, serum and milk inactivate QACs by adsorption; the colloidal protein in serum has an adsorbing surface of about $1 \text{ m}^2/\text{ml}$. A three- to fourfold increase in the concentration of a QAC is required for activity in the presence of colloidal or particulate organic matter. Cotton gauze adsorbs QACs (Kundsin & Walter, 1957). Cellulosic and synthetic materials used in containers or cleaning utensils, such as sponges and mops, also inactivate QACs by adsorption (Maurer, 1985). Anionic soaps and synthetic detergents inactivate by chemical reaction between the molecules which carry opposite electric charges. Many nonionic detergents (e.g. polysorbate 80) also inactivate QACs; calcium, magnesium, ferric and possibly aluminium ions reduce activity.

Adverse effects

The quaternary ammonium compounds are popular disinfectants and sanitizers because of their freedom from toxicity and other undesirable effects. The chronic oral toxicity of dilute solutions is low, but human death may be caused by swallowing a concentrated solution. Skin irritation and sensitization are reported occasionally.

Cement, synthetic rubbers and aluminium may be damaged by quaternary ammonium disinfectants, especially if an antirust compound has been added to the solution.

Applications

The quaternary ammonium compounds are suitable for disinfection of clean surfaces and are widely used as detergent-sanitizers. Lack of toxicity enables them to be used as sanitizers in the dairying, food production and catering industries as an alternative to chlorine compounds but the latter generally retain their established position.

QACs are not recommended for routine cleaning in hospitals but a high level of activity against pathogenic staphylococci may be useful if these bacteria are found to be colonizing or infecting patients. They are unreliable skin disinfectants because microorganisms may be trapped between the surface of the skin and the inactive side of the molecular film. However, a product containing cetrimide and chlorhexidine is an effective wound cleanser.

STRONG OXIDIZING AGENTS

Chlorine dioxide, peracetic acid, peroxygen biocide and hydrogen peroxide form a diverse group of chemical compounds which are used particularly for their sporicidal activity. They are highly reactive and the solutions may be unstable. Each has a broad spectrum of biocidal action, which includes bacterial spores.

Chlorine dioxide

Chlorine dioxide (ClO_2) is a stronger oxidizing agent than other chlorine disinfectants. It also differs from them as it does not give rise to hypochlorous acid and does not combine with ammonia or organic nitrogen compounds to produce amines. Chlorine dioxide is prepared by mixing dilute solutions of chlorine and sodium chlorite. Strong solutions are not prepared because explosion might occur. The dilute solutions, containing 4–5 per cent w/v of the active agent, may be stabilized by addition of boron compounds.

The bactericidal activity of chlorine dioxide is similar to that of other chlorine disinfectants and the sporicidal action is independent of pH over the range 6–10. Applications include water treatment, where it is useful for removing tastes and odours by breaking down phenolic compounds. It is used to control slime in paper pulp processing. The use of gaseous chlorine dioxide as a sterilizing agent is discussed in Chapter 7.

Peracetic acid

Pure peracetic acid ($CH_3CO.OOH$) is a colourless liquid, miscible with water and organic solvents. It has a pungent odour and is highly irritant. A 40 per cent w/w solution of peracetic acid is prepared commercially from acetic acid and hydrogen peroxide, with sulfuric acid as catalyst.

Peracetic acid is more active than is hydrogen peroxide against bacteria and their spores (Baldry, 1983). Sporicidal activity is retained, even at subzero temperatures, and biocidal activity is maintained in the presence of organic material (Block, 1991).

Solutions of peracetic acid of up to 3 per cent v/v concentration are used as disinfectants or sterilants. A 2 per cent v/v concentration may be used as an aerosol. The relative humidity should be around 80 per cent if peracetic acid is in the vapour phase (Portner & Hoffman, 1968). Activity is greater at lower pH levels; the usual range for efficacy is pH 5 to 8.

Apart from irritancy, solutions tend to be corrosive and the vapour is toxic, although easily removed from a ventilated area. If heated above its flash point of 56°C, peracetic acid presents a fire and explosion hazard (Block, 1991). It should be stored in its original containers, with vented caps to prevent pressure build-up, and at temperatures below 30°C.

Peracetic acid has long been used in germfree animal facilities. More recently, it has found application in the food and beverage industries, particularly as a terminal disinfectant or sterilant. It is also used in an enclosed, buffered system (Steris system) as a liquid sterilant for medical equipment, such as endoscopes (Block, 1991).

Peroxygen biocide

Potassium peroxymonosulfate (20.4 per cent) with sodium chloride (1.5 per cent) in a buffered, low pH, detergent formulation has an activity equivalent to 9.75 per cent available chlorine. It is marketed as a powder or 1 per cent solution under the brand name 'Virkon'. The inorganic surfactant in the formulation is 90 per cent biodegradable.

The peroxygen system is active against a wide range of microorganisms including bacteria, fungi, mycoplasmas and viruses, particularly the latter. It is of low toxicity to humans and animals and is less corrosive to textile fabrics and to a variety of materials, such as stainless steel, anodized aluminium and various plastics, than is sodium hypochlorite at equivalent concentration.

This detergent/disinfectant is currently recommended for cleaning and disinfecting industrial animal and agricultural facilities, especially in situations where viruses may present a challenge. However, HIV in blood was not inactivated on exposure to 'Virkon' for 10 minutes (Druce et al,

1993). Furthermore, Broadley et al (1993) reported that 'Virkon' has poor antimycobacterial activity.

Hydrogen peroxide

Hydrogen peroxide (H_2O_2) is a slow oxidizing agent. Dilute solutions are unstable, especially in the presence of tissue which contains the enzyme catalase. Concentrated solutions containing 90 per cent w/v H_2O_2, which are prepared electrochemically using inert containers and piping, are stable. These may be diluted to 3–6 per cent w/v for disinfection and the container may be opened daily without loss of the peroxide. A 6 per cent solution withstands heating. There are no toxic decomposition products.

There is some activity against most types of microorganisms but enteric viruses and bacterial spores require a high concentration for lethal action. An initial lag in the rate of sporicidal action may be shortened by an increase in the concentration or temperature. Fungi are relatively resistant.

Uses that have been proposed for hydrogen peroxide include spray disinfection of mechanical ventilators (Ayliffe et al, 1993), acrylic resin implants, plastic eating utensils and soft contact lenses. The absence of toxicity is attractive to the food industry and hydrogen peroxide is used to disinfect cartons which are aseptically filled with 'sterilized' milk (Swartling & Lindgren, 1968). The use of hydrogen peroxide in the vapour phase for decontaminating surfaces of enclosed spaces is discussed in Chapter 7.

REFERENCES

Ahrenholz D H, Marxen L. Simmons R L 1979 Depression of human neutrophil function by povidone iodine: a mechanism for the effect of betadine in *E. coli* peritonitis. Federation Proceedings 38: 1427

Archer G T L 1945 Bactericidal effect of mixtures of ethyl alcohol and water. British Medical Journal 2: 148–151

Ayliffe G A J 1996 Recommendations for the control of methicillin-resistant *Staphylococcus aureus* (MRSA). Division of Emerging and other Communicable Diseases Surveillance and Control, World Health Organization, p 1–28

Ayliffe G A J, Coates D, Hoffman P N 1993 Chemical disinfection in hospitals, 2nd edn. Public Health Laboratory Service, London

Baldry M G C 1983 The bactericidal, fungicidal and sporicidal properties of hydrogen peroxide and peracetic acid. Journal of Applied Bacteriology 54: 417–423

Benson W G 1984 Case report. Exposure to glutaraldehyde. Journal of the Society of Occupational Medicine 34: 63–64

Bergan T, Lystad A 1971 Antitubercular action of disinfectants. Journal of Applied Bacteriology 34: 751–756

Berkelman R L, Holland B W, Anderson R L 1982 Increased bactericidal activity of dilute preparations of povidone-iodine solutions. Journal of Clinical Microbiology 15: 635–639

Best M, Sattar S A, Springthorpe V S, Kennedy M E 1990 Efficacies of selected disinfectants against *Mycobacterium tuberculosis*. Journal of Clinical Microbiology 28: 2234–2239

Blair A, Saracci R, Stewart P A, Hayes R B, Shy C 1990 Epidemiologic evidence on the relationship between formaldehyde exposure and cancer. Scandinavian Journal of Work, Environment and Health 16: 381–393

Block S S 1991 Peroxygen compounds. In: Block S S (ed) Disinfection, sterilization, and preservation, 4th edn. Lea & Febiger, Philadelphia, ch 9, p 167

Bloomfield S F, Smith-Burchnell C A, Dalgleish A G 1990 Evaluation of hypochlorite-releasing disinfectants against the human immunodeficiency virus (HIV). Journal of Hospital Infection 15: 273–278

Broadley S J, Furr J R, Jenkins P A, Russell A D 1993 Antimycobacterial activity of 'Virkon'. Journal of Hospital Infection 23: 189–197

Burge P S 1989 Occupational risks of glutaraldehyde. British Medical Journal 299: 342

Clark R P 1983 Formaldehyde in pathology departments. Journal of Clinical Pathology 36: 839–846

Collins F M 1986 Kinetics of the tuberculocidal response by glutaraldehyde in solution and on an inert surface. Journal of Applied Bacteriology 61: 87–93

Dally K A, Hanrahan L P, Woodbury M A, Kanarek M S 1981 Formaldehyde exposure in nonoccupational environments. Archives of Environmental Health 36: 277–284

Davies G E, Francis J, Martin A R, Rose F L, Swain G 1954 1: 6-di-4'-chlorophenyldiguanidohexane ('Hibitane'). Laboratory investigation of a new antibacterial agent of high potency. British Journal of Pharmacology and Chemotherapy 9: 192–196

Death J E, Coates D 1979 Effect of pH on sporicidal and microbicidal activity of buffered mixtures of alcohol and sodium hypochlorite. Journal of Clinical Pathology 32: 148–153

Denton G W 1991 Chlorhexidine. In: Block S S (ed) Disinfection, sterilization, and preservation, 4th edn. Lea & Febiger, Philadelphia, ch 16, p 283–285

Drew R T, Laskin S, Kuschner M, Nelson N 1975 Inhalation carcinogenicity of alpha halo ethers. 1. The acute inhalation toxicity of chloromethyl methyl ether and bis (chloromethyl) ether. Archives of Environmental Health 30: 61–69

Druce J D, Jardine D, Locarnini S A, Birch C J 1995 Susceptibility of HIV to inactivation by disinfectants and ultraviolet light. Journal of Hospital Infection 30: 167–180

Goodall R R, Goldman J, Woods J 1968 Stability of chlorhexidine solutions. Pharmaceutical Journal 200: 33–34

Hanson P J V, Gor D, Jeffries D J, Collins J V 1989 Chemical inactivation of HIV on surfaces. British Medical Journal 298: 862–864

Jachuck S J, Bound C L, Steel J, Blain P G 1989 Occupational hazard in hospital staff exposed to 2 per cent glutaraldehyde in an endoscopy unit. Journal of the Society of Occupational Medicine 39: 69–71

Joubert P, Hundt H, Du Toit P 1978 Severe Dettol (chloroxylenol and terpineol) poisoning. British Medical Journal 1: 890

Klein M, Deforest A 1963 The inactivation of viruses by germicides. Chemical Specialities Manufacturers Association Proceedings 49: 116–118

Kundsin R B, Walter C W 1957 Investigations on adsorption of benzalkonium chloride U.S.P. by skin, gloves, and sponges. Archives of Surgery 75: 1036–1042

Lowbury E J L, Lilly H A 1973 Use of 4% chlorhexidine detergent solution (Hibiscrub) and other methods of skin disinfection. British Medical Journal 1: 510–515

Lustig F W 1963 A fatal case of hexachlorophane ('pHisoHex') poisoning. Medical Journal of Australia 1: 737

Maibach H 1975 Glutaraldehyde: cross-reactions to formaldehyde? Contact Dermatitis 1: 326–327

Maurer I M 1985 Hospital hygiene, 3rd edn. Edward Arnold, London

Mwaniki D L, Guthua S W 1992 Occupational exposure to glutaraldehyde in tropical climates. Lancet 340: 1476–1477

Norbäck D 1988 Skin and respiratory symptoms from exposure to alkaline glutaraldehyde in medical services. Scandinavian Journal of Work, Environment & Health 14: 366–371

O'Connor D O, Rubino J R 1991 Phenolic compounds. In: Block S S (ed) Disinfection, sterilization, and preservation, 4th edn. Lea & Febiger, Philadelphia, ch 12, p 214

Orringer E P, Mattern W D 1976 Formaldehyde-induced hemolysis during chronic hemodialysis. New England Journal of Medicine 294: 1416–1420

Partanen T 1993 Formaldehyde exposure and respiratory cancer — a meta-analysis of the epidemiologic evidence. Scandinavian Journal of Work, Environment and Health 19: 8–15

Portner D M, Hoffman R K 1968 Sporicidal effect of peracetic acid vapour. Applied Microbiology 16: 1782–1785

Price P B 1939 Ethyl alcohol as a germicide. Archives of Surgery 38: 528–542

Prince D L, Prince H N, Thraenhart O, Muchmore E, Bonder E, Pugh J 1993 Methodological approaches to disinfection of human hepatitis B virus. Journal of Clinical Microbiology 31: 3294–3304

Rosenberg A, Alatary S D, Peterson A F 1976 Safety and efficacy of the antiseptic chlorhexidine gluconate. Surgery, Gynecology & Obstetrics 143: 789–792

Russell A D 1994 Glutaraldehyde: current status and uses. Infection Control and Hospital Epidemiology 15: 724–733

Russell A D, Furr J R 1977 The antibacterial activity of a new chloroxylenol preparation containing ethylenediamine tetraacetic acid. Journal of Applied Bacteriology 43: 253–260

Saitanu K, Lund E 1975 Inactivation of enterovirus by glutaraldehyde. Applied Microbiology 29: 571–574

Sanderson K V, Cronin E 1968 Glutaraldehyde and contact dermatitis. British Medical Journal 3: 802

Shere L, Kelley M J, Richardson J H 1962 Effect of bromide-hypochlorite bactericides on microorganisms. Applied Microbiology 10: 538–541

Stonehill A A, Krop S, Borick P M 1963 Buffered glutaraldehyde. A new chemical sterilizing solution. American Journal of Hospital Pharmacy 20: 458–465

Swartling P, Lindgren B 1968 The sterilizing effect against Bacillus subtilis spores of hydrogen peroxide at different temperatures and concentrations. Journal of Dairy Research 35: 423–428

Wear J B Jr, Shanahan R, Ratliff R K 1962 Toxicity of ingested hexachlorophene. Journal of the American Medical Association 181: 587–589

Wlodkowski T J, Speck W T, Rosenkranz H S 1975 Genetic effects of povidone-iodine. Journal of Pharmaceutical Sciences 64: 1235–1237

Yodaiken R E 1981 The uncertain consequences of formaldehyde toxicity. Journal of the American Medical Association 246: 1677–1678

11. Principles of chemical disinfection

Aqueous solutions of antimicrobial agents were associated with two landmarks in the prevention of hospital-acquired infection during the nineteenth century. In 1847, Semmelweiss showed that the incidence of puerperal sepsis in a maternity hospital in Vienna could be reduced if the doctors rinsed their hands in chloride of lime between performing post mortem examinations and attending to their living patients. His recommendation did not receive full cooperation from the doctors and hospital authorities but Lister's method of antiseptic surgery, reported in the British Medical Journal in 1867, fared better. He achieved a dramatic reduction in post-operative infection, which previously killed up to 50 per cent of surgical patients, by disinfecting instruments with 5 per cent phenol and spraying a 2.5 per cent solution on the wound and adjacent skin. Chemical disinfection of instruments was replaced by sterilization when the emphasis shifted from antiseptic to aseptic surgery.

The purpose of this chapter is to explain the principles that govern the selection of liquid chemicals and their effective use in present-day roles. The susceptibility of different types of microorganisms, the factors influencing effectiveness of the disinfectants in use, the methods of evaluation and the importance of a hospital disinfection policy will be discussed.

MECHANISMS OF MICROBIOCIDAL ACTION

Chemicals that are used for disinfection of inanimate objects or intact body surfaces are selected for their rapid biocidal action against susceptible microorganisms and may be termed general protoplasmic poisons. It is difficult to identify any particular component or structure of the cell as the primary target of a rapidly lethal action. However, initial damage to the bacterial cell membrane resulting in the loss of important cell constituents, such as purines, pyrimidines, ribose, amino acids and potassium, has been demonstrated in studies on chlorhexidine, quaternary ammonium compounds, phenols and alcohols. These are commonly termed 'membrane active' disinfectants. Glutaraldehyde on the other hand, appears to seal the cell membrane against leakage of intracellular components.

Membrane active disinfectants

The bacterial cell membrane regulates the uptake of essential nutrients, including amino acids, and prevents the escape from the cell of vital protein and nucleic acid precursors. It is also the site of action of respiratory enzymes and coenzymes and of systems involved in the synthesis of cell wall components including peptidoglycan, which maintains the shape and integrity of the cell.

Investigations by Hugo & Longworth on the effects of chlorhexidine on Gram-positive and Gram-negative bacteria, and their conclusions regarding the mechanisms of bacteriostatic and bactericidal action, have been summarized by Hugo (1992).

Chlorhexidine is strongly adsorbed to the surface of *Staphylococcus aureus* and *Escherichia coli*, reducing the negative charge on the cells. The subsequent changes in cell structure or metabolism depend on the concentration of chlorhexidine in the solution. Leakage of cytoplasmic constituents occurs at bacteriostatic concentrations below 0.05 per cent w/v. Studies with the electron microscope show that the bacteria are transformed into 'ghost' cells. They may be revived by restoration to favourable conditions for growth but eventually die if stasis is maintained until the loss of essential components can no longer be replenished. The rate of leakage from the membrane-damaged cells increases as the concentration of chlorhexidine is raised until rapid bactericidal action commences. Leakage then ceases abruptly as chlorhexidine penetrates to the interior of the cells and changes indicative of precipitation or coagulation within

the cytoplasm can be observed by electron microscopy (Hugo, 1992).

Support for the conclusion that the cell membrane is the primary site of action of chlorhexidine has been provided by studies on protoplasts and spheroplasts, produced from Gram-positive and Gram-negative bacteria respectively. These are fragile cells which have been deprived partially or completely of their rigid cell wall component (peptidoglycan). They can survive only in a suspending fluid containing a high concentration of sucrose to balance the osmotic pressure within the cytoplasm; they lyse on dilution with water. Treatment with a low concentration of chlorhexidine causes them to lyse while they are still in the protective solution. A bactericidal concentration precipitates proteins in the cell membrane and lysis does not occur even when the suspending fluid is diluted.

The mechanism of action of quaternary ammonium disinfectants closely resembles that of chlorhexidine in the pattern of leakage at bacteriostatic, and precipitation of cell contents at bactericidal, concentrations (Davies et al, 1968). Inhibition of respiration, probably through action on the cytochrome system, by cetyltrimethylammonium bromide has been reported (Wiseman, 1971). Gram-negative bacteria, especially *Pseudomonas* spp., tend to be more resistant than are Gram-positive bacteria to the disinfectant action because of the presence of lipoproteins, lipopolysaccharides and phospholipids in their cell walls (Maris, 1995).

Gram-positive bacteria are more sensitive to membrane-active disinfectants than are the Gram-negative species because of differences in cell wall composition. Gram-negative bacteria are relatively resistant because they contain complex lipoproteins and lipopolysaccharides which impede access of antibacterial agents to the underlying membrane. If these cell wall components are disaggregated and magnesium ions removed by treatment with ethylenediamine tetraacetic acid (EDTA) the susceptibility of the Gram-negative bacteria is greatly increased (Russell & Furr, 1977).

Aldehydes

Glutaraldehyde and formaldehyde are alkylating agents which probably owe their ability to kill spores to reaction with nucleic acids as well as with proteins. If protoplasts and spheroplasts are treated with glutaraldehyde, they fail to lyse on dilution of the protective medium. This indicates the hardening of the cell membrane (Munton & Russell, 1970; 1973) or cell wall (McGucken & Woodside, 1973). Glutaraldehyde at low concentrations inactivates poliovirus and echovirus by reacting with capsid proteins (Chambon et al, 1992). Aldehydes can cross link amino groups (Russell, 1994).

Halogens

The halogen-based disinfectants are oxidizing agents, chlorine being stronger than iodine. Evidence for the role of oxidation in the bactericidal action is provided by the conversion of about 90 per cent of iodine which has been taken up by the cells to inactive iodide (Brandrick et al, 1967). However, a role for the direct halogenation of cell constituents is indicated by the fact that hydrogen peroxide and potassium permanganate, which are the stronger oxidizing agents, are less efficient bactericides. The killing action of chlorine is mediated mainly through hypochlorous acid (HOCl).

SUSCEPTIBILITY OF MICROORGANISMS

Vegetative bacteria

Gram-positive and Gram-negative bacteria are readily killed by all types of hospital grade disinfectants. However, some species of Gram-negative bacteria are capable of survival and growth in phenolic, quaternary ammonium and biguanide disinfectants if the solutions are too dilute, stale or have been inactivated by mixture or contact with incompatible materials. Species of *Klebsiella, Proteus, Serratia* and *Pseudomonas* have been isolated frequently from contaminated disinfectants and in outbreaks of infections caused by them. These bacteria owe their ability to grow in diluted disinfectants or in water containing traces of organic and inorganic impurities to simple nutritional requirements and the ability to multiply at ambient temperatures (Favero et al, 1971). In contrast, Gram-positive *Listeria monocytogenes* was found to be more susceptible to a quaternary ammonium compound of modern formulation than to sodium

hypochlorite, although either could be used as an effective sanitizer in dilute solution (Mustapha & Liewen, 1989).

The natural tendency towards resistance of Gram-negative bacteria to disinfectants which damage the cell membrane is associated with relative inaccessibility of the membrane. The cell wall of *Pseudomonas aeruginosa* is especially protective because it is rich in magnesium and more complex than that of the enteric bacteria. The resistance of Gram-negative bacteria also varies with the conditions in which they have grown. *Burkholderia cepacia* which has grown in water or a dilute disinfectant at ambient temperature undergoes a dramatic decrease in resistance when re-exposed to the disinfectant after a single laboratory subculture in nutrient broth at 37°C (Bassett et al, 1970). The pH of the disinfectant may also determine whether bacterial multiplication occurs. A pseudomonad which was isolated from a solution containing a quaternary ammonium compound and chlorhexidine that had been diluted in the hospital with distilled water (pH 6) was easily killed by the same disinfectant concentration when prepared with tap water in the laboratory at pH 7.2. This is close to the optimum pH for activity of cationic disinfectants (Bassett, 1971a).

The possibility of increased resistance in Gram-negative bacteria as a result of repeated exposure to disinfectants and of a relationship to multi-antibiotic resistance have been investigated. Both are considered unlikely because disinfectants act as general protoplasmic poisons, and operation of the mutation-selection process that may lead to antibiotic resistance would not be expected. However, a considerable amount of evidence that some of the increased resistance may have a genetic basis has accumulated since Gillespie et al (1967) reported that 10 out of 13 strains of *Proteus mirabilis* isolated from patients who had received numerous applications of chlorhexidine for urinary catheterization had minimum inhibitory concentrations (m.i.c.) of 125–500 μg/ml. Stickler & Thomas (1980) examined 802 isolates of Gram-negative bacteria causing urinary tract infections in patients who were subject to extensive contact with chlorhexidine for urinary catheterization. Strains of *E. coli* were uniformly sensitive but some strains of *Proteus, Providencia* and *Pseudomonas* were above the normal m.i.c. range for cationic disinfectants and also for several antibiotics.

Laboratory investigations have confirmed that an increase in the resistance of certain Gram-negative bacteria to chlorhexidine can occur if they are serially subcultured in gradually increasing concentrations of the disinfectant. Stickler (1974) observed significant increases in the minimum inhibitory concentration of chlorhexidine for two strains of *P. mirabilis* from 20 μg/ml to 200 μg/ml and 800 μg/ml. Prince et al (1978) also obtained an increase in the resistance of strains of *Proteus*, *Pseudomonas* and *Serratia* to chlorhexidine. With *Proteus*, the resistance was lost after further sub-cultures without the disinfectant but it was stable in *Pseudomonas* and *Serratia*. A slight increase in resistance to benzalkonium chloride was also de-tected. A similar experiment with povidone-iodine did not produce any strains with increased resist-ance to this compound. Stickler et al (1987) chal-lenged isolates, e.g. species of *Pseudomonas*, *Proteus* and *Klebsiëlla*, from the urines of spinally injured patients with chlorhexidine (200 μg/ml) in a catheterized bladder model by a simulated bladder washout technique. Bacteria on the wall of the bladder were embedded in protective polysaccha-ride (glycocalyx) and the effect of irrigation with chlorhexidine was minimal and temporary. Mini-mum inhibitory concentrations for chlorhexidine ranged from 4 μg/ml for a sensitive (control) strain of *E. coli* to 1280 μg/ml for *P. mirabilis*.

In view of these findings, the possibility of increased resistance, acquired during repeated exposure to chlorhexidine or quaternary am-monium compounds, cannot be ruled out. Martin (1969) reported that none of 205 isolates of *Pro-teus*, including the most resistant species *P. mirabilis*, survived exposure to 0.02 per cent w/v chlorhexidine, the lowest concentration used in practice. However, O'Flynn & Stickler (1972) reported that 39 per cent of 45 strains of *P. mirabilis* which were isolated from patients were resistant to this concentration.

As mentioned before, some of the isolates of *Proteus*, *Providencia* and *Pseudomonas* which were relatively resistant to chlorhexidine (Stickler & Thomas, 1980) were also resistant to several antibiotics. However, Russell (1972) had found that two strains of *P. aeruginosa* which were resistant to several antibiotics were as susceptible as antibiotic sensitive strains to chlorhexidine, cetrimide, glutaraldehyde, chloroxylenol and lysol.

Studies on plasmid-bearing *S. aureus*, *B. cepacia*, *P. aeruginosa* and *Alcaligenes xylosoxidans* have con-firmed the existence of genes which determine increased resistance to chlorhexidine and QACs. Townsend and co-workers (1983; 1984) demon-strated that plasmids carrying gentamicin resist-ance in methicillin-resistant *S. aureus* (MRSA) also encoded resistance to QACs. In their review of the genetic basis of antimicrobial resistance in *S. aureus*, Lyon & Skurray (1987) identified three distinct plasmids capable of transferring resistance to QACs. On the other hand, Nagai & Ogase (1990) did not find any evidence for plasmids in isolates of Gram-negative bacilli *B. cepacia* and *A. xylosoxidans* which were resistant to both chlorhexidine and a QAC. Resistance was neither lost by treatment of the microbial cells with acri-dine orange nor transferable to *E. coli*. Because of the cross resistance, the suggestion by these workers was that a common mechanism, probably related to decreased membrane permeability, was responsible for the increased resistance.

Genetically conferred bacterial resistance to chlorhexidine and QACs does not pose a problem in practice because the recommended in-use con-centrations of disinfectants generally greatly exceed the observed m.i.c. values, even for the most resistant bacterial strains. Moreover, vancomycin-resistant enterococci and multidrug-resistant tu-bercle bacilli are as sensitive to commonly used dilutions of disinfectants as are the antibiotic-sensitive strains of these species (Rutala, 1996).

Acid-fast bacteria

These include *Mycobacterium tuberculosis*, *Myco-bacterium avium* and other human pathogens. The organisms have a high lipid content, including waxes, which impedes penetration of aqueous solutions unless they contain a high concentration of soap or detergent, as in some phenolics (Hegna, 1977). Best et al (1990) investigated the efficacy of disinfectants against *M. tuberculosis* in suspension and carrier tests in the presence and absence of sputum. Ethanol (70 per cent v/v) was effective only in suspension tests and in the absence of sputum.

Phenol and chlorine (10 000 p.p.m.) were efficacious, as was 2 per cent glutaraldehyde provided contact time was extended (Collins, 1986).

Bacterial spores

While bacterial spores are killed by aldehyde and halogen disinfectants, high concentrations and prolonged exposures may be necessary (Coates, 1996; Sagripanti & Bonifacino, 1996). Glutaraldehyde is a more effective sporicide than is formaldehyde (Sagripanti & Bonifacino, 1996). Whereas the sporicidal activity of chlorine-releasing compounds is considerably reduced in the presence of a low level of blood (Coates, 1996), the rapid sporicidal action of peracetic acid is virtually unaffected by organic material (Coates, 1996; Rutala, 1996). Suspension tests have been used for these investigations. The AOAC sporicidal carrier test has been criticized as inaccurate and non-reproducible (Miner et al, 1995).

Viruses

Although incapable of multiplication outside host cells, viruses can survive in the environment. The extent to which a particular virus survives depends on such variables as its concentration and the temperature, humidity and nature of its milieu. When suspended in 10 per cent serum, HIV can remain infectious for weeks; and, even when dried on coverslips, HIV cultures retain infectivity for several days (van Bueren et al, 1994). The survival of HIV has been attributed, in part, to the presence of a lipid envelope (Damjanovic, 1987). Viruses with lipid envelopes are classed as lipophilic viruses. Examples are herpes, influenza and the measles virus. However, although the lipid envelope confers environmental protection, lipophilic viruses are more susceptible to chemical disinfectants than are the viruses without envelopes. The latter are classed as hydrophilic viruses and include coxsackie, echovirus and the hepatitis viruses. Aldehydes and the halogens are most effective against this group.

Prions

Prions are resistant to most chemical disinfectants including those with broad spectrum activity, such as peracetic acid (Taylor, 1991) and the aldehydes. Exposure to sodium hypochlorite at a concentration of 2 per cent (20 000 p.p.m.) available chlorine for 1 hour is recommended for effective decontamination of these agents (Kimberlin et al, 1983; Taylor, 1986). Taylor et al (1994) confirmed this for the BSE agent but found that sodium hypochlorite, and not sodium dichloroisocyanurate, must be used as the chlorine-releasing compound. Treatment with 1M sodium hydroxide for 1 hour has also been recommended and is less corrosive to metals (Brown et al, 1986; Rosenberg et al, 1986). However, prion inactivation by 1M or 2M sodium hydroxide for either 1 or 2 hours has been shown to be incomplete (Tamai et al, 1988; Tateishi et al, 1988; Taylor et al, 1994).

Table 11.1 Appropriate disinfectants for particular microorganisms

Types of microorganisms	Effective chemical disinfectants (alphabetical order)
Gram-positive bacteria (non-sporing)	Any potent bactericide
Gram-negative bacteria (particularly *Proteus*, *Klebsiella*, *Pseudomonas*)	Alcohols Halogens (chlorine, iodine) Phenolics (clear soluble type with high level of activity; not chloroxylenols)
Acid-fast bacilli (*M. tuberculosis*)	Alcohols (suspensions) Aldehydes Halogens Phenolics (some clear soluble formulations)
Bacterial spores	Aldehydes (prolonged exposure) Halogens (strong solutions) Peracetic acid (e.g. Steris system, Nu-Cidex)
Viruses — hydrophilic and lipophilic groups	Aldehydes Halogens (strong solutions) Peracetic acid
Viruses — lipophilic group only	Alcohols (suspensions) Chlorhexidine Phenolics (clear soluble type) QACs
Prions	Chlorine (20 000 p.p.m. for 1 h) with sodium hypochlorite as chlorine-releasing agent
Fungi	Aldehydes Halogens (strong solutions) Phenolics

Fungi

These eucaryotic, usually multicellular organisms present special problems in disinfection as all vegetative cells and spores must be killed to prevent regrowth. Antifungal agents are more often fungistatic than fungicidal and species susceptibility varies widely. Alkaline glutaraldehyde has antifungal activity (Gorman & Scott, 1977), and hypochlorites may control growth in some situations. The filamentous fungi that cause tinea (ringworm) in humans and animals are inaccessible to disinfectants because they are located within the keratinized skin scales shed into the environment.

Appropriate types of chemical disinfectants for use against the different groups of microorganisms are shown in Table 11.1.

FACTORS AFFECTING IN-USE EFFECTIVENESS

Each type of chemical disinfectant has a characteristic potential for biocidal action which is determined by its antimicrobial spectrum and mechanism of action. However, its efficiency in the conditions of use may be influenced, often adversely, by many factors. Some of these relate to the number and condition of the microorganisms and others to changes in the effective concentration of the disinfectant.

Number of microorganisms

Chemical disinfection has a low margin of safety and the rate of killing often slows in the later stages, producing tailing curves. Low initial contamination levels, which may be achieved by precleaning the articles or surfaces to be disinfected, are therefore very important.

Conditions of growth

The conditions in which natural populations of microorganisms have grown is usually unknown. However, certain Gram-negative bacteria, such as the pseudomonads, are more resistant to disinfectants when they have grown in water or some other nutritionally deficient medium, such as

dilute disinfectant, at ambient temperature than when they have been cultured in a laboratory medium at 37°C (Bassett et al, 1970). Bacteria that are actively multiplying in the logarithmic phase of population growth are usually more susceptible than are physiologically old cells of the stationary phase.

Accessibility of microorganisms

Dried or clotted blood, pus, excreta, oil films or milk residues can protect microorganisms from effective contact with liquid disinfectants. Proteins are coagulated or precipitated by alcohols and hardened by aldehydes. Virus particles or their infective nucleic acid core may be protected by accompanying particulate matter (Salk & Gori, 1959) or by hardening of the protein coat when they are treated with formalin to prepare a killed vaccine (Gard, 1959). Moisture is always essential for antimicrobial action; microorganisms are not killed by dried disinfectant residues on floors (Ayliffe et al, 1966) or blankets (Rubbo et al, 1960).

Some articles harbour contaminants in pores, crevices or cracks, such as may occur in wood (Gilbert & Watson, 1971), concrete and damaged metalware, or between closely mated metal surfaces (e.g. hinged instruments). The human skin has a population of resident bacteria which multiply between the outer layers of the keratinized epithelium and cannot be reached by disinfectants.

Concentration of disinfectant

The rate of killing increases with the concentration of the antimicrobial agent. The magnitude of the effect is expressed by the concentration coefficient (n), which is calculated from the equation $k = tc^n$, where k is a death rate constant, c is the concentration and t is the time of disinfection (minutes) for a specified reduction in the viable count. For many types of disinfectants the concentration coefficient is unity, so that halving the concentration doubles the time. Phenols, however, have an unusually high coefficient (up to 6) so that a small change in concentration results in a large difference in killing time, as shown in Figure 11.1.

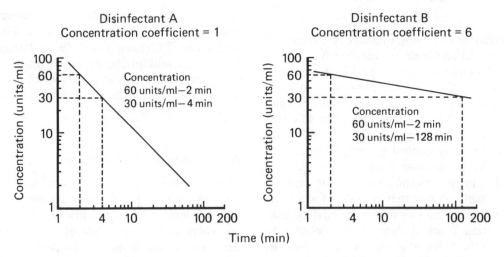

Fig. 11.1 Influence of concentration on the time required for biocidal action of a disinfectant (A) with a low concentration coefficient and (B) with a high concentration coefficient.

Temperature

Chemical disinfectants are commonly used at room temperature but some are suitable for use in conjunction with hot cleaning processes.

$$\text{Temperature coefficient} = \frac{\text{Time to kill at } x°C}{\text{Time at } (x + 10°C)}$$

The term 'to kill' implies, as usual, some specified degree of reduction in viable microorganisms. Temperature coefficients range from 2 to 14. Alkaline glutaraldehyde has a temperature coefficient of 4, so that a 10°C increase in temperature effects a fourfold reduction in the time to kill. Phenols have coefficients of 2–6. The sporicidal activity of sodium hypochlorite is increased by more than 50 per cent when the temperature is raised by 10°C. A temperature coefficient may apply within a limited temperature range only.

Hydrogen ion concentration (pH)

The effect of pH on bactericidal action may be exerted on the disinfectant, the microorganisms or both. Quaternary ammonium compounds and chlorhexidine are active as cations. The optimum pH for their action is on the alkaline side of neutrality because this increases the number of negatively charged groups on the proteins of the

bacterial surface with which the antibacterial agent may combine. The activity of phenols is generally favoured by an acid pH although they may be active under alkaline conditions in the presence of certain solubilizers (Prindle, 1983).

Glutaraldehyde is more stable at acid pH but far more microbiocidal at alkaline pH. However, this difference in biocidal activity becomes negligible as the temperature is raised above 40°C (Russell, 1994). As pH increases over the range of 1 to 8 so does the microbiocidal activity of glutaraldehyde. However, no differences in the chemical nature or structure of the aldehyde could be detected over this pH range (Holloway & Dean, 1975). The increased activity of glutaraldehyde with increasing pH is attributed to the formation of more binding sites for glutaraldehyde on the cell surfaces of microorganisms (Russell, 1994).

The halogen-based disinfectants are most active in the pH range of 6–8. The active form of chlorine disinfectants is unionized hypochlorous acid and ionic forces are not involved in the reaction of the disinfectant with microorganisms. Hypochlorite anions, which predominate in alkaline solutions, are virtually devoid of activity. The relationship between pH and per cent of Cl_2, HOCl and OCl^- is shown in Table 11.2. Iodine, in the form I_2, is also active in neutral or acid solutions.

Table 11.2 Influence of pH on availability of undissociated hypochlorous acid, the active agent in chlorine disinfection

pH	%Cl$_2$	% HOCl	%OCl
4	0.5	99.5	0
5	0	99.5	0.5
6	0	96.5	3.5
7	0	72.5	27.5
8	0	21.5	78.5
9	0	1.0	99.0
10	0	0.3	99.7

Formulation

Most disinfectants are used as aqueous solutions but some skin disinfectants contain a high concentration (60–80 per cent v/v) of ethyl or isopropyl alcohol, which contributes to the immediate biocidal action and promotes penetration of skin furrows and folds. Alcoholic solutions of formaldehyde and glutaraldehyde are not always more active than their aqueous solutions of similar strength (Willard & Alexander, 1964; Rubbo et al, 1967).

Phenolic disinfectants contain surface active agents to promote solubility of the active compounds. Quaternary ammonium compounds are also formulated with detergents but only nonionic types are compatible and the activity of the final formula must be confirmed by microbiological tests. Chlorhexidine is not used as a detergent-sanitizer but is formulated as a bactericidal skin cleanser (Lowbury & Lilly, 1973). An excess of the active agent is required to ensure that sufficient (1 per cent w/v) is available for biocidal action. The compatibility of detergents for combination with chlorine disinfectants and iodophors must also be verified. Unauthorized mixing of different disinfectants may result in inactivation.

The antibacterial spectrum of phenolic formulations is influenced by the types and amounts of phenols used. Some are more active against Gram-positive and others against Gram-negative bacteria.

Organic matter

Soluble, colloidal or particulate organic material, such as blood, serum, pus, faeces and oils or fats, which may be introduced into diluted solutions by the articles being treated, inactivates all disinfectants to some extent (Gélinas & Goulet, 1983). The effect is greatest with quaternary ammonium compounds, which are adsorbed to colloidal and particulate material, and halogen disinfectants, which are converted to inactive chloride or iodide by oxidative reactions. Phenolics are less susceptible to inactivation by organic matter but those prepared from synthetic alkyl and halogenated phenols are affected more seriously than are the crude coal tar formulations containing cresols and xylenols. Aldehydes are partially inactivated by reaction with proteins. Allowance must be made for inactivation by soiling materials when determining the concentration of a disinfectant to be recommended for use on objects or surfaces that have not been cleaned.

Cellulosic and synthetic materials

Cotton materials and a wide range of synthetics may come in contact with disinfectants in the form of cotton wool, gauze dressing, cleaning cloths, sponges or mops and plastic containers for storage or use of the disinfectant. Both types of material reduce the activity of the surface active quaternary ammonium compounds and chlorhexidine by adsorption but other disinfectants are not affected significantly (Maurer, 1985).

CONTAMINATED DISINFECTANTS

This term may appear to be a contradiction. However, a large quantity of published literature concerning the survival and growth of bacteria in diluted disinfectants, including reports of associated hospital-acquired infections, had accumulated over three decades (Lowbury, 1951; Bean & Farrell, 1967; Bassett, 1971b). The types of microorganisms and disinfectants involved and the likely causes of contamination are now well known. However, despite widespread dissemination of information and advice, the problem continues to occur (Barry et al, 1984; Newman et al, 1984; Sautter et al, 1984; Panlilio et al, 1992). The problem is avoidable if recommended precautions, which are set out in Table 11.3, are taken.

Table 11.3 Bacterial contamination of disinfectants

Causes	Remedies
Inaccurate dilution (Maurer, 1985)	Give clear instructions for preparation
Contaminated water used for preparing dilutions (Guinness & Levey, 1976; Morris et al, 1976; Wishart & Riley, 1976)	Check bacteriological quality of distilled or deionized water
Unclean containers (Cockcroft et al, 1965; Burdon & Whitby, 1967; Thomas et al, 1972; Ayliffe et al, 1993)	Avoid 'topping up'; discard unused solution, wash and sterilize or disinfect bottles or other containers before refilling with freshly prepared solution
Incompatible containers, soaps, detergents, hard water (Maurer, 1985)	Consult disinfectant manufacturer about compatibilities
Unsuitable closures (Lowbury, 1951; Anderson & Keynes, 1958; Linton & George, 1966; Simmons & Gardner, 1969)	Do not use cork stoppers or caps with cork or plastic liners
Unfavourable pH of solution (Bassett, 1971a; Ayliffe et al, 1993)	Check pH of solution (e.g. with QAC, chlorhexidine, sodium hypochlorite)
Stale solution (Maurer, 1985)	Prepare solutions daily
Inactivation by organic matter, cotton or plastics (Kundsin & Walter, 1957; Plotkin & Austrian, 1958; Malizia et al, 1960; Lee & Fialkow, 1961; Maurer, 1985)	Prevent or allow for inactivation by rayon, cotton wool or gauze swabs, cotton mops and synthetic sponges, brushes or mops
Recommended concentration very low (e.g. 0.02% chlorhexidine for bladder irrigation)	Purchase sterile solution

Contamination is most often encountered in dilute solutions of quaternary ammonium compounds, chlorhexidine, synthetic phenolic disinfectants and in creams or emulsions containing these compounds. However, contamination of an iodophor with *P. aeruginosa* during production has been reported (Berkelman et al, 1984). The contaminants, which are invariably Gram-negative bacilli, include *P. aeruginosa*, *B. cepacia* and species of *Proteus*, *Klebsiella*, *Alcaligenes*, *Serratia* and *Enterobacter*. The microorganisms are opportunistic

pathogens, common in hospital environments, which may cause serious or fatal illness in patients who are abnormally susceptible to infection as a result of natural disorders of the immune system or medical treatment. If they are introduced into the solution during preparation or use, their non-exacting nutritional requirements enable them to multiply, producing cell populations up to 10^7/ml within 2 days at room temperature in stale water or disinfectants. A strain of *P. aeruginosa* was found to utilize benzalkonium chloride as a carbon source when the solution was buffered with ammonium acetate, which served as a nitrogen source (Adair et al, 1969). Unused solutions in stock bottles may become contaminated as well as those that have been used. Dilute solutions of some disinfectants at the concentration required (e.g. 0.02 per cent w/v chlorhexidine) are now available commercially in suitable volumes for a single use. Chlorhexidine and quaternary ammonium disinfectants are sterilized by autoclaving. Skin swabs impregnated with a QAC solution are stable to gamma radiation but chlorhexidine solutions are decomposed by this process.

IN-USE TEST

The simple In-use test described by Maurer (1985) should be used regularly in hospitals to detect heavy contamination of disinfectants before they cause infection of patients. A 1 ml sample of the solution to be tested is added to 9 ml of a suitable diluent which contains an appropriate inactivator for the type of disinfectant. Ten drops, each of 0.02 ml volume, of the diluted sample are placed on each of two nutrient agar plates; one is incubated at 37°C for 3 days and the other at room temperature for 7 days. Five or more colonies on either plate indicate a problem that requires investigation. The method is illustrated in Figure 11.2.

Contamination usually results from faults in the preparation or use of the disinfectant. The type or brand should not be changed unless a fault cannot be found. A pass result in the In-use test demonstrates that the liquid disinfectant is unlikely to be a reservoir of infection but it does not prove that the articles that were treated by it have been disinfected. The test should be performed frequently when a new product or method of use has been

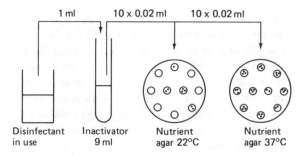

1 ml   10 x 0.02 ml   10 x 0.02 ml

Disinfectant   Inactivator   Nutrient   Nutrient
in use   9 ml   agar 22°C   agar 37°C

Fig. 11.2 Diagram of procedure of an In-use test for detecting bacterial multiplication in a chemical disinfectant.

introduced into the hospital policy, but the intervals may be extended when confidence in a product and its correct use has been established.

EVALUATION OF DISINFECTANTS

The complete profile of a chemical disinfectant includes information about the types and species of susceptible microorganisms, the influence of organic matter and other materials or conditions of use on its performance, and advice concerning any adverse effects on materials or personnel. These aspects have already been discussed; the types of microbiological tests that are used to investigate the rate of biocidal action and determine effective concentrations of a disinfectant for use will be outlined in this section. Chemical disinfectants cannot be evaluated on the basis of the quantity of active agent because this does not allow for changes in biocidal activity that may result from interaction with other components of the formulation or from the influence of dilution, pH, organic matter and other materials.

Microbiological tests require technical skill, combined with regular practice, and should be performed only in manufacturers' quality control laboratories, authorized independent laboratories or the laboratory of a regulatory authority. Disinfectant testing in hospitals should be limited to performance of the In-use test described earlier in this chapter.

All disinfectants intended for use on inanimate objects, intact skin or mucous membranes must be tested for biocidal action; reversible growth inhibition (biostasis) has no relevance to the evaluation of disinfectants.

Expression of disinfectant concentrations

As all tests are performed on one or more specified concentrations of the disinfectant and the recommendations for its use are stated in terms of concentration and time, it is important that the different ways in which concentrations (or dilutions) may be expressed are understood.

Per cent weight/weight (w/w)

The available chlorine content of a powdered chlorine disinfectant, in a pure state or mixed with inactive substances, is expressed as grams per 100 g of the powder. The concentration of alcohol in an alcohol-water mixture may also be expressed as per cent w/w. The commonly recommended concentration of 70 per cent ethyl alcohol originally referred to w/w; 70 per cent w/w is equivalent to 77 per cent v/v and 80 per cent v/v is recommended for most uses.

Per cent weight/volume (w/v)

The concentration of aldehydes, chlorhexidine and QACs is expressed as per cent w/v (grams of active agent per 100 ml of solution). This method should be used for concentrated stock solutions and also for use-dilutions. If a 20 per cent w/v chlorhexidine stock solution is diluted by a factor of 1 in 200 v/v, the concentration in the diluted solution is 0.1 per cent w/v.

Per cent volume/volume (v/v)

Phenolic formulations and other disinfectants which contain several active ingredients are diluted by volume. The dilution factor may be expressed as per cent v/v, 1 in X or 1:X. Per cent v/v refers to ml of concentrated solution per 100 ml of diluted solution. One in X means that 1 ml of the concentrated solution is made up to a total volume of X ml. One:X means that 1 ml of the concentrated solution is added to X ml of diluent, making a total volume of X + 1 ml. The label on a diluted solution should identify the original solution and indicate which method has been used to express the dilution.

The calculations involved in the preparation of dilute solutions may be tedious or time-consuming.

The following formula may be helpful: if the concentrated solution contains X per cent (w/v or v/v) of the active substance and a more dilute solution containing Y per cent is required, y ml of the concentrated solution should be measured and diluted to a final volume of x ml. For example, if X is 10 per cent w/v and 1 per cent is desired, 1 ml of X would be made up to a total volume of 10 ml.

Bactericidal tests

A bactericidal test must include the following sequence of steps:

1. The test organism is exposed to a suitable concentration of the disinfectant
2. Samples are taken at specified times and added immediately to a diluent or culture medium containing the appropriate disinfectant inactivator
3. The treated samples are cultured for surviving microorganisms.

General purpose disinfectants are subjected to tests against selected Gram-positive and Gram-negative species by methods that are officially recognized or recommended by the regulatory authority. The following description of reagents and techniques has general application. A more detailed description of some standard tests will then be presented.

Test organisms

Specified strains of *S. aureus*, *P. aeruginosa*, *Proteus vulgaris* and *E. coli* are usually recommended. A single species, or one Gram-positive and one Gram-negative species, may be selected if a preliminary bactericidal or bacteriostatic screening test is carried out to ascertain which is most resistant to the disinfectant to be tested. Other species or strains of bacteria that are causing contamination or infection in a hospital may be included.

Preparation of inoculum

The test organisms are preserved as freeze-dried (lyophilized) cultures in sealed glass ampoules.

These are opened, as required, to inoculate nutrient agar slopes which are incubated for 24 hours. The slopes may be kept in the refrigerator for one month as working stock cultures. A synthetic broth (Wright & Mundy, 1960) is recommended for preparing a series of daily subcultures to be used in the tests. Any freshly prepared culture from the fifth to the fifteenth in a series may be used in a test.

The 24 hour broth culture may be used without further treatment; however, it is usually filtered, if necessary, to remove slime and centrifuged to eliminate remaining constituents of the culture medium. The washed bacteria are resuspended in hard water (342 p.p.m. hardness) to which autoclaved yeast or serum may be added to simulate dirty conditions of use. Finally, the suspension is shaken with glass beads on a Vortex mixer and a viable count is set up immediately before performing the test.

Suspension tests and surface tests

The suspension of bacteria may be added directly to the disinfectant or dried on small carriers made from glass, stainless steel or porcelain, as appropriate to the articles or surfaces on which the disinfectant will be used. Although suspension tests may favour the disinfectant because the bacteria are uniformly exposed, they give the most reproducible results. The level of challenge can be adjusted to represent the conditions of use by varying the size of the inoculum and the type and amount of organic matter included. In a capacity test (Cantor & Shelanski, 1951), the disinfectant is challenged repeatedly by successive additions of the bacterial suspension until its capacity to kill has been exhausted.

Surface disinfection tests are more realistic than are suspension tests in simulating the conditions of use but the reagents and conditions are more difficult to standardize and the results are less reproducible. A serious disadvantage of surface disinfection tests is that they do not distinguish between bactericidal action and the removal of bacteria from the carriers during immersion in the disinfectant, diluent or inactivator. Controlling the number of bacteria exposed to the disinfectant is also difficult.

Disinfectant inactivators

The validity of a disinfectant test depends on immediate termination of the bactericidal action in samples which have been taken for detecting or enumerating surviving bacteria. It is also necessary to prevent bacteriostatic action in the recovery medium by the small amount of disinfectant that is carried over by the sample. If the survivors are to be assayed by plate counts, the appropriate inactivator is added to the diluent that is used to prepare dilutions of the sample for counting. The recovery medium contains the inactivator if the samples are added to it directly.

A nonionic detergent, such as polysorbate 80 (Tween 80) may be used, alone at a high concentration or at a lower concentration in combination with lecithin, to inactivate quaternary ammonium compounds, chlorhexidine and substituted (synthetic) phenolic compounds. Egg lecithin or soya bean lecithin of 90 per cent purity should be used; it is insoluble in water but may be dispersed by mixing with the warm detergent and added before the solution is made up to volume. Lecithin produces cloudiness in the medium which may interfere with the detection of growth by turbidity.

Sodium thiosulfate inactivates chlorine and iodine disinfectants but is inhibitory to staphylococci; the concentration in the recovery medium should not exceed 0.1 per cent w/v (Kayser & van der Ploeg, 1965; Gross et al, 1973). Green & Litsky (1974) added 0.1 per cent sodium sulfite to an agar medium and found it less toxic than is thiosulfate to the bacteria. However, low concentrations of chlorine and iodine are inactivated by the proteins in nutrient broth, without the need for addition of a specific inactivator (MacKinnon, 1974).

Disinfectants containing formaldehyde or glutaraldehyde are difficult to inactivate because the excess sodium bisulfite that is required inhibits growth of bacteria and germination of spores. Glycine (1 per cent w/v) was superior to other inactivators of glutaraldehyde which were tested by Gorman & Scott (1976). However, Cheung & Brown (1982) found that 1 per cent glycine failed to inactivate 0.5 per cent w/v alkaline glutaraldehyde and recommended that a glycine concentration of at least 2 per cent w/v should be used

to inactivate 2 per cent glutaraldehyde effectively.

Every test must include controls to demonstrate that the disinfectant has been inactivated and that the inactivator does not kill or inhibit the test organism.

Preparation of disinfectant

The concentrations or dilutions of the disinfectant to be tested may be based on the manufacturer's recommendations for use but a preliminary trial is usually required to determine a suitable range for testing. The solutions should be prepared on the day of the test unless the effect of ageing is to be investigated. Distilled water or WHO standard hard water (342 p.p.m.) is used for preparing the solutions; tap water is unsuitable because it contains chemicals which may precipitate some disinfectants (e.g. chlorhexidine).

Recovery of surviving bacteria

The medium used to culture bacteria that have survived exposure to the disinfectant, but have probably been damaged, must be especially favourable for growth and free from traces of inhibitory substances. A good quality meat broth or nutrient agar is commonly used. A non-toxic inactivator (e.g. a nonionic detergent) may be included in a liquid recovery medium. A low incubation temperature (32°C) may increase the number of survivors recovered. The cultures should be incubated for 48 hours.

The killing of all the microorganisms added to the disinfectant cannot be proven. Bactericidal tests may be designed to follow the killing process by plate counts until the dilutions yield counts that are no longer accurate. A reduction of 99.9999 per cent (six logarithms) of the inoculum can be determined provided the initial bacterial count was at least 10^9 per ml of disinfectant. If this level is reached within 30 minutes, the performance is usually deemed to be satisfactory. A death rate curve may be prepared by plotting a series of survivor counts against the times at which the samples were taken.

An alternative system uses the Most Probable Number (MPN) method of estimating the number of viable bacteria. An equal volume of the sample (e.g. 0.02 ml) is added to each tube in a set of replicates containing the liquid recovery medium. When some positive and some negative cultures are observed in a set, it is probable that the volume of sample added to each positive tube contained an average of one survivor. The per cent kill can be calculated from the number of bacteria added to the disinfectant. The MPN method is more sensitive than are plate count methods for detecting the end point but it does not measure the progress of the bactericidal action. A death rate curve cannot be prepared by this method but the overall reduction can be calculated.

British Standard quantitative suspension tests

The first British Standard quantitative suspension test was designed for the evaluation of the QACs and published in 1960 (BS 3286). The performance of this test is illustrated in Figure 11.3. It was designed when the necessity to use disinfectant inactivators in order to distinguish bactericidal action from the high level of bacteriostatic activity that is characteristic of dilute QACs was first appreciated. The test is applicable to other bactericides, such as chlorhexidine and synthetic phenolics, and also to tests for sporicidal action if the contact times are extended. The inactivator for these disinfectants contains 2 per cent lecithin and 3 per cent nonionic detergent (e.g. polysorbate 80). A protocol for controls to demonstrate that inactivation has been achieved and that the inactivator itself is not bacteriostatic is included. The test may be performed with or without the inclusion of an organic matter challenge and on suspensions of selected Gram-positive and Gram-negative bacteria, as appropriate to the intended use of the product to be tested. If a series of samples is taken from a dilution of the disinfectant containing 5×10^8 to 5×10^9 bacteria per ml at the start of the test, a death rate curve may be prepared from the colony counts on the agar-containing recovery medium and reduction factors up to 10^6 (99.9999 per cent kill) can be verified.

The test for quaternary ammonium disinfectants was revised in 1984 (BS 6471). The aim is to determine the antimicrobial value of QAC-containing formulations as the greatest dilution (lowest concentration) of the product that, under the described test conditions, will reduce the microbial population to a colony count not greater than 0.01 per cent of that in the control. The principle of the test is the same as in the original Standard but a single test organism (*E. coli* ATCC 11229, NCIB

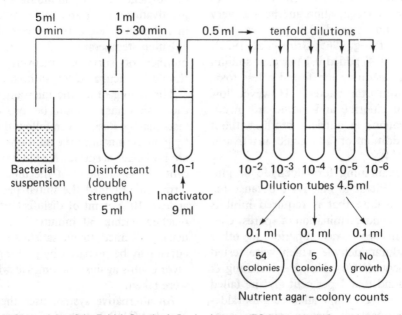

Fig. 11.3 Diagram of procedure of the British Standards Institution test (BS 3286, 1960) for evaluation of disinfectants by a quantitative suspension test.

9517) and a single contact time of 600 ± 5 seconds are specified. The challenge medium is a diluted broth culture of the test organism to which an equal volume of horse serum has been added. One ml is added to 9 ml of each dilution of the disinfectant and also to two control tubes containing 9 ml diluent alone. At the end of the exposure period, 1 ml of each mixture is added to 9 ml of inactivator and the surviving bacteria are counted as colony-forming units on agar plates. If the potency of the product to be tested is not known, a series of dilutions is tested to determine the dilution that will achieve the objective of reducing the colony count to 0.01 per cent of the control. An amendment to BS 6471 concerns the standards of repeatability and reproducibility of the test. The performance of the product is compared with standard dilutions of dodecyldimethyl-2-phenoxyethyl-ammonium bromide (75 mg/l and 125 mg/l), the reference QAC.

Kelsey-Sykes test (Kelsey & Maurer, 1974)

The Kelsey-Sykes test is a triple challenge capacity test, designed to determine concentrations of a disinfectant that will be effective in clean and dirty conditions. The disinfectant is challenged by three successive additions of a bacterial suspension;

during the course of the test, which takes just over 30 minutes to perform, the concentration of the disinfectant is reduced by half and organic matter (autoclaved yeast cells) builds up to a final concentration of 0.5 per cent (dry weight). Thus it simulates conditions that are relevant to many uses in hospitals and laboratories. A single test organism may be selected from *S. aureus* NCTC 4163, *P. aeruginosa* NCTC 6749, *P. vulgaris* NCTC 4635 and *E. coli* NCTC 8196 by comparing the minimum inhibitory concentration of the disinfectant for each organism. *P. aeruginosa* NCTC 6749 is usually most resistant to chlorhexidine and QACs but *S. aureus* NCTC 4163 may be more resistant to phenolics. BS 6905 (1987, 1993) gives the test details. Figure 11.4 illustrates the procedure.

The three sets of five replicate cultures corresponding to each challenge are incubated at 32°C for 48 hours and growth is assessed by turbidity. Sets that contain two or more negative cultures are recorded as a negative result. The disinfectant passes at the dilution tested if negative results are obtained after the first and second challenges. The third challenge is not included in the pass/fail criterion but positive cultures serve as an inbuilt control, showing that the recovery medium is capable of growing small numbers of bacteria which have actually been exposed to the disinfectant. If

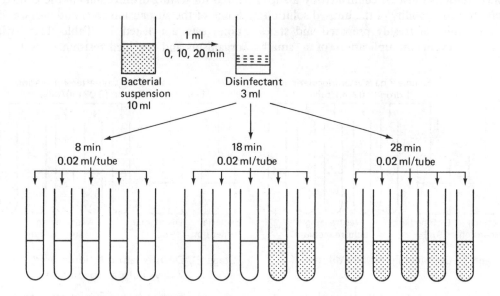

Fig. 11.4   Diagram of procedure of the Kelsey-Sykes capacity test for general disinfectants (Kelsey & Maurer, 1974).

Table 11.4 Specimen result of a Kelsey-Sykes test on a clear soluble phenolic with *P. aeruginosa* as test organism in the presence of yeast (dirty conditions)

Concentration (% v/v)	Inoculum (count per ml)	Challenge No. 1	2	3	Result
1.0	2×10^9	+++++	+++++	+++++	Fail
1.5	2×10^9	----+	--+++	+++++	Pass
2.0	2×10^9	-----	-----	----+	Pass

there are no positive cultures after the third challenge, a lower concentration of the disinfectant should be tested.

In product development tests, three concentrations of the disinfectant should be run simultaneously and separate tests are required for each organism in both clean and dirty conditions. All the tests must be repeated on three separate days with freshly prepared bacterial suspensions and freshly diluted disinfectant, and all of the tests must be successful. Specimen results are shown in Table 11.4.

Test for Stability and Long-term Effectiveness (Maurer, 1969)

Recommended concentrations based on the Kelsey-Sykes test apply only to freshly prepared solutions but if the solutions are likely to be kept for more than 24 hours, the effectiveness of these concentrations must be confirmed by a supplementary test for stability of the unused solution and for the ability of freshly prepared and stale solutions to prevent multiplication of a small

number of bacteria that may have survived the short-term exposure. *P. aeruginosa* NCTC 6749 is used as the test organism.

Sufficient disinfectant solution is prepared for two tests. One portion is inoculated immediately and tested for growth after holding for 7 days at room temperature. The other portion is kept at room temperature for 7 days and then inoculated with a freshly prepared suspension of test organism. It is also tested for growth 7 days after inoculation. If growth is detected, a higher concentration of the disinfectant must be tested in the same way. The test for stability and long-term effectiveness is illustrated in Figure 11.5.

AOAC disinfectant tests

Methods approved by the Association of Official Analytical Chemists (AOAC) are officially recognized for testing disinfectants in the United States. Some of the suspension tests and surface disinfection tests are listed in Table 11.5, with test organisms and specified resistance levels.

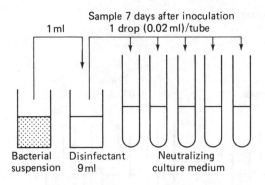
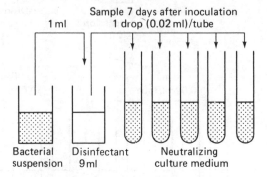

Fig. 11.5 Diagram of procedure in Maurer's test for stability and long-term effectiveness of chemical disinfectants (Maurer, 1969).

Table 11.5 Approved tests of the Association of Official Analytical Chemists (Beloian 1995)

Name of test	Type of test	Test organisms	Resistance standard
Phenol coefficient methods	Suspension	*S.* Typhi ATCC 6539 *S. aureus* ATCC 6538 *P. aeruginosa* ATCC 15442	Phenol, 1:90, 1:100 Phenol, 1:60, 1:70 Phenol, 1:80, 1:90
Hard surface carrier test methods	Surface (disposable glass carriers)	*S.* Choleraesuis ATCC 10708 *S. aureus* ATCC 6538 *P. aeruginosa* ATCC 15442	As above
Chlorine (available) germicidal equivalent concentration	Suspension (capacity test)	*S.* Typhi ATCC 6539 and/or *S. aureus* ATCC 6538	Sodium hypochlorite 200, 100 & 50 p.p.m. available chlorine
Sporicidal activity	Surface (porcelain cylinders, silk suture loops)	*B. subtilis* ATCC 19659 *C. sporogenes* ATCC 3584	H chloric acid, 2.5N
Tuberculocidal activity	Surface (porcelain cylinders)	*M. smegmatis* PRD No. 1 (presumptive test) *M. bovis* (BCG) (confirmative test)	Phenol, 1:50, 1:75
Fungicidal activity	Suspension (conidia)	*T. mentagrophytes* (e.g. ATCC 9533)	Phenol, 1:60, 1:70

Phenol coefficient methods

The principle of the phenol coefficient test is derived from the Rideal-Walker test which, when it was introduced in 1908, had the distinction of being the earliest quantitative test for evaluation of the coal tar phenolic disinfectants in use at that time. However, with a single test organism, no provision for neutralization of bacteriostatic effects and no organic matter challenge, the Rideal-Walker test was inadequate for the evaluation of QACs and other disinfectants which exert bacteriostatic activity in high dilution. The AOAC test takes account of these deficiencies by the addition of two test organisms which are better representatives than is the original *Salmonella* Typhi of causative agents of infection today, and by the inclusion of disinfectant inactivators in the recovery medium. Organic matter is limited to the proteins and peptones in nutrient broth. 'Letheen broth' containing inactivators lecithin (0.7 g/l) and polysorbate 80 (5 g/l) is the usual recovery medium but nutrient broth or thioglycollate broth (also with inactivators) may be used. In separate tests, the bacterial cultures are added to standard dilutions of pure phenol and several dilutions of the disinfectant that is being tested. After contact times of 5, 10 and 15 minutes, samples are trans-

ferred to the recovery medium by a standard wire loop. When the positive and negative cultures have been recorded, the result of the test is expressed as a phenol coefficient, calculated by dividing the denominator expressing the greatest dilution (lowest concentration) of the disinfectant that kills the test inoculum in 10 minutes but not in 5 minutes by the dilution of phenol that gives the same result. For example, if a 1:350 dilution of the product matches the performance of a 1:90 dilution of phenol, the phenol coefficient would be 350/90 = 3.89, reported as 3.9.

Hard surface carrier test methods

In order to confirm the efficiency of a disinfectant dilution derived from the phenol coefficient test in practice, a use-dilution surface disinfection test must be performed. Three test organisms are used, *S.* Typhi being replaced by *S.* Choleraesuis. The disposable (single use) borosilicate glass carriers are prepared for use by first rinsing in water and ethyl alcohol. They are then immersed in water and sterilized by autoclaving. The carriers are cooled before immersion in one of the bacterial cultures. The inoculated cylinders are drained on a filter paper mat and dried at 37°C for 40 minutes before the test is begun. They are then added singly to tubes containing the disinfectant dilution. After a contact time of 10 minutes, each is transferred to the appropriate recovery medium and incubated for the prescribed time. A result showing no growth in all 10 tubes confirms the result of the phenol coefficient test. If any carrier produces growth, the test must be repeated using a lower dilution (higher concentration) of the test disinfectant.

Chlorine (available) germicidal equivalent concentration

The test for chlorine (available) germicidal equivalent concentration applies specifically to the use of chlorine-based disinfectants on previously cleaned, nonporous surfaces. Alone among the AOAC repertoire, it is a capacity test in which a volume of the disinfectant is challenged by successive additions of the test cultures, *S.* Typhi or *S. aureus*. The test is carried out by making, in turn, ten successive additions of the test culture to each of three standard solutions of sodium hypochlorite at concentrations 200, 100 and 50 p.p.m. available chlorine. One minute after each addition, a sample is transferred to the subculture medium and the next addition is made, 1.5 minutes after the preceding one. The disinfectant, at the recommended concentration, is then tested in the same way. For equivalence in disinfecting activity to 200 p.p.m. available chlorine, the product must yield negative cultures in the same number of consecutive tubes in the subculture series as does the 200 p.p.m. standard. The same applies to the 100 p.p.m. and 50 p.p.m. standards. The validity of the tests depends on the resistance of the test culture being such that the 50 p.p.m. standard yields at least one negative culture and the 200 p.p.m. standard yields one positive culture.

Sporicidal activity

The sporicidal test utilizes two species of spore-forming bacteria, one being aerobic and the other anaerobic (see Table 11.5). Each is dried on 30 silk suture loops and 30 porcelain cylinders, making 120 carriers in all. The spores should survive 2–20 minutes in the standard (2.5 N)

hydrochloric acid. The inoculated carriers are added in six groups of five to separate tubes of the disinfectant under test and transferred individually after a contact time of 2 minutes to the appropriate subculture medium. They are incubated at 37°C for 21 days. If no growth has occurred after this time, the tubes are heated at 80°C for 20 minutes and re-incubated for a further three days. A claim for sporicidal activity is supported if there are no more than two out of 120 positive cultures; sterilization can be claimed only if all cultures from the two test spores on both types of carriers are negative. If the test is carried out on a gaseous disinfectant, the dried inoculated carriers should be rehydrated by immersion for a short time in water before testing.

Tuberculocidal activity

The tuberculocidal test is performed in two parts, a presumptive test against *Mycobacterium smegmatis* then a confirmatory test in which *Mycobacterium bovis* (BCG) is the test organism. In the first test, 30 or more inoculated porcelain cylinders are separately immersed for 10 minutes in each of three widely spaced disinfectant dilutions; the per cent of negative cultures obtained from each dilution is plotted on a graph and the best-fitting line is extrapolated to 99 per cent kill. The corresponding dilution is used in the confirmative test. In the latter, groups of ten inoculated carriers are tested against standard phenol dilutions and the product that is being tested for a contact time of 10 minutes. All carriers from 1:50 phenol should yield negative cultures and those from 1:75 phenol should produce positive cultures. The maximum dilution (lowest concentration) of the disinfectant that kills *M. bovis* (BCG) on ten carriers is considered to be safe for tuberculocidal disinfection.

Fungicidal activity

Microconidia produced by *Trichophyton mentagrophytes*, of concentration 5×10^6 per ml, are used in the fungicidal test. They should survive a 10 minute exposure to 1:70 dilution of phenol and be killed by the 1:60 dilution. The spores are added to dilutions of the fungicide for 5, 10 and 15 minutes and the highest dilution that kills them in 10 minutes would be expected to disinfect inanimate surfaces contaminated with pathogenic fungi.

The foregoing descriptions of some of the AOAC tests do not contain the details of the preparation of the test cultures, culture media, apparatus and procedure that must be strictly observed in the performance of these tests (Beloian, 1995).

Virucidal tests

The requirements for laboratory testing of virucides are discussed by Chen (1991). These include the careful control of variables, such as times and temperatures, and the implementation of dilution or other procedures to overcome the problem of residual toxicity of the disinfectant in samples tested for inactivation. Of course, the complete inactivation of viruses cannot be tested because different (and unknown) numbers of viruses initiate infection in different hosts. For practical reasons, prototype viruses, e.g. representing the lipophilic or hydrophilic groups, are generally selected for testing. Above all, the results should be interpretable in terms of the practical applications of the virucide.

Suspension tests have generally been favoured because many viruses are inactivated by drying but interest in surface disinfection tests has been stimulated by concern about viral infections which may be spread by hands or fomites. A surface test has been designed by Tyler & Ayliffe (1987) and used to compare the action of several disinfectants against herpes simplex 1 virus and poliovirus (Tyler et al, 1990). In this test, the virus is grown in a monolayer of baby hamster kidney cells, incubated in Eagle's medium supplemented with tryptose phosphate broth and calf serum. After separation of the virus from the cells by sonication and centrifugation, $10\mu l$ amounts of the suspension containing 3×10^9 plaque-forming units, are dried on coverslips. An initial count is set up and the inoculated coverslips are placed singly in 5 ml of disinfectant for 1, 5 or 10 minutes. After removal, the coverslips are rinsed briefly, sonicated to disperse the virus evenly, and assayed. In a preliminary study, the results of the test showed that 2 per cent w/v alkaline glutaraldehyde and 70 per cent v/v ethanol or isopropanol were effective against herpes virus within one minute. Hypochlorite (2500 p.p.m. available chlorine) and povidone-iodine (1 per cent available iodine) were slower, requiring 5 minutes, and disinfectants containing phenols, QACs, or chlorhexidine were ineffective in 10 minutes. Alcohols above 95 per cent were also ineffective.

This surface test has also been used to investigate the action of alcohol and glutaraldehyde on cell-free and cell-associated HIV, in the presence or absence of dried serum (Hanson et al, 1989). The cell-free virus was inactivated by 1 per cent and 2 per cent (w/v) glutaraldehyde within one minute; 2 per cent glutaraldehyde inactivated it in serum in 2 minutes but 1 per cent was ineffective. Neither 70 per cent v/v industrial methylated spirits nor ethyl alcohol was effective and could not be recommended for surface disinfection of HIV. While 2 per cent glutaraldehyde was effective, it should not be allowed to decrease in concentration or become stale.

Springthorpe et al (1986) and Lloyd-Evans et al (1986) carried out a collaborative study, using suspension and surface tests, of the action of several common disinfectants on rotaviruses. The disinfectants were challenged by the inclusion of peptone or diluted infant faeces in the virus suspension. After exposure to the disinfectant for one minute, the action was stopped by dilution and surviving virus was estimated by plaque assay. Glass, stainless steel, smooth and rough plastic discs were inoculated with the virus suspension for the surface disinfection test. The time of contact was 1 minute and, after addition of a broth diluent to stop the action, the virus was eluted by sonication and assayed. In a comparison of results from the two tests, 2 per cent glutaraldehyde, 70 per cent ethyl alcohol and 70 per cent isopropyl alcohol were effective against rotavirus but the other disinfectants tested were unreliable or ineffective in the suspension test. Glutaraldehyde was also effective in the surface disinfection test but the alcohols were ineffective.

POLICIES FOR DISINFECTION IN HOSPITALS

The concept of formulating a policy for the selection and application of chemical disinfectants in hospitals was introduced by Kelsey & Maurer

(1967). Their recommendations have been frequently repeated and reemphasized (Maurer, 1985; Ayliffe et al, 1993) and are now widely practised to achieve the benefits of greater efficiency and reduced cost (Rutala, 1996).

The development of a policy to suit a particular hospital is initiated by conducting a comprehensive survey of all departments and preparing a list of products that are currently purchased and the purposes for which they are used. The concentrations in use should also be noted. The list provides a basis for eliminating the use of disinfectants when:

1. Sterilization is required
2. Disinfection by hot water or steam can be carried out
3. The use of an antimicrobial agent is unnecessary.

All instruments that penetrate tissues or blood vessels, or come in contact with delicate mucous membranes or wounds, must be sterilized. Some types of articles can be disinfected by pasteurization; this method should also be used for disinfection of manual and mechanical cleaning equipment (e.g. mops, buckets and the tanks of wet scrubbing machines) and of stock bottles when they are refilled with diluted disinfectants. Situations in which the use of a chemical disinfectant is unnecessary are exemplified by the general cleaning of the hospital environment. It has been demonstrated by Ayliffe et al (1967) and other investigators that the benefit of including an antibacterial agent in the cleaning solution is restricted to the short period of wet contact. Residual disinfectant which may remain on the floor is inactive in the dry state and does not retard the rate or decrease the level of recontamination in areas where uncontrolled movement of people and equipment occurs. Much of the equipment used in hospital wards, including infant incubators, can also be rendered safe by efficient cleaning unless it has been used by an infected patient.

The next step towards the development of a policy is to itemize the purposes for which a chemical disinfectant is required. These may be divided into three categories:

1. Disinfection of hospital equipment
2. Disinfection of the hospital environment
3. Disinfection of skin and mucous membranes.

The selection of an appropriate type of disinfectant for each purpose, and the concentration at which it should be used, can now be made. No single type is suitable for all purposes but the aim is to reduce the number of products and different concentrations to a minimum.

Disinfection of hospital equipment

A phenolic disinfectant is appropriate for decontamination of used instruments (with the exception of those which are contaminated with blood or exudates that may contain hepatitis viruses or HIV) and for use in discard jars in bacteriological laboratories. When the presence of the above viruses is considered to be a risk, a chlorine disinfectant used at a concentration of 0.5–1 per cent (5000–10 000 p.p.m.) available chlorine is recommended (e.g. disinfection of blood-stained articles that withstand the high concentration). Alkaline glutaraldehyde should be substituted for metal instruments.

Disinfection with glutaraldehyde is also recommended for endoscopic instruments, such as bronchoscopes and gastroscopes, in the short time available between the use of the same instrument for successive patients. These instruments may be sterilized in the Steris system by peracetic acid in about 20 minutes. When time is available, endoscopes may be sterilized by ethylene oxide or gas plasma. The immersion of endoscopes in 2 per cent glutaraldehyde for 3 hours is an acceptable means of sterilization, if no other alternative is available (Ayliffe et al, 1993). A weak chlorine disinfectant (125 p.p.m.) is used for infant incubators after use by an infectious infant.

Disinfection of the hospital environment

A phenolic disinfectant or a chlorine compound is suitable, depending on the types of microorganisms that are likely to be present, for disinfection of floors, walls, furniture and fittings in areas where immunodeficient or other susceptible patients are nursed and for contaminated areas in other locations. Phenolics are usually recommended but a strong chlorine preparation (5000–10 000 p.p.m.) should be used for cleaning up blood spills. Lower concentrations of available chlorine (e.g. 500 p.p.m.) are adequate for disinfecting beds, baths or taps and 200 p.p.m. is sufficient for sanitization of cleaned benches in the hospital kitchen. Ethyl alcohol, at the usual concentration of 80 per cent v/v, may be used on clean trolley tops and similar surfaces that have been physically cleaned.

Disinfection of skin and mucous membranes

Bactericidal skin cleansers containing chlorhexidine, povidone-iodine (PVP-I) or triclosan may be used for hygienic handwashing; the purpose is to kill and remove transient contaminants. Alcoholic chlorhexidine may be used as a rinse or 'rub' between patients if the hands have not been contaminated or visibly soiled.

Alcoholic chlorhexidine, alcoholic PVP-I or aqueous PVP-I are used to reduce resident skin bacteria to low levels on surgeons' hands and patients' operation sites. Povidone-iodine, which has a broader spectrum of antimicrobial action than has chlorhexidine, may be more effective for use on venepuncture sites.

Hexachlorophene skin cleanser had been widely used for neonatal antistaphylococcal skin care but usage has declined dramatically since its systemic toxicity was discovered. Chlorhexidine and triclosan are used as replacements.

Weak aqueous solutions of chlorhexidine gluconate may be used for irrigation of the bladder; alcohols are too toxic to be used on mucous membranes. Disinfection of skin and mucous membranes is discussed in Chapter 12.

Administration of a disinfection policy

The successful implementation of a disinfection policy depends on the provision of information to the staff throughout the hospital, especially persons who are responsible for putting it into practice or supervising others who do so. The responsibility for preparing dilutions should be centralized and placed under the supervision of a pharmacist. The solutions that are distributed to wards and departments should be ready for use

and clearly labelled to identify the type of disinfectant. The concentration should be stated as weight/volume (w/v) whenever possible; if this cannot be done, the identity of the concentrated solution should be stated, together with the degree of dilution by volume (v/v). All of the precautions which have been discussed in this chapter should be taken during the preparation and use of the solutions to avoid access of bacterial contaminants and prevent their multiplication. Fresh solutions should be prepared daily, whenever possible, or presterilized solutions should be used.

Selection of types and brands of disinfectants

The disinfection policy should include clear directions concerning the types and brands of products which have been selected for use. An alternative product may be nominated in the policy but changes should not be made unless they are authorized by the Infection Control Committee. Hospital staff at several levels and in many departments are subject to pressure from manufacturers' representatives to try a new product but the claims should be validated by an expert before a disinfectant that is performing satisfactorily, as indicated by regular In-use tests, is replaced. Even if In-use tests have revealed that a solution has supported growth of bacteria, the cause may be found in the methods of preparation or use and might not be due to a deficiency in the product.

It is sometimes difficult for hospital staff to interpret the information that is provided by the manufacturer to validate a new product and the advice of a microbiologist who understands the method of evaluation should be sought. The matter may be clarified easily if a standard requirement for the performance of hospital grade disinfectants is in existence. Any disinfectant which has passed the Kelsey-Sykes capacity test, conducted in an authorized testing laboratory, will give a satisfactory performance of bactericidal action at the concentrations recommended for use in clean and dirty conditions. The selection of a type or brand can then be made on the basis of other properties, such as compatibility with materials with which it may come in contact during use or the risk of harm to the user or the articles treated. Cost-effectiveness is usually the deciding factor if two products appear to be similar in other respects. It is most unwise for bacteriologists to attempt the occasional evaluation of products in hospital laboratories because special skills and regular practice are required.

REFERENCES

Adair F W, Geftic S G, Gelzer J 1969 Resistance of *Pseudomonas* to quaternary ammonium compounds 1. Growth in benzalkonium chloride solution. Applied Microbiology 18: 299–302

Anderson K, Keynes R 1958 Infected cork closures and the apparent survival of organisms in antiseptic solutions. British Medical Journal 2: 274–275

Ayliffe G A J, Coates D, Hoffman P N 1993 Chemical disinfection in hospitals, 2nd edn. Public Health Laboratory Service, London

Ayliffe G A J, Collins B J, Lowbury E J L 1966 Cleaning and disinfection of hospital floors. British Medical Journal 2: 442–445

Ayliffe G A J, Collins B J, Lowbury E J L, Babb J R, Lilly H A 1967 Ward floors and other surfaces as reservoirs of hospital infection. Journal of Hygiene 65: 515–536

Barry M A, Craven D E, Goularte T A, Lichtenberg D A 1984 *Serratia marcescens* contamination of antiseptic soap containing triclosan: implications for nosocomial infection. Infection Control 5: 427–430

Bassett D C J 1971a The effect of *p*H on the multiplication of a pseudomonad in chlorhexidine and cetrimide. Journal of Clinical Pathology 24: 708–711

Bassett D C J 1971b Common-source outbreaks. Proceedings of the Royal Society of Medicine 64: 980–986

Bassett D C J, Stokes K J, Thomas W R G 1970 Wound infection with *Pseudomonas multivorans*. A water-borne contaminant of disinfectant solutions. Lancet i: 1188–1191

Bean H S, Farrell R C 1967 The persistence of *Pseudomonas aeruginosa* in aqueous solutions of phenols. Journal of Pharmacy and Pharmacology 19 (Suppl): 183S–188S

Beloian A 1995 Disinfectants. In: Cunniff P A (ed) Official methods of analysis of AOAC International, 16th edn. AOAC International, Arlington, vol I, ch 6

Berkelman R L, Anderson R L, Davis B J et al 1984 Intrinsic bacterial contamination of a commercial iodophor solution: investigation of the implicated manufacturing plant. Applied and Environmental Microbiology 47: 752–756

Best M, Sattar S A, Springthorpe V S, Kennedy M E 1990 Efficacies of selected disinfectants against *Mycobacterium tuberculosis*. Journal of Clinical Microbiology 28: 2234–2239

Brandrick A M, Newton J M, Henderson G, Vickers J A 1967 An investigation into the interaction between iodine and bacteria. Journal of Applied Bacteriology 30: 484–487

Brown P, Rohwer R G, Gajdusek D C 1986 Newer data on the inactivation of scrapie virus or Creutzfeldt-Jakob disease virus in brain tissue. Journal of Infectious Diseases 153: 1145–1148

BS 3286 1960 Method for laboratory evaluation of disinfectant activity of quaternary ammonium compounds by suspension test procedure. British Standards Institution, London

BS 6471 1984 Determination of the antimicrobial value of QAC disinfectant formulations. British Standards Institution, London

BS 6905 1987 (R1993) British Standard Method for Estimation of concentration of disinfectants used in dirty conditions in hospitals by the modified Kelsey-Sykes test. British Standards Institution, London

van Bueren J, Simpson R A, Jacobs P, Cookson B D 1994 Survival of human immunodeficiency virus in suspension and dried onto surfaces. Journal of Clinical Microbiology 32: 571–574

Burdon D W, Whitby J L 1967 Contamination of hospital disinfectants with *Pseudomonas* species. British Medical Journal 2: 153–155

Cantor A, Shelanski H A 1951 A 'capacity' test for germicidal action. Soap and Sanitary Chemicals 27: 133–135

Chen J H S 1991 Methods of testing virucides. In: Block S S (ed) Disinfection, sterilization, and preservation, 4th edn. Lea & Febiger, Philadelphia, ch 62, p 1076

Cheung H Y, Brown M R W 1982 Evaluation of glycine as an inactivator of glutaraldehyde. Journal of Pharmacy and Pharmacology 34: 211–214

Chambon M, Bailly J-L, Peigue-Lafeuille H 1992 Activity of glutaraldehyde at low concentrations against capsid proteins of poliomyelitis type 1 and echovirus type 25. Applied and Environmental Microbiology 58: 3517–3521

Coates D 1996 Sporicidal activity of sodium dichloroisocyanurate, peroxygen and glutaraldehyde disinfectants against *Bacillus subtilis*. Journal of Hospital Infection 32: 283–294

Cockcroft W H, Roberts F J, Davis F A 1965 Contamination of bactericidal agents. Canadian Medical Association Journal 93: 820–821

Collins F M 1986 Kinetics of the tuberculocidal response by alkaline glutaraldehyde in solution and on an inert surface. Journal of Applied Bacteriology 61: 87–93

Damjanovic V 1987 What makes human immunodeficiency virus (HIV) resistant to dry heat inactivation? Journal of Hospital Infection 10: 209–211

Davies A, Bentley M, Field B S 1968 Comparison of the action of Vantocil, cetrimide and chlorhexidine on *Escherichia coli* and its spheroplasts and the protoplasts of Gram positive bacteria. Journal of Applied Bacteriology 31: 448–461

Favero M S, Carson L A, Bond W W, Petersen N J 1971 *Pseudomonas aeruginosa*: growth in distilled water from hospitals. Science 173: 836–838

Gard S 1959 Theoretical considerations in the inactivation of viruses by chemical means. Annals of the New York Academy of Sciences 83: 638–648

Gélinas P, Goulet J 1983 Neutralization of the activity of eight disinfectants by organic matter. Journal of Applied Bacteriology 54: 243–247

Gilbert R J, Watson H M 1971 Some laboratory experiments on various meat preparation surfaces with regard to surface contamination and cleaning. Journal of Food Technology 6: 163–170

Gillespie W A, Lennon G G, Linton K B, Phippen G A 1967 Prevention of urinary infection by means of closed drainage into a sterile plastic bag. British Medical Journal 3: 90–92

Gorman S P, Scott E M 1976 Evaluation of potential inactivators of glutaraldehyde in disinfection studies with *Escherichia coli*. Microbios Letters 1: 197–204

Gorman S P, Scott E M 1977 A quantitative evaluation of the antifungal properties of glutaraldehyde. Journal of Applied Bacteriology 43: 83–89

Green B L, Litsky W 1974 The use of sodium sulfite as a neutralizer for evaluating povidone-iodine preparations. Health Laboratory Science 11: 188–194

Gross A, Cofone L, Huff M B 1973 Iodine inactivating agent in surgical scrub testing. Archives of Surgery 106: 175–178

Guinness M, Levey J 1976 Contamination of aqueous dilutions of Resiguard disinfectant with *Pseudomonas*. Medical Journal of Australia 2: 392

Hanson P J V, Gor D, Jeffries D J, Collins J V 1989 Chemical inactivation of HIV on surfaces. British Medical Journal 298: 862–864

Hegna I K 1977 An examination of the effect of three phenolic disinfectants on *Mycobacterium tuberculosis*. Journal of Applied Bacteriology 43: 183–187

Holloway C E, Dean F H 1975 ^{13}C-NMR study of aqueous glutaraldehyde equilibria. Journal of Pharmaceutical Sciences 64: 1078–1079

Hugo W B 1992 Disinfection mechanisms. In: Russell A D, Hugo W B, Ayliffe G A J (eds) Principles and practice of disinfection, preservation and sterilization, 2nd edn. Blackwell Scientific Publications, Oxford, ch 9, p 187

Kayser A, van der Ploeg G 1965 Growth inhibition of staphylococci by sodium thiosulphate. Journal of Applied Bacteriology 28: 286–293

Kelsey J C, Maurer I M 1967 The choice of disinfectants for hospital use. Monthly Bulletin of the Ministry of Health 26: 110–114

Kelsey J C, Maurer I M 1974 An improved (1974) Kelsey-Sykes test for disinfectants. Pharmaceutical Journal 213: 528–530

Kimberlin R H, Walker C A, Millson G C et al 1983 Disinfection studies with two strains of mouse-passaged scrapie agent. Guidelines for Creutzfeldt-Jakob and related agents. Journal of the Neurological Sciences 59: 355–369

Kundsin R B, Walter C W 1957 Investigations of adsorption of benzalkonium chloride U.S.P. by skin, gloves, and sponges. Archives of Surgery 75: 1036–1042

Lee J C, Fialkow P J 1961 Benzalkonium chloride — source of hospital infection with Gram-negative bacteria. Journal of the American Medical Association 177: 708–710

Linton K B, George E 1966 Inactivation of chlorhexidine ('Hibitane') by bark corks. Lancet i: 1353–1355

Lloyd-Evans N, Springthorpe V S, Sattar S A 1986 Chemical disinfection of human rotavirus-contaminated inanimate surfaces. Journal of Hygiene 97: 163–173

Lowbury E J L 1951 Contamination of cetrimide and other fluids with *Pseudomonas pyocyanea*. British Journal of Industrial Medicine 8: 22–25

Lowbury E J L, Lilly H A 1973 Use of 4% chlorhexidine detergent solution (Hibiscrub) and other methods of skin disinfection. British Medical Journal 1: 510–515

Lyon B R, Skurray R 1987 Antimicrobial resistance of *Staphylococcus aureus*: genetic basis. Microbiological Reviews 51: 88–134

McGucken P V, Woodside W 1973 Studies on the mode of action of glutaraldehyde on *Escherichia coli*. Journal of Applied Bacteriology 36: 419–426

MacKinnon I H 1974 The use of inactivators in the evaluation of disinfectants. Journal of Hygiene 73: 189–195

Malizia W F, Gangarosa E J, Goley A F 1960 Benzalkonium chloride as a source of infection. New England Journal of Medicine 263: 800–802

Maris P 1995 Modes of action of disinfectants. In: Scientific and technical review. Disinfectants: actions and applications. Office International des Épizooties, Paris, 14 (1): 47–55

Martin T D M 1969 Sensitivity of the genus *Proteus* to chlorhexidine. Journal of Medical Microbiology 2: 101–108

Maurer I M 1969 A test for stability and long term effectiveness in disinfectants. Pharmaceutical Journal 203: 529–534

Maurer I M 1985 Hospital hygiene, 3rd edn. Edward Arnold, London

Miner N A, Mulberry G K, Starks A N, et al 1995 Identification of possible artifacts in the Association of Official Analytical Chemists Sporicidal Test. Applied and Environmental Microbiology 61: 1658–1660

Morris S, Gibbs M, Hansman D, Smyth N, Cosh D 1976 Contamination of aqueous dilutions of Resiguard disinfectant with *Pseudomonas*. Medical Journal of Australia 2: 110–111

Munton T J, Russell A D 1970 Effect of glutaraldehyde on protoplasts of *Bacillus megaterium*. Journal of General Microbiology 63: 367–370

Munton T J, Russell A D 1973 Interaction of glutaraldehyde with spheroplasts of *Escherichia coli*. Journal of Applied Bacteriology 36: 211–217

Mustapha A, Liewen M B 1989 Destruction of *Listeria monocytogenes* by sodium hypochlorite and quaternary ammonium sanitizers. Journal of Food Protection 52: 306–311

Nagai I, Ogase H 1990 Absence of role for plasmids in resistance to multiple disinfectants in three strains of bacteria. Journal of Hospital Infection 15: 149–155

Newman K A, Tenney J H, Oken H A, Moody M R, Wharton R, Schimpff S C 1984 Persistent isolation of an unusual *Pseudomonas* species from a phenolic disinfectant system. Infection Control 5: 219–222

O'Flynn J D, Stickler D J 1972 Disinfectants and Gram-negative bacteria. Lancet i: 489–490

Panlilio A L, Beck-Sague C M, Siegal J D et al 1992 Infections and pseudoinfections due to povidone-iodine solution contaminated with *Pseudomonas cepacia*. Clinical Infectious Diseases 14: 1078–1083

Plotkin S A, Austrian R 1958 Bacteremia caused by *Pseudomonas* sp. following the use of materials stored in solutions of a cationic surface-active agent. American Journal of Medical Sciences 235: 621–627

Prince H N, Nonemaker W S, Norgard R C, Prince D L 1978 Drug resistance studies with topical antiseptics. Journal of Pharmaceutical Sciences 67: 1629–1631

Prindle R F 1983 Phenolic compounds: In: Block S S (ed) Disinfection, sterilization, and preservation, 3rd edn. Lea & Febiger, Philadelphia, ch 9, p 197

Rosenberg R N, White C L, Brown P et al 1986 Precautions in handling tissues, fluids, and other contaminated materials from patients with documented or suspected Creutzfeldt-Jakob disease. Annals of Neurology 19: 75–77

Rubbo S D, Gardner J F, Webb R L 1967 Biocidal activities of glutaraldehyde and related compounds. Journal of Applied Bacteriology 30: 78–87

Rubbo S D, Stratford B C, Dixson S 1960 'Self-sterilization' of chemically treated blankets. Medical Journal of Australia 2: 330–332

Russell A D 1972 Comparative resistance of R$^+$ and other strains of *Pseudomonas aeruginosa* to non-antibiotic antibacterial agents. Lancet ii: 332

Russell A D 1994 Glutaraldehyde: current status and uses. Infection Control and Hospital Epidemiology 15: 724–733

Russell A D, Furr J R 1977 The antibacterial activity of a new chloroxylenol preparation containing ethylenediamine tetraacetic acid. Journal of Applied Bacteriology 43: 253–260

Rutala W A 1996 APIC guideline for selection and use of disinfectants. American Journal of Infection Control 24: 313–342

Sagripanti J-L, Bonifacino A 1996 Comparative sporicidal effects of liquid chemical agents. Applied and Environmental Microbiology 62: 545–551

Salk J E, Gori J B 1959 A review of theoretical, experimental, and practical considerations in the use of formaldehyde for the inactivation of poliovirus. Annals of the New York Academy of Sciences 83: 609–637

Sautter R L, Mattman L H, Legaspi R C 1984 *Serratia marcescens* meningitis associated with a contaminated benzalkonium chloride solution. Infection Control 5: 223–225

Simmons N A, Gardner D A 1969 Bacterial contamination of a phenolic disinfectant. British Medical Journal 2: 668–669

Springthorpe V S, Grenier J L, Lloyd-Evans N, Sattar S A 1986 Chemical disinfection of human rotavirus: efficacy of commercially-available products in suspension tests. Journal of Hygiene 97: 139–161

Stickler D J 1974 Chlorhexidine resistance in *Proteus mirabilis*. Journal of Clinical Pathology 27: 284–287

Stickler D J, Clayton C L, Chawla J C 1987 The resistance of urinary tract pathogens to chlorhexidine bladder washouts. Journal of Hospital Infection 10: 28–39

Stickler D J, Thomas B 1980 Antiseptic and antibiotic resistance in Gram-negative bacteria causing urinary tract infection. Journal of Clinical Pathology 33: 288–296

Tamai Y, Taguchi F, Miura S 1988 Inactivation of the Creutzfeldt-Jakob disease agent. Annals of Neurology 24: 466–467

Tateishi J, Tashima T, Kitamoto T 1988 Inactivation of the Creutzfeldt-Jakob disease agent. Annals of Neurology 24: 466

Taylor D M 1986 Decontamination of Creutzfeldt-Jakob disease agent. Annals of Neurology 20: 749

Taylor D M 1991 Resistance of the ME7 scrapie agent to peracetic acid. Veterinary Microbiology 27: 19–24

Taylor D M, Fraser H, McConnell I et al 1994 Decontamination studies with the agents of bovine spongiform encephalopathy and scrapie. Archives of Virology 139: 313–326

Thomas M E M, Piper E, Maurer I M 1972 Contamination of an operating theatre by Gram-negative bacteria. Examination of water supplies, cleaning methods and wound infections. Journal of Hygiene 70: 63–73

Townsend D E, Ashdown N, Greed L C, Grubb W B 1984 Analysis of plasmids mediating gentamicin resistance in methicillin-resistant *Staphylococcus aureus*. Journal of Antimicrobial Chemotherapy 13: 347–352

Townsend D E, Greed L, Ashdown N, Grubb W B 1983 Plasmid-mediated resistance to quaternary ammonium compounds in methicillin-resistant *Staphylococcus aureus*. Medical Journal of Australia 2: 310

Tyler R, Ayliffe G A J 1987 A surface test for virucidal activity of disinfectants: preliminary study with herpes virus. Journal of Hospital Infection 9: 22–29

Tyler R, Ayliffe G A J, Bradley C 1990 Virucidal activity of disinfectants: studies with the poliovirus. Journal of Hospital Infection 15: 339–345

Willard M, Alexander A 1964 Comparison of sterilizing properties of formaldehyde-methanol solutions with formaldehyde-water solutions. Applied Microbiology 12: 229–233

Wiseman D 1971 The effect of cetyltrimethylammonium bromide on the cytochrome system of *Escherichia coli*. Journal of Pharmacy and Pharmacology 23 (Suppl): 257S–258S

Wishart M M, Riley T V 1976 Infection with *Pseudomonas maltophilia* hospital outbreak due to contaminated disinfectant. Medical Journal of Australia 2: 710–712

Wright E S, Mundy R A 1960 Defined medium for phenol coefficient tests with *Salmonella typhosa* and *Staphylococcus aureus*. Journal of Bacteriology 80: 279–280

FURTHER READING

Cremieux A, Fleurette J Methods of testing disinfectants. In: Block S S (ed) 1991 Disinfection, sterilization, and preservation, 4th edn. Lea & Febiger, Philadelphia, ch 57, p 1009

Reybrouck G Evaluation of the antibacterial and antifungal activity of disinfectants. In: Russell A D, Hugo W B, Ayliffe G A J (eds) 1992 Principles and practice of disinfection, preservation and sterilization, 2nd edn. Blackwell Scientific Publications, Oxford, ch 4, p 114

12. Disinfection of living tissue

The role of human hands in the transmission of infectious disease in hospitals and in the community was recognized before the establishment of microbiology as a science. Historical aspects have been reviewed by Laufman (1989). The role of skin bacteria, whether as transient surface contaminants or the more deeply situated indigenous resident flora, is no less important today, especially in hospitals where infected or colonized patients are the major reservoir of nosocomial infection and the hands of hospital staff are the principal mode of spread (Maki, 1989). Aspects to be covered in this chapter include the microbial flora of human skin and mucous membranes, the antimicrobial agents and formulations which may be used to remove transient surface contaminants or to reduce the resident bacteria to a safe level and the procedures that are recommended in different situations. Particular attention is given to hygienic handwashing, surgical skin disinfection and neonatal skin care in hospitals. The importance of handwashing in food hygiene and other areas of community health is included and the methods of evaluating skin disinfectants are discussed.

The roles of disinfection and antisepsis in this context need to be clarified. The term skin disinfectant should be used for preparations that are applied to intact, healthy skin to prevent the transmission of transient or resident skin bacteria from person to person or from a patient's operation site to underlying tissues. Rapid bactericidal action against a broad range of bacteria is required for skin disinfection.

Antiseptics are agents that are applied, usually in more dilute solutions, to mucous membranes or injured tissues to prevent the multiplication of microbial contaminants to a level that may cause clinical infection. This objective may be achieved by continuing bacteriostatic action if the natural host defence mechanisms are operative but bactericidal action is preferred.

MICROBIAL FLORA OF SKIN AND MUCOUS MEMBRANES

Bacteria are the major components of the microbial flora of skin and mucous membranes but fungi, protozoa and viruses may also be present. Anaerobic bacteria are found in the sebaceous follicles of the skin and are particularly prevalent on the mucous membranes lining the gastrointestinal and genital tracts. In general, the microbial flora of mucous membranes differ from skin flora in being of greater density and diversity.

Skin flora

The microbial flora of the skin consist of resident, multiplying bacteria and transient, contaminating microorganisms. Gram-positive cocci and Gram-positive rod-shaped bacteria predominate but Gram-negative rods also occur, particularly in moist skin folds, on areas subject to contamination by intestinal bacteria and on the hands.

Some of the bacterial flora on the skin are not easily classified as either resident or transient. This applies, for example, to the Gram-negative rods found on the skin of the hands. Knittle et al (1975) reported that, although Gram-negative bacteria were transient on the hands of some nurses, there was evidence for their persistence with active multiplication on the hands of others. Guenthner et al (1987) showed that, after a hygienic hand wash with soap and water, Gram-negative bacilli could be recovered from about 50 per cent of the washed hands. Furthermore, the Gram-negative bacilli were apparently not transients remaining after a single wash since they could not be removed by five consecutive hand washes. These authors proposed that the term 'transitional' be applied to those bacteria remaining on the hands after a single hygienic hand wash and requiring multiple hand washes for removal.

Resident skin flora

The criterion of resident status for a microorganism is the ability to multiply between the loosening outer layers of the epidermis or within the skin glands. Healthy sweat glands are free of microorganisms, as are their secretions until they become contaminated by bacteria on the skin surface. The inner two-thirds of hair follicles are also free of microorganisms but bacteria are found in the outer regions of the follicle and particularly around the openings where their growth is supported by the lipid-rich secretions of sebum. The sebaceous follicles harbour anaerobic bacteria (Pecora et al, 1968; Montes & Wilborn, 1970).

Microbial species are classed as major residents if they are found regularly in all persons. If restricted in distribution and found only infrequently and irregularly, they are regarded as minor residents. Major residents of the skin include species of Gram-positive cocci belonging to the genera *Staphylococcus* and *Micrococcus* and species of Gram-positive rods belonging to the genera *Corynebacterium* and *Propionibacterium*.

The coagulase-negative staphylococci are especially prominent on the skin. Among these, *Staphylococcus epidermidis* is a major and widely distributed component of skin flora. This species can act as an opportunistic pathogen causing infections associated with indwelling medical devices and prostheses. Another major resident and opportunistic pathogen, *S. hominis*, shows a preference for the axillae, arms, perineum and legs, while *S. capitis* occurs mainly on the scalp, face, neck and ears. *S. haemolyticus* may be regarded as a minor resident of the skin, occupying a variety of niches (Kloos & Schleifer, 1986). The species of *Staphylococcus* which prefers anaerobic conditions of growth, *S. saccharolyticus*, frequently inhabits the skin of the forehead and, less frequently, that of the back and arms (Evans et al, 1978). Micrococci found primarily on the skin include the yellow-pigmented species, *Micrococcus luteus* and *M. varians*.

The coryneform group of Gram-positive rods include lipophilic and non-lipophilic types. Both types inhabit the skin. *Corynebacterium* spp. occur particularly where apocrine sweat is secreted, on the scalp and skin around the eyes and in the axillae, groin and toe webs. Their growth is promoted by moisture, as can be demonstrated by experimental occlusion of the skin beneath a plastic wrapping. The penicillin-resistant species of *Corynebacterium*, *Corynebacterium jeikeium* and *C. urealyticum*, have been reported as colonizing the skin of hospitalized patients. The groin was the most frequent site of colonization but both species were also isolated from the other areas sampled, the axillae and periumbilical area of the abdominal wall. *C. jeikeium* was more prevalent in males whereas *C. urealyticum* was much more prevalent in the female patients (Soriano et al, 1988). The aerobic coryneform, *Brevibacterium epidermidis*, also contributes to the indigenous flora of the skin (Pitcher & Noble, 1978). The natural habitat of the anaerobic Gram-positive rod, *Propionibacterium acnes*, is the sebaceous follicle, where the lipid secretions and anaerobic conditions are ideal for its growth. This species is associated with acne but is also found on normal skin.

Yeasts and yeast-like fungi form part of the resident flora on cutaneous, as well as mucosal, surfaces. However, the major pathogenic yeast, *Candida albicans*, is rarely encountered on the skin unless associated with lesions or diseased skin. Yeasts which do occur commonly on cutaneous surfaces include *C. parapsilosis*, *C. glabrata*, *C. krusei* and *C. guilliermondii* (Odds, 1988). *Malassezia* spp. inhabit skin sites where their lipid requirement is supplied by lipid-rich secretions from pilosebaceous glands (Marcon & Powell, 1992).

Transient skin flora

The composition of the transient flora is not constant as it depends on the sources from which it is derived; namely, from other persons, colonized body cavities (e.g. oral cavity or intestine), inanimate objects or the environment. Some species may be opportunistic pathogens but many are nonpathogenic. *Staphylococcus aureus* is regarded as a transient contaminant on the hands which acquire it from resident sites in the nose or on the perineum, scalp or beard. *S. aureus* has been found on the hands of 29 per cent of nurses in a general hospital and 78 per cent of those in a hospital specializing in skin diseases (Ayliffe et al, 1988).

Most transient contaminants remain on the skin for a limited time only, depending on their capacity for survival and the rate of removal by friction, washing or disinfection. Gram-positive bacteria survive better than do Gram-negative bacteria. Among the latter, species of *Acinetobacter* and *Enterobacter* survive for longer than do *Escherichia coli*, *Proteus vulgaris* and *Pseudomonas aeruginosa*, whereas *Klebsiella* spp. vary in their survival ability with epidemic strains surviving better than non-epidemic strains (Casewell & Desai, 1983; Ayliffe et al, 1988).

Although the usual source of *Acinetobacter* spp. is the environment, these Gram-negative rods are also often isolated from the skin, especially of hospital inpatients (Al-Khoja & Darrell, 1979), and from the hands of hospital nurses (Guenthner et al, 1987). They are resistant to many antibiotics and an important cause of nosocomial infections e.g. bacteraemias and infections of surgical sites and the respiratory and urinary tracts.

Gram-negative rods of the family Enterobacteriaceae which are commonly recovered from the skin of the hands include *E. coli*, *Serratia marcescens* and species of the genera *Citrobacter*, *Enterobacter*, *Klebsiella* and *Proteus*. Pseudomonads, mainly *P. aeruginosa*, are also found on the hands (Guenthner et al, 1987). The skin of the perineum and groin is particularly subject to contamination by faecal flora, e.g. *E. coli* and other enteric bacteria, as well as by anaerobes such as *Clostridium perfringens*.

Viruses may occur as transient contaminants, despite their inability to replicate or survive for long outside their specific host cells. They may also resist removal by ordinary handwashing procedures (Eggers, 1989).

Flora of the mucous membranes

The indigenous flora of the throat and nasopharynx include nonhaemolytic species of *Streptococcus*, nonpathogenic species of *Neisseria* and *Corynebacterium* and coagulase-negative species of *Staphylococcus*. This area may also be the site of carriage of, or infection by, pathogenic species of each of these genera. However, the major site for the carriage of *S. aureus* is the anterior nares;

coagulase-negative staphylococci and *Corynebacterium* spp. are also found in the nose.

The oral cavity provides for an even greater diversity of microorganisms, in addition to the four major genera listed above. Included in the range are anaerobic and facultatively anaerobic Gram-positive rods of the genus *Lactobacillus*; strictly anaerobic Gram-negative rods of the genera *Bacteroides, Porphyromonas, Prevotella* and *Fusobacterium*; the anaerobic, Gram-positive *Peptostreptococcus* as well as branching, Gram-positive filamentous bacteria and fastidious Gram-negative rods, curved rods and helical forms. The anaerobic flora are particularly associated with such sites as the gingival crevices and are isolated, in mixed cultures, from dental abscesses.

The predominant yeast in the mouth is *C. albicans*, (Odds, 1988). This species may be responsible for serious mucocutaneous and systemic diseases, especially in those with impaired immunity.

In the genital tract, *Corynebacterium* spp. and coagulase-negative staphylococci are found associated with the mucous membranes in both sexes. In the post-pubertal female, anaerobic and facultatively anaerobic species of *Lactobacillus* predominate in the vagina and cervix. The lactic acid produced by these bacteria maintains a low pH in the vagina, which serves to restrict the occurrence and range of other microbial colonizers. However, acid-tolerant *C. albicans* is a common isolate and a frequent cause of vaginal discharge (Goldacre et al, 1979). In addition, the vagina supports an anaerobic flora, mainly Gram-negative bacilli and *Peptostreptococcus*. *E. coli* and the enteric streptococci (*Enterococcus*) occur less frequently as transients in this site.

BACTERICIDAL AGENTS AND FORMULATIONS

An ideal skin disinfectant would fulfil the following requirements:

1. Freedom from adverse skin reactions, including removal of lipids (perceived as dry skin), irritation, toxic or allergic dermatitis
2. Absence of dermal absorption resulting in systemic toxicity

3. Ability to penetrate crevices, skin folds or other skin structures
4. Rapid broad-spectrum action against Gram-positive and Gram-negative bacteria; activity against viruses or bacterial spores may also be desired
5. Retention of activity in the presence of skin secretions, blood, mucus or faeces
6. Residual or cumulative action due to retention of the active agent on the skin.

Although it is desirable, in the interests of efficiency and economy, to minimize the types and numbers of products that are used in a hospital or other health care facility, no single antimicrobial agent or formulation is likely to meet all of these requirements. Ethyl and isopropyl alcohol, chlorhexidine, povidone-iodine (PVP-I) and triclosan (Irgasan DP300) are the main agents in present day use for skin disinfection. They are available as aqueous solutions, alcoholic solutions or bactericidal skin cleansers. Nonmedicated soaps or detergents may be adequate for routine handwashing in situations where the presence of pathogenic microorganisms is unlikely but bactericidal agents are required in hospitals where patients who are colonized by pathogens or are abnormally susceptible to infection are nursed. Rapidly acting bactericides are also needed in microbiological laboratories. The general nature, properties and main uses of the agents listed above have been presented in Chapter 10; aspects pertaining to their use for disinfection of living tissues will be elaborated on here.

Alcohols

Ethyl and isopropyl alcohols are rapidly bactericidal to Gram-positive and Gram-negative bacteria. They inactivate mycobacteria in suspension as well as many viruses, including some from the non-enveloped (hydrophilic) group. However, ethyl alcohol at 70 per cent v/v concentration has been shown to be incapable of inactivating cell-free HIV within 10 minutes (Hanson et al, 1989). Alcohols must be diluted with sufficient water to facilitate their antimicrobial action, which is dependent on protein denaturation. This applies whether the alcohol is used as the sole disinfectant or as the solvent in a preparation of a nonvolatile bactericide. Ethyl alcohol is generally used at 70–80 per cent v/v and isopropyl alcohol at 60–70 per cent v/v. The activity of alcohols is lost on evaporation and they exert no residual effect.

Chlorhexidine

Chlorhexidine, as the digluconate salt, is generally acknowledged as a versatile and widely used skin disinfectant by virtue of its capacity for immediate, residual and cumulative action on skin bacteria, combined with low toxicity by topical application. Although its spectrum of activity does include the Gram-negative bacteria, it is slightly less active against Gram-negative than against Gram-positive bacteria; some of the Gram-negative rods have shown increased resistance to dilute aqueous solutions (see Ch. 11). Lipophilic viruses, such as respiratory syncytial virus (Platt & Bucknall, 1985), are rapidly inactivated but hydrophilic viruses are usually resistant. The bactericidal activity of chlorhexidine is not reduced by blood which may soil the surgeon's gloved hand (Lowbury & Lilly, 1974; Ulrich, 1981). It is inactivated on the skin by the use of hand creams which contain anionic detergents (Walsh et al, 1987; Benson et al, 1990).

After extensive use for two decades in the United Kingdom, other European countries and Canada, chlorhexidine was approved by the Food and Drug Administration (FDA) in the United States for use as a hygienic hand wash, surgical scrub and preoperative tincture (Rosenberg et al, 1976). Alcoholic solutions contain 0.5 to 1 per cent w/v chlorhexidine in 60 to 70 per cent isopropyl or ethyl alcohol. Aqueous solutions contain up to 4 per cent w/v chlorhexidine. Weaker solutions (0.02–0.05 per cent w/v) are used for application to mucous membranes (e.g. bladder irrigation). As the weak aqueous solutions are liable to contamination and growth of Gram-negative bacteria, such as *Proteus*, *Klebsiella*, *Pseudomonas* and *Serratia*, they should be obtained commercially as sterile products packed in volumes designed for single use. Formulations containing ethyl or isopropyl alcohol are generally more active than are aqueous solutions of similar strength. The inclusion of emollients, such as glycerol or resins, is necessary

in alcoholic solutions if they are intended for repeated use on the hands in lieu of handwashing with a bactericidal skin cleanser. Chlorhexidine is widely used as a bactericidal skin cleanser at a concentration of 4 per cent w/v for hygienic and surgical handwashing. The high concentration ensures that at least 1 per cent is available for bactericidal action. A small amount of alcohol may be included in water-based preparations to prevent growth of Gram-negative contaminants. Montefiori et al (1990) showed that both the chlorhexidine formulations they tested efficiently inactivated cell-free HIV within 15 seconds. One was a detergent formulation containing 4 per cent chlorhexidine and 4 per cent isopropyl alcohol; the other consisted of 0.5 per cent chlorhexidine in 70 per cent isopropyl alcohol with emollients. The former was also completely effective at a 1:100 dilution while the latter was effective at a 1:5 dilution. The findings indicate that, when used in accordance with manufacturers' instructions (i.e. undiluted for 15 seconds), these chlorhexidine formulations are effective for the disinfection of hands after contact with HIV-containing materials. A preparation consisting of chlorhexidine combined with silver sulfadiazine is used for topical applications.

Povidone-iodine

Povidone-iodine (PVP-I) is a water soluble powder containing 10 per cent w/w available iodine. A 10 per cent w/v solution of the powder has an available iodine content of approximately 1.0 per cent, which is released gradually as the free (elemental) iodine is used up. There may be an increase in the rate of antimicrobial activity on dilution of the 10 per cent (full-strength) solution to 1.0 − 0.1 per cent solutions because of the release of iodine from the PVP-I complex (Berkelman et al, 1982). However, Davis et al (1985) warned that dilution of PVP-I predisposes the disinfectant to significant inactivation by organic material. The broad-spectrum biocidal activity includes Gram-positive and Gram-negative bacteria, bacterial spores, lipophilic and hydrophilic viruses and yeasts (including *C. albicans*). Povidone-iodine has some sporicidal action on the skin but it is relatively slow. A detergent-based surgical scrub, containing 7.5

per cent povidone-iodine, and an aqueous antiseptic solution containing 1.0 per cent are widely used; alcoholic solutions of PVP-I are also available. The iodophor has a high level of immediate action on transient and resident skin bacteria but it lacks residual action because the iodine is inactivated by skin secretions. Cumulative action, resulting from regular use, has been demonstrated but is slightly inferior to that of chlorhexidine.

Hexachlorophene

This phenolic compound is active against Gram-positive bacteria, including *S. aureus*, but is inactive against Gram-negative bacteria and yeasts, which may grow in the emulsion. Bactericidal action on the skin is initially slow, taking up to one hour to become detectable, but residual and cumulative action is good. However, because of its neurotoxicity, hexachlorophene is now rarely used.

Triclosan

Triclosan is a diphenyl ether, known commercially as Irgasan DP300. It is active against Gram-positive bacteria and also against Gram-negative bacteria but less so against *P. aeruginosa* (O'Connor & Rubino, 1991). At bacteriostatic concentrations, triclosan prevents the uptake of essential amino acids; at bactericidal concentrations, it causes disorganization of the cytoplasmic membrane leading to leakage of the cell contents (O'Connor & Rubino, 1991). The use of triclosan in deodorants and germicidal soaps (at a 1 per cent w/v concentration) is well established (Larson, 1995). The concentration of triclosan used in antibacterial cleansers ranges from 1 per cent (Brady et al, 1990; Webster et al, 1994) to 1.5 to 2 per cent w/v (Bartzokas et al, 1987a, b). It is also formulated as a 1 per cent w/v concentration in combination with povidone-iodine at 5 per cent w/v concentration (Faogali et al, 1995).

Nonmedicated soaps and detergents

Solid and liquid soaps and synthetic anionic detergents are weak and selective in their antibacterial action, which is usually bacteriostatic. Their role in handwashing is limited to the removal of transient skin contaminants and as vehicles for bactericidal skin cleansers containing more potent disinfectants. Only nonionic or amphoteric detergents are compatible with chlorhexidine but triclosan may also be formulated with soap or with anionic detergents.

Some detergent cleansers that do not contain any potent bactericidal agents have been found to be superior to nonmedicated liquid or bar soaps for the removal of skin bacteria, achieving up to 41.5 per cent reduction of skin bacteria, compared with 81.2 per cent for a 4 per cent chlorhexidine skin cleanser (Lilly & Lowbury, 1974). An emulsion containing 6 per cent fatty components was better tolerated by nursing staff who had skin problems than a liquid soap in regular use.

ADVERSE REACTIONS TO SKIN DISINFECTANTS

The incidence of skin irritation, hypersensitivity reactions and systemic toxicity which may be associated with frequent application of antibacterial agents to skin or mucous membranes may not be assessed, and may even remain undetected, until the chemical has been in use for several years. The assessment of irritancy is subjective; for example, a trial of two batches of bar soap that were identical except for having either one or two holes punched through the centre, resulted in approximately half of the participants in the survey favouring one lot, while the rest expressed a preference for the other lot (Blank, 1969). A sensation of dry skin results from the removal of oils by detergents or alcohol. Chemical damage to the skin is manifested by reddening and soreness; it may be caused by the strongly alkaline soaps or detergents in some disinfectants. Although a successful skin disinfectant must have a low incidence of hypersensitivity reactions, it is always likely that a few individuals will be allergic to the active agent or accompanying detergents, so that alternative products should be made available to the users. Patients receiving only a single treatment before surgery are unlikely to become sensitized except by molecular iodine or, to a less extent, iodophors.

Alcohols

Ethyl, isopropyl and n-propyl alcohols are toxic

and are unsuitable for application to mucous membranes. When alcohol alone, or an alcoholic solution of another disinfectant, is intended for frequent application to the hands, the inclusion of skin conditioners is necessary. As alcohol exerts its effects on the skin by removal of the natural lipids, repetitive use leads to a sensation of dryness.

Chlorhexidine

A low potential for skin irritation and allergic sensitization is a prominent feature of chlorhexidine (Rosenberg et al, 1976; Gardner & Gray, 1983). However, there are some situations in which the use of chlorhexidine is contraindicated. Haematuria has been reported after bladder irrigation with 0.02 per cent w/v aqueous chlorhexidine but this has also occurred with other irrigating solutions and can be avoided by limiting the volume of each instillation to 25 ml (Pearman, 1971). Chlorhexidine does not delay healing when applied to wounds (Saatman et al, 1986). It should never be used in surgery on the middle ear because it may cause sensorineural deafness (Bicknell, 1971). Risks of similar magnitude are associated with brain surgery. The occurrence of sclerosing peritonitis in 11 out of 162 patients on continuous ambulatory peritoneal dialysis was reported by Junor et al (1985); this complication resulted from leakage of a small volume of the alcoholic solution into the peritoneal cavity through spraying a faulty connecting system during exchange of the bag. In 1989, Okano et al described six surgical cases in which urticaria, dyspnoea and anaphylactic shock resulted from hypersensitivity to chlorhexidine that was applied to the face, vagina or urethral orifice. Of 108 similar cases reported in Japan, nine involved anaphylactic shock; in these also, chlorhexidine had been applied to mucous membranes of the vagina or urinary bladder. However, a concentration of 0.05 per cent w/v was considered to be safe.

Povidone-iodine

Povidone-iodine has replaced strong solutions of free iodine for skin disinfection as it is less irritant and less likely to cause hypersensitive reactions. The colour of the solutions may discourage their use for handwashing but the stains can be removed from skin and textiles. Povidone-iodine has been shown to be capable of causing alteration of DNA (Wlodkowski et al, 1975) and the detergent carrier may be cytotoxic, killing leukocytes (Rodeheaver et al, 1982). All iodine preparations are absorbed percutaneously and across mucous membranes (Laufman, 1989); they may cause hyperiodinism (Connolly & Shepherd, 1972), and hypothyroidism in very-low-birthweight infants has been reported (Smerdely et al, 1989). The instillation of povidone-iodine, as a powder or spray, into surgical wounds has been a subject of controversy. Gilmore & Sanderson (1975) reported a decrease in postoperative infections with no sign of bacterial resistance or other harmful effects. Morgan (1979) and others also reported a significant decrease. However, several investigators (Pollock & Evans, 1975; Galland et al, 1977; De Jong et al, 1982; Rodeheaver et al, 1982) found no evidence of a decrease in wound infection and Rodeheaver et al (1982) concluded that any benefit from application of povidone-iodine to wounds or into the peritoneal cavity did not justify the risks involved. Hulka (1965) demonstrated by experiments using guinea pigs that injection of an iodophor skin preparation into the peritoneal cavity caused inflammation of the lining of the bowel and resulted in death of some of the animals.

Hexachlorophene

Acute oral toxicity of hexachlorophene has been manifested on several occasions when hospital patients, who had been given the emulsion for use in the shower, mistook it for milk of magnesia and ingested it, possibly because it was presented in a drinking cup (Wear et al, 1962; Lustig, 1963). Chronic systemic toxicity, resulting from dermal absorption, was not recognized until hexachlorophene emulsions had been used for 20 years for bathing newborn infants as well as for disinfection of the hands of hospital staff. The toxicity was revealed only when long-term animal feeding tests were performed to assess the safety of hexachlorophene as a potential food preservative. The laboratory rats developed paralysis in the limbs and the white matter in the brain showed spongiform encephalopathy, indicative of oedema. The mean blood level associated with the brain changes in the animals was 1.2 μg/ml (Kimbrough & Gaines, 1971; Kimbrough, 1973). Blood levels ranging from 0.009–0.646 μg/ml in newborn infants at the end of their hospital stay confirmed the evidence for dermal absorption (Curley et al, 1971). Excessive blood levels and clinical symptoms, including convulsions, have occurred in premature infants of low birth weight and those with abnormal or diseased skin (Kopelman, 1973; Powell et al, 1973). The death of 36 healthy infants was caused by a gross error in the formulation of a hexachlorophene-containing dusting powder; the 'baby powder' contained 6.3 per cent hexachlorophene (Martin-Bouyer et al, 1982). Severe symptoms or death have occurred in adults and children after a hexachlorophene emulsion had been applied to burned skin (Larson, 1968; Mullick, 1973). Neither significant blood levels nor clinical symptoms have occurred during its use on normal full-term infants (Alder et al, 1972; Plueckhahn, 1973) or on the hands of doctors and nurses (Butcher et al, 1973). Nonetheless, availability of hexachlorophene has been restricted to medical prescription in the United States.

Triclosan

This compound is not known to cause photoallergenic dermatitis, as are related compounds. Although triclosan can be absorbed through intact skin, it is nonallergenic and nonmutagenic with short-term use (Larson, 1995). Opposite findings have been reported for product acceptability of triclosan compared to 4 per cent chlorhexidine. Bendig (1990) found that adverse reactions occurred with triclosan but not with chlorhexidine. In contrast, Webster (1992) reported that triclosan caused significantly less damage to the hands of staff than did chlorhexidine. However, both the triclosan concentrations and the detergent formulations differed in the two studies. Oral toxicity is not a problem because triclosan is very poorly absorbed from the gastrointestinal tract. Indeed, triclosan has found applications in the area of oral health care.

EVALUATION OF SKIN DISINFECTANTS

The efficacy of skin disinfectants cannot be determined by in vitro tests, although a preliminary test of this type may serve to screen products that are grossly deficient in bactericidal activity. Most methods for testing products for disinfection of the hands of surgeons and nurses involve the cooperation of volunteers who may be drawn from hospital personnel; or, if appropriate, to the intended use of the product, from industrial premises or the community. Tests must be relevant to the intended use of the product and amenable to statistical interpretation (Rotter, 1988; Larson, 1990; Rotter, 1990). The result may be compared with suitable reference formulations, such as non-medicated soap for bactericidal skin cleansers or 60 per cent v/v isopropyl alcohol for alcoholic solutions, that are tested at the same time. Different products, designated for the same use, may also be compared with one another.

Products that are intended for hygienic hand disinfection are tested for activity against transient skin contaminants; a selected species of a readily identifiable Gram-positive or Gram-negative bacterium is usually applied to the skin because the natural contaminants vary in type and may not be numerous. *E. coli* ATCC 11229 is generally favoured but *S. marcescens* ATCC 133880 is also used in the United States. Products that are intended for surgical disinfection of hands and operation sites must be tested for their capacity to reduce the total skin flora to a low level that is unlikely to cause exogenous or endogenous infection of a patient's wound. These tests are performed on the hands of volunteers but preoperative estimation of the number and types of skin bacteria adjacent to the incision site and also in the wound prior to closure may provide some information about the likelihood of wound infection (Garibaldi et al, 1988).

As bacteria cannot be directly counted on the skin, evaluation of the efficiency of skin disinfection must be based on the number that can be recovered by a standard procedure. Samples are taken from the test site on the skin by the use of a fluid containing a surface active agent and appropriate disinfectant inactivators. The number of colony-forming units is determined in samples taken before and after the disinfection procedure has been performed and the result is expressed as per cent reduction or, more commonly, the equivalent $\log_{10}$ reduction factor. A factor of 2.5–3.0 is expected in tests for hygienic hand disinfection and a higher level (3.0–4.0) for tests for reduction of the resident flora (Rotter et al, 1986).

The ultimate test for efficacy of a disinfection procedure would be a survey of its effect on the incidence of nosocomial infection. However, it is difficult to separate the effect of handwashing from many other factors that influence the incidence of infection unless an epidemic is in progress or the endemic rate is unusually high. Rotter (1990) has estimated that two groups, each of 2500 patients, would be required to demonstrate a 50 per cent reduction in hand-transmitted infections from an incidence of 2 per cent to 1 per cent.

The following methods for evaluating the efficacy of skin disinfectants against the transient or resident skin bacteria are currently used.

Tests against transient contaminants

Two similar, but not identical, tests are used in the United Kingdom and several European countries. They are referred to as the Birmingham model and the Vienna model respectively and have been subjected to a collaborative trial (Rotter et al, 1986). The Vienna model is accepted as a standard test in several European countries, including Austria and Germany.

Vienna model (Rotter et al, 1986)

Fifteen volunteers are required. A broth culture of *E. coli* ATCC 11229 is used as contaminant. The original test is suitable for alcoholic formulations only as 60 per cent v/v isopropanol is the reference standard. However, the recent introduction of a soap-and-water wash as a standard allows disinfectant-detergents to be tested (Ayliffe, 1992). Tests on the product and standard are carried out on the same subjects on the same day. The sequence of steps is clearly defined:

1. The hands are washed with plain soap and water for 2 minutes and dried on a paper towel
2. The hands are contaminated with the suspension of test organism by immersion to the middle of the palms for 5 seconds,

drained and dried in air for 3 minutes, while held horizontally and rotated to avoid accumulation of inoculum at finger tips
3. Samples are taken for the initial count; the finger tips are rubbed and kneaded for 1 minute in 10 ml of sampling fluid, contained in a 9 cm petri dish
4. The *E. coli* culture is reapplied (as above)
5. The disinfection procedure is performed on the standard preparation or the product to be tested; two successive 3 ml amounts are rubbed over both hands, with attention to interdigital areas, finger tips and under the nails, for a total time of 1 minute
6. The finger tips are sampled (as above)
7. Dilutions of samples taken before and after the disinfection procedure are plated on casein soy agar, with fresh pipettes and careful rinsing at each dilution step. The plates are incubated at 36°C for 20 hours.

Birmingham model (Ayliffe et al, 1978; 1988)

Ten to 15 volunteers with intact skin and short finger nails are required. The artificial contaminant is *E. coli* ATCC 11229, as in the Vienna model. Two reference standards are used: non-medicated bar soap for bactericidal skin cleansers and 60 per cent v/v isopropyl alcohol for alcoholic solutions.

1. The hands are washed with soap and water and dried on two paper towels
2. The palmar surface of each finger tip on both hands is inoculated with a 0.02 ml drop of the test organism; opposing fingers and thumbs are rubbed together for 40 seconds and allowed to dry in air for a further 80 seconds
3. Two minutes after application of the test organism, the fingers and thumbs are sampled by rubbing vigorously on glass beads (3–5 mm diameter) in a bowl containing 100 ml sampling fluid for 1 minute; 2×0.5 ml of undiluted broth and 5×0.02 ml of tenfold dilutions are transferred to the surfaces of well-dried blood agar plates, which are incubated at 37°C for 18 hours

4. The test bacterial culture is reapplied for 2 minutes
5. The reference formulation is applied to the hands which are rubbed together as follows: 5 strokes each; rubbing back and forth, palm to palm; right palm over left dorsum and left palm over right dorsum; palm to palm with fingers interlaced; knuckles of left hand worked into right palm and vice versa (simultaneously); rotational rubbing of right thumb clasped in left palm and left thumb in right palm; rotational rubbing of clasped fingers of right hand in palm of left hand, and fingers of left hand in palm of right hand. The whole procedure is repeated three times for aqueous solutions and until the hands are dry for alcoholic solutions. The total time is 30 seconds
6. The hands are rinsed with running water and dried on two paper towels for tests on soaps and detergents; for testing alcohols they are dried in air for a further 30 seconds
7. The sampling procedure and viable counts are repeated.

The entire procedure is then repeated with the product under investigation. In a supplementary test for residual action, 10 hand washes with the product are performed in 6 hours by the same method of application. After the last application, the palmar surfaces of the finger tips and thumbs of both hands are inoculated with the *E. coli* broth culture and the fingers are rubbed together for 40 seconds. Paired fingers and thumbs are sampled 2, 4, 8, 16 and 32 minutes after inoculation and survivor counts are performed.

In assessing the differences between the Vienna and Birmingham tests, it has been pointed out by Ayliffe (1989) that the latter is more stringent because the inoculum is rubbed on to the skin, instead of being allowed to dry in air. Lilly & Lowbury (1978) found that an inoculum of *S. aureus* was more easily removed when spread and allowed to dry than when it was rubbed on the skin (2 per cent survival and 29.4 per cent survival respectively). The use of a second test organism, e.g. *S. aureus*, is recommended as *E. coli* tends to die out on drying (Ayliffe, 1989; Ayliffe et al, 1990). A similar method for testing hand disinfectants against a multiply-resistant strain of *Klebsiella* sp. is described by Casewell et al (1988); this test also includes the step of rubbing the inoculum on the skin and incorporates a test for residual action of the disinfectant. A modification of the test protocol, in which the finger tips are inoculated with suspensions of vaccine-strain poliovirus, bacteriophages of *E. coli* or bovine rotavirus, may be used for assessing virucidal activity (Bellamy et al, 1993; Davies et al, 1993). In these tests, the alcohols performed best.

Tests against resident skin flora

The main difference between tests for reduction of transient skin contaminants and those that are designed to evaluate the effect of antimicrobial agents against the natural resident bacterial flora is the extension of the latter to determine residual and cumulative action in addition to the immediate effect. The resident flora are sampled to estimate the initial bacterial count and the final count after a disinfection procedure has been carried out. As in the tests against transient contaminants, the validity of the tests depends on the use of appropriate inactivators for the type of product that is to be tested. The nonionic detergent polysorbate 80 (Tween 80) is combined with lecithin to inactivate chlorhexidine, hexachlorophene and triclosan; sodium thiosulfate, up to a maximum concentration of 1 per cent w/v, inactivates povidone-iodine but may be inhibitory to staphylococci. Most sampling methods are derived from the serial basin technique of Price (1938) but are carried out on a smaller scale.

Method of Lowbury, Lilly & Bull (1963)

This method has been used consistently by the authors over a 20 year period to investigate new products as they were introduced between 1960 and 1980; it has also been used frequently by other investigators.

The number of volunteers required for the Latin square design of the test is no more than six. On the first day, the subjects scrub with a nylon brush in running water for 2 minutes and then use the allotted preparation. On days 2 and 3, they repeat the procedure for a total of six times. After the sixth treatment, gloves are worn for 1 hour and then removed. The gloves are rinsed by addition of 100 ml of sampling fluid containing inactivators and the hands are also rinsed in 100 ml in the following manner: three strokes each, palm to palm; right palm over left dorsum; left palm over right dorsum; and three strokes with fingers interlaced. The hands are rinsed in the fluid between each set of three strokes. Sampling is carried out after the first and sixth treatments. Pour plates are prepared from aliquots of the undiluted glove washing and tenfold dilutions of the hand washings. After incubation at 37°C for 24 hours, the difference in colony counts before and after the test procedure is expressed as per cent or $\log_{10}$ reduction. Hand counts are carried out between tests to monitor the return of the subjects' normal flora before the next product is tested.

FDA method (Rosenberg et al, 1976)

This test was devised to evaluate the efficacy of the three chlorhexidine formulations (aqueous solution, skin cleanser and tincture) that were officially approved for use in American hospitals. Like the Lowbury test, it assesses immediate and persistent effects. Before tests on the products commence, 30 test subjects are selected from a panel of volunteers on the basis of producing counts between 1.5×10^6 and 4×10^6 on each hand on three successive days in the week prior to the test.

In the test week, the hands and two-thirds of the forearm are rinsed for 30 seconds with soap and warm water at 35–40°C and the nails are cleaned. Six-minute scrubs with 10 ml of the product to be tested are performed 11 times, finishing on day 5. Samples are taken after the first wash (day 1), the second wash (day 2) and final wash (day 5). On each day, a glove is placed on the left hand of each subject and a different person is sampled at times from 1 to 6 hours. Sampling is carried out by introducing 75 ml of fluid containing disinfectant inactivators into the glove, the wrist being secured by the subject. The gloved hand is massaged thoroughly for 1 minute and an aliquot of the fluid is removed for dilution and counting. Approximately 80 per cent of the bacteria on the skin are recovered by one wash with this fluid (Peterson, 1973). The result of the test is calculated in the usual way. The criterion for acceptability of subjects for the FDA test has been criticized as it excludes as many suitable volunteers as are accepted (Spradlin, 1980).

METHODS OF SKIN DISINFECTION

Hygienic handwashing

The purpose of hygienic handwashing is to kill and remove pathogenic microorganisms that may be present on the hands as transient surface contaminants. These may be acquired from hospital patients by doctors, nurses and other persons who care for them in wards, nurseries, intensive care units and diagnostic departments. Persons who work in community health care facilities, such as medical and dental clinics, nursing homes, microbiological laboratories or in the food production and catering industries must also be aware of the need for, and importance of, handwashing. The procedure is usually for the protection of other individuals but may be for self-protection of the worker in some situations.

Compliance with handwashing policy

Surveys with electronic monitors have shown that hospital staff, including physicians, are found to wash their hands much less frequently than is claimed (Broughall et al, 1984; Ayliffe et al, 1988; Maki, 1989). In some hospital areas, such as intensive care wards and nurseries, it may be necessary for a nurse to wash up to 40 times in a single work shift (Maki, 1989). A lower frequency may be satisfactory in other situations, where the patients are unlikely to be colonized or infected. Excessive frequency (e.g. 100 times on the same day) may result in damage to the hands, particularly the fingers, leading to an increase in the number of bacteria and failure of disinfectants to reduce it (Ojajärvi et al, 1977; Larson et al, 1986a). Kolari et al (1989) have reported that an emulsion cleanser containing 6 per cent fat was a favourable alternative to liquid soap for use by hospital staff with skin problems. The first prerequisite for achieving compliance with the hospital policy is the generous provision of handwashing facilities wherever they are needed. Wash basins and sinks should be fitted with foot operated or photoelectrically operated taps of a non-splashing type. Dispensers for liquid cleansing agents, including those that contain bactericidal agents, must be emptied and thoroughly cleaned before recharging with fresh solution (Rahman, 1988) and, if bar soap is provided, a draining rack is essential to prevent contamination with Gram-negative bacteria. Nail brushes should not be provided; if an individual requires a brush, it should be provided in sterile condition and removed after a single use. Interventions to improve hand-washing compliance have generally resulted in a temporary improvement only. Educational efforts proved to be of little benefit but feedback based on compliance observations fared better (Dubbert et al, 1990; Larson, 1995).

Regardless of frequency, the hands must always be washed thoroughly, with meticulous attention to all areas including the nails and interdigital spaces, with vigorous rubbing. A number of situations in which handwashing is essential have been listed (Garner and Favero, 1985):

1. Prolonged and intense contact with any patient
2. Before taking care of particularly susceptible patients (e.g. immunocompromised persons or newborn infants)
3. Before performing invasive procedures
4. Before and after touching wounds
5. After situations when microbial contamination of the hands is likely to occur (e.g. contact with mucous membranes, blood, body fluids, secretions and excretions)
6. After touching inanimate objects that are likely to be contaminated (e.g. urine measuring devices)
7. Between contacts with different patients in a high-risk unit or during the care of one such patient.

Handwashing is also an integral component of the personal hygiene of hospital staff.

Handwashing policies and procedures

The use of nonmedicated soaps and detergents, in solid or liquid forms, is efficacious in removing most transient contaminants from the hands. However, bactericidal skin cleansers are recommended for use by hospital staff who are known to carry strains of *S. aureus*, coagulase-negative staphylococci or Gram-negative rods on the hands some or all of the time (Maki, 1989). The immediate effect of a short hand wash with plain soap or detergent is a sharp increase in the bacterial count (Lowbury et al, 1963; Lilly & Lowbury, 1978). This is attributed to increased shedding of bacteria-carrying skin scales; it does not occur when a bactericidal skin cleanser is used. All products that are intended for use on the hands must be suitable for repetitive use and the time taken for the procedure must be practical; 15 seconds is recommended (Montefiori et al, 1990). Shorter washing (e.g. 7–10 seconds) is unsafe. The efficiency of the procedure is influenced by the amount of the handwashing preparation that is used. At least 3 to 5 ml is necessary (Larson et al, 1987; Geiss & Heeg, 1992). The thoroughness of the washing procedure may be as important as is which product is chosen (Ayliffe et al, 1988).

Rapid immediate action is the main requirement for a bactericidal hand cleanser. Residual action on bacteria that may be acquired by the worker between handwashings can be demonstrated by artificial inoculation of the fingers with bacteria (e.g. *E. coli*) after a series of washes and measurement of the rate at which the number decreases; however, the benefit of residual action in relation to hygienic handwashing has been questioned (Ayliffe et al, 1988). Products containing chlorhexidine (4 per cent w/v) or povidone-iodine (available iodine 0.75 per cent) are effective in achieving a $\log_{10}$ reduction factor of 2.5–3.0 of an artificial contaminant in a 30 second handwash, whereas triclosan gives a $\log_{10}$ reduction factor of 2.0 which is no better than that of non-medicated soaps (Ayliffe et al, 1988). Faogali et al (1995) found that 1 per cent triclosan had only a small cumulative action after 5 days of continuous use.

Hygienic handwashing should be supplemented by the wearing of gloves in some situations; e.g. those involving invasive procedures, touching open wounds, or when there is risk to the wearer of contact with blood (Garner & Favero, 1985). The gloves should then be removed before touching objects, such as patients' records or a telephone, and the hands should always be washed to remove traces of blood that may have penetrated through pinholes or other defects. Handwashing is completed by drying the hands on clean paper towels or by means of a hot air drier. Several investigations (Meers & Leong, 1989; Matthews & Newsom, 1987; Maki, 1989) have failed to find a significant difference in efficiency or safety but the time required for drying by hot air is likely to discourage handwashing unless paper towels are provided as an alternative for more rapid drying.

Ethyl or isopropyl alcohol, appropriately diluted with sufficient water for maximum bactericidal action, or an alcoholic preparation containing 0.5 per cent w/v chlorhexidine gluconate, may be used as an alternative to handwashing if skin emollients are included in the formulation. Bartzokas et al (1983) showed that a solution containing 2 per cent triclosan was equivalent to 60 per cent isopropyl alcohol and slightly better than alcoholic chlorhexidine. These formulations are applied directly to clean hands without washing and drying. They may be used between handwashings to kill pathogenic microorganisms acquired from patients (Larson et al, 1986b). Alcohols have the advantages of being time-saving, as they can be rubbed into the hands while moving on to the next task or patient, and economical (Mackintosh & Hoffman, 1984; Daschner, 1988; Maki, 1989). Alcoholic solutions are recommended for all hygienic hand cleansing in some European countries (Rotter et al, 1986). They may also be used in any situation where handwashing facilities are not available. A $\log_{10}$ reduction factor of 3.0–4.0 can be achieved by alcoholic solutions which are rubbed into the hands until they have dried on the skin (Ayliffe et al, 1988); chlorhexidine prolongs the effect as its retention on the skin confers residual activity.

Surgical skin disinfection

Reduction of the resident bacteria on the hands of the surgical team and the operation site to the lowest possible level is required to prevent exogenous and endogenous wound infections. Similar disinfectants to those used for hygienic handwashing are effective but extended treatment (2–5 minutes) and regular use are required for the combination of immediate, residual and cumulative action. Detergent formulations containing chlorhexidine, or povidone iodine are usually used although alcohols (e.g. 60 per cent v/v n-propanol) are more effective (Ayliffe, 1992). Alcoholic chlorhexidine and aqueous or alcoholic povidone-iodine are used for disinfection of the operation site immediately prior to incision; alcoholic chlorhexidine may also be used on the surgeon's hands after preliminary washing with soap and water.

Surgical disinfection of hands

Although gloves are worn by members of the surgical team, disinfection is necessary because microscopic pinholes are common and accidental tearing may occur (Walter & Kundsin, 1969). The effectiveness of 4 per cent w/v chlorhexidine skin cleanser was established by Lowbury & Lilly (1973) and has been confirmed by many investigators (Rosenberg et al, 1976; Peterson et al, 1978). Comparative evaluations of the immediate effect of a single 2 minute wash and the cumulative action of repeated use of chlorhexidine, povidone-iodine and hexachlorophene skin cleansers are shown in Table 12.1. The value of triclosan for surgical disinfection has not been firmly established (Bendig, 1990).

Chlorhexidine preparations, in regular use, are slightly superior to those containing povidone-

Table 12.1 Per cent reduction of resident skin flora after single use (immediate effects) and repeated use (cumulative effects) of skin disinfectants

Usage	Chlorhexidine		Povidone-iodine		Hexachlorophene	
Single use	86.7[1]	99.9[2]	68.0[1]	97.3[2]	51.1[1]	83.3[2]
Repeated use	99.2	99.98	99.7	99.2	98.4	99.0

[1] Lowbury & Lilly, 1973
[2] Peterson et al, 1978

iodine or hexachlorophene; povidone-iodine would be more effective against viruses but is more likely than chlorhexidine to cause irritation. A foam containing 1 per cent w/v chlorhexidine with 50 per cent alcohol has been reported as being similar to the detergent preparation in its immediate and cumulative effects (Beeuwkes & de Rooij, 1986). An alcoholic formulation containing 0.5 per cent w/v chlorhexidine, with skin conditioners, or an alcoholic preparation containing 1 per cent w/v triclosan, may be used as an alternative to the detergent preparation, after precleansing with plain soap which has been removed by rinsing (Larson et al, 1990). The alcoholic preparations achieved 97.9 per cent reduction of the resident flora after a single application and 99.7 per cent reduction on repeated use (Lowbury et al, 1974). In a two-phase procedure, in which repeated handwashing with a detergent preparation was followed by a single 2 minute application of the alcoholic solution, a final maximum reduction factor of 99.98 per cent was achieved. In a later study, Lilly et al (1979) reversed the order of the two phases and found that a minimum survivor level of 0.02 per cent was reached in the alcohol phase and no further reduction occurred when this was followed by a chlorhexidine detergent wash. If a non-antiseptic detergent was used instead, a large increase in the recovered bacteria occurred. The conclusion was drawn that the alcohol, with or without chlorhexidine, was capable of reaching an equilibrium level beyond which no further reduction of the resident flora could be achieved. The view was that this level is reached when the bacteria emerging from the deeper skin layers balance those being killed. In a study of surgical hand disinfection, Babb et al (1991) found that the efficacy of the four chlorhexidine scrubs tested varied considerably, despite the similarity of their constituents.

Involvement of the surgeon's hands in the genesis of postoperative infection may be infrequent but imperfections in the gloves could provide access of pathogenic bacteria to the wound if the surgeon is a heavy carrier of *S. aureus*, haemolytic streptococci or coagulase-negative staphylococci. Bactericidal agents are especially recommended in orthopaedic surgery and neurosurgery where organisms on the hands are most likely to cause infection through defects in gloves (Maki, 1989).

Methods that may be used for detection of pinholes in gloves have been described by Paulssen et al (1988).

Disinfection of operation sites

Preoperative disinfection for elective surgery is performed in two stages:

1. Cleansing the operation site, locally or by showering or bathing the whole body on admission of the patient to hospital on the day before the operation
2. Final disinfection of the operation site in the operating room.

The removal of hair is no longer recommended. When necessary, hair can be cut with scissors or removed with depilatory cream (Frost et al, 1989). When shaving is essential for operations on hair areas, it should be performed wet immediately before surgery to prevent the development of infection by skin bacteria at abraded sites (Leclair et al, 1988; Mackenzie, 1988; Laufman, 1989). Chlorhexidine or, less frequently, povidone-iodine skin cleansers may be used for whole body bathing but studies spread over a decade have yielded equivocal results concerning its effect on the number of bacteria that can be recovered from the skin after washing and on the incidence of postoperative infection.

Showering with chlorhexidine skin cleanser has been compared with nonmedicated soap in most studies, but comparison with povidone-iodine has also been made. Swedish workers (Brandberg & Andersson, 1981) showed that a single shower with chlorhexidine reduced the number of aerobic bacteria on the skin of volunteers while nonmedicated soap increased it. Brandberg et al (1981) also found that repeated showers with chlorhexidine skin cleanser reduced the incidence of postoperative infection after operations involving the groin from 17.5 per cent to 8 per cent. Leigh et al (1983) confirmed lowering of the bacterial count in the anal region but found no difference in the infection rate. In 1983, Ayliffe et al compared the effect of a single preoperative shower with chlorhexidine with that of ordinary soap on the incidence of infection in a study of 5536 patients and concluded from the figures of 5.4 per cent in the chlorhexidine group and 4.9 per cent in the control group that the bactericidal agent conferred no advantage. Another large study, conducted by the European Working Party on Control of Hospital Infections (Rotter et al, 1988), reported a similar result although the patients in this study had two showers, one on the preceding day and the second on the day of operation. Newsom & Rowland (1988) also found no reduction in the incidence of wound infection after cardiovascular surgery. Neither did Brady et al (1990) for whole-body washing in 1 per cent triclosan, although MRSA carriage and infections were highly significantly reduced.

A similar number of favourable reports on the advantages of chlorhexidine showering over povidone-iodine or over nonmedicated soap have been published. Hayek et al (1987) compared chlorhexidine detergent cleanser with a placebo formulation and also with bar soap in a group of 2000 patients. A postoperative wound infection rate associated with two showers was 7.2 per cent in the chlorhexidine group, compared with 10 per cent in the groups using the placebo or bar soap, a reduction of 30 per cent. These figures applied to clean surgery; the incidence of staphylococcal infections was reduced from 4.0–5.3 per cent to 2.6 per cent. Garibaldi and others (Garibaldi, 1988; Garibaldi et al, 1988), who used intraoperative wound contamination as a basis for evaluation, found 43 per cent negative cultures with chlorhexidine, 16 per cent with povidone-iodine and 6 per cent with a germicidal soap containing trichlorocarbanilide. The groups in this study were not large enough for comparison of infection rates. Another small scale study (Kaiser et al, 1988) on patients who showered on two occasions found chlorhexidine to be superior to povidone-iodine for reducing the colony count on the skin of patients undergoing coronary surgery. Byrne et al (1990) used ten volunteers to ascertain the optimum number of showers for maximum level of skin disinfection and confirmed that one shower or bath is not enough; they recommended a maximum of three to allow for less efficient performance by patients.

In contrast to views on the merits of precleaning procedures, the final preparation of the operation site before incision is more clearly defined. Davies et al (1978) found that 70 per cent v/v ethyl alcohol, 0.5 per cent w/v chlorhexidine in water or ethyl alcohol and aqueous or alcoholic povidone-iodine (1 per cent available iodine) reduced the bacterial flora of the skin of the abdomen by 99 per cent within 5 minutes. Alcoholic solutions are seen as more effective than aqueous solutions of the same antimicrobial agents. In hospitals where the use of alcohol in the operating room is regarded as a potential fire hazard, aqueous povidone-iodine is preferred to aqueous chlorhexidine. However, there should be no hazard if the alcoholic preparation is used correctly; the amount used should be adequate to keep the site wet for the recommended time and should then be allowed to evaporate completely before electrocautery or laser instruments are switched on. Pooling of excess liquid beneath the patient should not be allowed to occur. Chlorhexidine in alcohol has some advantages over povidone-iodine which may be toxic to tissue in the open wound. However, povidone-iodine has a special application in orthopaedic surgery where spores of *C. perfringens*, which occur in the bowel, may be present on the skin. An aqueous solution should be applied as a wet compress for 15–30 minutes (Lowbury et al, 1964; Drewett et al, 1972). Povidone-iodine may also be more effective than chlorhexidine for disinfection of the umbilicus and in other situations where its superior activity against Gram-negative bacteria or yeasts is required.

Neonatal skin care

Hexachlorophene emulsions or creams were applied to the skin of newborn infants over a long period, prior to 1970, to curtail the spread of staphylococcal infection among normal and premature infants. After the discovery of the harmful effects of bathing premature infants or those with skin abnormalities with emulsions or dusting powder containing hexachlorophene, alternative bactericides were used including triclosan and chlorhexidine. Webster et al (1994) reported that the use of 1 per cent w/v triclosan as handwashing agent eliminated endemic MRSA from a neonatal intensive care unit over a 12-month period. The authors also commented that the in-use performance of triclosan is superior to that predicted by in vitro laboratory tests on its efficacy.

A 4 per cent chlorhexidine detergent cleanser, diluted 1 in 80, was found to be equivalent in efficiency to hexachlorophene emulsion in a study that included 2000 infants (Tuke, 1975). A similar study of 3500 infants by Maloney (1975) using a 1 in 10 dilution of the chlorhexidine detergent cleanser also reported no adverse reactions. Hnatko (1977) and Fares et al (1977) concluded that chlorhexidine was an acceptable substitute for hexachlorophene. A more extensive investigation by Gongwer et al (1980) involving neonatal rhesus monkeys was designed to test for the possibility of dermal absorption and brain changes. The monkeys were bathed daily over a long period with chlorhexidine detergent cleanser containing double strength chlorhexidine and no evidence was found of absorption or adverse effects. Alder et al (1980) compared dusting powders containing 0.33 per cent hexachlorophene and 1.0 per cent chlorhexidine and found them to be equally effective in preventing colonization of the skin by S. aureus; 87 infants were dusted with each powder once a day and the umbilical and perineal areas were treated at each napkin change. Samples of venous blood showed only low or undetectable amounts of chlorhexidine. Absence of dermal absorption was confirmed by Oneill et al (1982) for a 1 in 10 dilution of chlorhexidine skin cleanser and by O'Brien et al (1984), who applied the full strength solution (4 per cent) to 100 babies, with total body washing on the first three days after birth.

A solution of chlorhexidine (0.5 per cent w/v in 70 per cent v/v ethyl or isopropyl alcohol) is commonly used to control colonization and infection of the umbilical cord in neonates (Bygdeman et al 1984; Nyström et al, 1985). Champagne et al (1984) reduced the frequency of isolation of coagulase-negative staphylococci in the blood of 38 colonized infants to a low level by the use of 70 per cent v/v isopropyl alcohol, followed by a 0.5 per cent w/v solution of chlorhexidine in 70 per cent ethyl alcohol.

Povidone-iodine and other iodine-containing preparations should not be used on newborn infants (premature or normal) because it has been shown to cause high levels of iodine in the urine, leading to hyperiodinism and hypothyroidism (Connolly & Shepherd, 1972; Smerdely et al, 1989).

Indwelling intravascular devices

Intravascular catheters are inserted, centrally or peripherally, in veins (central venous catheters) or arteries (arterial catheters), to provide access to the bloodstream for nutrients or therapeutic agents. Colonization of the tip or within the lumen of the catheter by bacteria or yeasts is often followed by local infection, bacteraemia and septicaemia. The microorganisms are usually transient or resident bacteria from the patient's skin; these include S. aureus, S. epidermidis, streptococci and Gram-negative rods, including species of Klebsiella and Pseudomonas (Elliott, 1988). If the patient has been treated with broad-spectrum antibiotics, these may select for multiresistant Gram-negative bacteria, penicillin-resistant corynebacteria, or Candida spp. which can cause fungaemia. Composition exerts an influence, e.g. bacteria adhere more readily to PVC than to a Teflon catheter. Once growth has been established, S. aureus and S. epidermidis, in particular, become entrapped in a slime layer, or glycocalyx. Such biofilms challenge the antimicrobial action of disinfectants by conferring protection on the microorganisms and so interfering with access of disinfectants to their microbial targets.

More than 90 per cent of all intravascular device-related bacteraemias, septicaemias and fungaemias are due to central venous and arterial catheters. Of these, the rate of infection is higher for central venous catheters than it is for arterial catheters (Maki et al, 1991). These complications are life-threatening, especially in patients who are already likely to be immunocompromised or debilitated.

Basic to the prevention of catheter-related infections are the prior disinfection of the insertion site and the use of skin disinfectants in follow-up care of the site. Important also are the cleaning and disinfection of the hands of the person inserting the catheter and the wearing of sterile gloves during the insertion procedure.

Maki et al (1991) conducted a large study, involving 668 catheters, on the comparative efficacy of three skin disinfectants in preventing infections associated with central venous and arterial catheters. The disinfectants tested were 10 per cent povidone iodine, 70 per cent isopropyl alcohol and 2 per cent aqueous chlorhexidine. Application to the insertion sites was by vigorous rubbing for about 30 seconds after which the sites were allowed to dry. Every 48 hours thereafter, the sites were treated again with the same disinfectant as was allocated and used initially. Chlorhexidine was associated with the lowest incidence of local catheter-related infection (2.3 per cent compared to 7.1 and 9.3 per cent for alcohol and povidone-iodine, respectively); and of catheter-related bacteraemia (0.5 per cent compared to 2.3 and 2.6 per cent for alcohol and povidone-iodine). The lowest incidence of infusion-related bacteraemia was also observed in the chlorhexidine group. Maki et al (1991) concluded that the use of 2 per cent chlorhexidine for skin disinfection of catheter-insertion sites and subsequent site care can substantially reduce the incidence of catheter-related infections. Aqueous 2 per cent chlorhexidine should, therefore, be used for catheter insertion and care rather than 10 per cent povidone-iodine or 70 per cent isopropanol. Of relevance to the efficacy of chlorhexidine are its residual activity and protein tolerance.

DISINFECTION OF MUCOUS MEMBRANES

Oral cavity

Chlorhexidine digluconate in aqueous form is used in dentistry for the control of dental plaque and gingivitis. It is available in 0.1 (or 0.12) and 0.2 per cent formulations as a mouthrinse and as a 1 per cent gel for application to the oral mucosa. Mouthwash preparations of povidone-iodine (with 0.05 per cent available iodine) and Listerine® have been shown to be at least as effective as is chlorhexidine in reducing gingivitis but they are not as effective against plaque (Fine, 1985; Axelsson & Lindhe, 1987).

A major disadvantage of chlorhexidine is its tendency to cause staining of tooth surfaces, fillings and the tongue on concentrated or prolonged usage. It may also cause desquamation and soreness of the mouth (Flötra et al, 1971) or the formation of white patches and ulcers on the gingivae and oral mucosa (Almqvist & Luthman, 1988). Another undesirable characteristic of chlorhexidine is its bitter taste. This is better tolerated in mouthrinses of 0.1 per cent, rather than 0.2 per cent, concentration (Hepsø et al, 1988).

The use of chlorhexidine for ongoing plaque control is not practical or advisable. However, chlorhexidine is of value for the control and prevention of plaque and gingivitis in certain situations. These include periods of interrupted oral hygiene after dental surgery when inflamed tissues hamper brushing (Greenstein, 1987). Chlorhexidine mouthwashes before and after the insertion of orthodontic appliances in patients with malocclusions can also play a role in suppressing caries-associated *Streptococcus mutans*. *S. mutans* otherwise tends to colonize the irregular sites and increases in number on insertion of the orthodontic appliances, thereby increasing the risk of caries in these patients (Lundström & Krasse, 1987). Chlorhexidine mouthwashes are particularly beneficial for maintaining oral hygiene in patients undergoing cytotoxic chemotherapy or radiation treatment. These patients often experience serious oral complications and infections during and after these treatments. Ferretti et al (1987) showed that rinsing the mouths of bone marrow transplant patients with 0.12 per cent chlorhexidine three times a day protected these immunosuppressed patients from oral infection and also resolved their mucositis and oral candidosis.

Urogenital tract

Urinary tract infections are a common complication of short-term indwelling catheterization after surgery and long-term intermittent or indwelling catheterization of geriatric and spinally injured patients, who have special problems. These have been reviewed by Stickler & Chawla (1987), Chawla et al (1988) and Stickler (1990). Mitchell & Gillespie (1964) reported that the incidence of urinary tract infections in catheterized patients was reduced by the use of preparations containing chlorhexidine for disinfection of the perineum and lower urethra and also by instillation of a 0.02–0.05 per cent (w/v) solution of aqueous chlorhexidine into the bladder through the catheter after emptying the drainage bag. However, the efficacy of chlorhexidine has declined because of the limited activity of dilute solutions against Gram-negative bacteria and increased resistance of *P. mirabilis*, *P. aeruginosa*, *Providencia stuartii* and *S. marcescens* following repeated exposure to chlorhexidine (Stickler & Thomas, 1980; Stickler et al, 1987a).

Studies on the urethral flora of spinally injured patients have shown that the bacterial flora consist predominantly of coagulase-negative staphylococci and diphtheroids on admission to hospital but these Gram-positive bacteria are replaced within a few days by Gram-negative rods that become firmly established and are difficult to eradicate (Kunin & Steele, 1985; Fawcett et al, 1986). This suggests that chlorhexidine may be selecting for these bacteria and that its use may therefore be counterproductive. Baillie (1987) tested 155 catheter specimens of urine and found that 74 of these yielded chlorhexidine-resistant bacteria. The concentration required for bactericidal action was increased when the strains were tested in urine, which was inhibitory to the action of chlorhexidine. Stickler et al (1987b), using a model bladder in which they simulated the bladder washout technique, demonstrated that bacteria also survived because they became embedded in a deposit of protective glycocalyx on the wall of the bladder.

Povidone-iodine, which has greater activity against Gram-negative bacteria, may be used as an alternative to chlorhexidine for disinfection of the periurethral area and for application to the catheter as a lubricant gel. Some reports have been favourable (Harrison, 1980; Cohen, 1985) but there is no evidence that it is more effective than is chlorhexidine in excluding Gram-negative bacteria from the urethra (Stickler & Chawla, 1987). Chawla et al (1988) suggest that further investigation of phenoxyethanol, which is slightly more active than is chlorhexidine against Gram-negative bacteria and has not been associated with increased resistance, might be worthwhile. However, the introduction of low-friction catheters coated with a lubricant containing povidone-iodine may help in overcoming the problem. Harper (1981) proposed topical use of a solution containing polymyxin and neomycin, alternating with one containing ethyl-enediamine tetraacetic acid (EDTA) and lysozyme, to avoid the development of resistant strains.

Instillation of antibacterial solutions into the bladder has also been subjected to revision of previous views. Davies et al (1987) found that neither chlorhexidine (0.02 per cent w/v) nor the saline control reduced the number of bacteria in the urine; five patients had overgrowth of *Proteus* after chlorhexidine and two had symptomatic infection. However, Pearman et al (1988) reported that a solution containing 0.01 per cent chlorhexidine gluconate, combined with EDTA and tris buffer, was equivalent to kanamycin/colistin in its effect. Stickler & Chawla (1987) tested several antibacterial agents and found that only phenoxyethanol was effective against *Providencia* and *Pseudomonas*.

Chlorhexidine, povidone-iodine and hydrogen peroxide have been used for disinfection of urine collected in drainage bags but the results of trials have been variable. Gillespie et al (1983) found that addition of chlorhexidine each time the bag was emptied kept the contents sterile but the frequency of infection was not reduced significantly. Schaeffer et al (1980) found that addition of 100 ml of 3 per cent stabilized hydrogen peroxide solution to the drainage bag would ensure an effective residual concentration of 0.6 per cent after 8 hours and that this was sufficient to kill a large mixed bacterial population in urine within 30 minutes. Sweet et al (1985) reported that addition of hydrogen peroxide reduced the level of contamination in the bag but did not reduce catheter-associated bacteriuria or the frequency of symptomatic urinary tract infection. However, the frequency of urinary tract infections caused by *P. mirabilis* during an outbreak among elderly patients was reduced from 63 per cent to 30 per cent when hydrogen peroxide was added to the drainage bag (Holliman et al, 1987; Seal & Holliman, 1988). In tests against *E. coli* and *P. aeruginosa* in simulated human urine, Yum et al (1988) suggested that the addition of a single tablet containing paraformaldehyde in a polymeric carrier would control these bacteria by maintaining a formaldehyde concentration of at least 90 μg/ml for 10 days. Winterbottom & Seal (1987) conducted tests which showed that air bubbles could rise up the tube from non-vented bags when they were nearly full and suggested that precautions should be taken to prevent transport of micro-organisms into the bladder by this mechanism.

Chawla et al (1988), acknowledging that urinary tract infection is still common in patients who receive long-term intermittent catheterization, have expressed the following views and recommendations:

1. Antiseptic barriers are easily penetrated by bacteria
2. Antiseptics should be used sparingly; soap and water is adequate for daily washing of the skin of the perineum and lower abdomen
3. There is no evidence that chlorhexidine prevents colonization of the lower urethra by Gram-negative pathogenic bacteria
4. Instillation of antiseptics into the bladder at each catheterization is not recommended; sterile saline may be used to remove debris and salts.

Chlorhexidine and, to a lesser extent, povidone-iodine have also been the subject of several investigations on disinfection of the perineum and vagina in obstetrics and gynaecological surgery. Calman & Murray (1956) gave an early indication that chlorhexidine may be suitable for these purposes and that it did not cause irritation or discomfort to midwifery patients. More detailed investigations (Byatt & Henderson, 1973; Duignan & Lowe, 1975) showed that a chlorhexidine detergent cleanser or a combination of chlorhexidine with the cationic surface active agent cetrimide was more effective than was chlorhexidine alone. This was attributed to the need to remove mucous secretions and fatty acid exudates that protected the perineal flora from effective contact with the bactericidal agents. Vorherr et al (1984; 1988) have conducted a series of studies in which they compared the efficiency of skin cleansers containing chlorhexidine, povidone-iodine and hexachlorophene. As in earlier investigations, their results favour the chlorhexidine preparation on the basis of marginal superiority over povidone-iodine with respect to disinfection of the perineum and groin of pregnant women and also because they found no evidence that chlorhexidine was absorbed through the vaginal mucosa, as are iodine and hexachlorophene (Vorherr et al, 1980). In a separate investigation of the effect of whole body showering with chlorhexidine on the incidence of postoperative infection in day surgery patients un-

dergoing vasectomy, Randall et al (1985) found that a shower within one hour before the operation and another on the following day reduced the infection rate from 17 per cent in a control group to 6.7 per cent in those treated.

Contaminated wounds

Antimicrobial agents, which may be disinfectants or antiseptics, are used to cleanse contaminated wounds of foreign material and to eliminate or prevent the multiplication of microorganisms that could lead to symptomatic infection. The agent that is selected should not impair the host defence mechanisms or impede the healing process. A cationic surface active agent, such as cetrimide, or a cetrimide-chlorhexidine formulation may be used for cleansing skin wounds. However, a suitable formulation of sodium hypochlorite, such as a modified Dakin's solution, is still considered most effective for the debridement of injured or dead tissue and foreign material (Laufman, 1989). Disinfectants that contain iodine-releasing compounds or those containing hexachlorophene should never be applied to injured tissues. The absorption of iodine into the blood upsets normal iodine metabolism and absorption of hexachlorophene results in the neurological damage that has been described in the section of this chapter on the systemic toxicity of disinfectants. Repeated bathing with hexachlorophene of children who had been born with a skin defect that necessitated the removal of a parchment-like outer membrane or who had accidental burn injuries resulted in their death (Mullick, 1973).

REFERENCES

Alder V G, Burman D, Simpson R A, Fysh J, Gillespie W A 1980 A comparison of hexachlorophane and chlorhexidine powders in prevention of neonatal infection. Archives of Disease in Childhood 55: 277–280

Alder V G, Burman D, Corner B D, Gillespie W A 1972 Absorption of hexachlorophane from infants' skin. Lancet ii: 384–385

Al-Khoja M S, Darrell J H 1979 The skin as the source of Acinetobacter and Moraxella species occurring in blood cultures. Journal of Clinical Pathology 32: 497–499

Almqvist H, Luthman J 1988 Gingival and mucosal reactions after intensive chlorhexidine gel treatment with or without oral hygiene measures. Scandinavian Journal of Dental Research 96: 557–560

Axelsson P, Lindhe J 1987 Efficacy of mouthrinses in inhibiting dental plaque and gingivitis in man. Journal of Clinical Periodontology 14: 205–212

Ayliffe G A J 1989 Standardization of disinfectant testing. Journal of Hospital Infection 13: 211–216

Ayliffe G A J 1992 Efficacy of handwashing and skin disinfection. Current Opinion in Infectious Diseases 5: 542–546

Ayliffe G A J, Babb J R, Quoraishi A H 1978 A test for 'hygienic' hand disinfection. Journal of Clinical Pathology 31: 923–928

Ayliffe G A J, Noy, M F, Babb J R, Davies J G, Jackson J 1983 A comparison of pre-operative bathing with chlorhexidine-detergent and non-medicated soap in the prevention of wound infection. Journal of Hospital Infection 4: 237–244

Ayliffe G A J, Babb J R, Davies J G, Lilly H A 1988 Hand disinfection: a comparison of various agents in laboratory and ward studies. Journal of Hospital Infection 11: 226–243

Ayliffe G A J, Babb J R, Davies J G et al 1990 Hygienic hand disinfection in three laboratories. Journal of Hospital Infection 16: 141–149

Babb J R, Davies J G, Ayliffe G A J 1991 A test procedure for evaluating surgical hand disinfection. Journal of Hospital Infection 18 Suppl B: 41–49

Baillie L 1987 Chlorhexidine resistance among bacteria isolated from urine of catheterized patients. Journal of Hospital Infection 10: 83–86

Bartzokas C A, Gibson M F, Graham R, Pinder D C 1983 A comparison of triclosan and chlorhexidine preparations with 60% isopropyl alcohol for hygienic hand disinfection. Journal of Hospital Infection 4: 245–255

Bartzokas C A, Corkill J E, Makin T 1987a Evaluation of the skin disinfecting activity and cumulative effect of chlorhexidine and triclosan handwash preparations on hands artificially contaminated with Serratia marcescens. Infection Control 8: 163–167

Bartzokas C A, Corkill J E, Makin T, Parry E 1987b Comparative evaluation of the immediate and sustained antibacterial action of two regimens, based on triclosan- and chlorhexidine-containing handwash preparations, on volunteers. Epidemiology and Infection 98: 337–344

Beeuwkes H, de Rooij S H 1986 Microbiological tests on operating-theatre staff of a new disinfectant foam based on 1% chlorhexidine gluconate. Journal of Hospital Infection 8: 200–202

Bellamy K, Alcock R, Babb J R, Davies J G, Ayliffe G A J 1993 A test for the assessment of 'hygienic' hand disinfection using rotavirus. Journal of Hospital Infection 24: 201–210

Bendig J W A 1990 Surgical hand disinfection: comparison of 4% chlorhexidine detergent solution and 2% triclosan detergent solution. Journal of Hospital Infection 15: 143–148

Benson L, LeBlanc D, Bush L, White J 1990 The effects of surfactant systems and moisturizing products on the residual activity of a chlorhexidine gluconate handwash using a pigskin substrate. Infection Control and Hospital Epidemiology 11: 67–70

Berkelman R L, Holland B W, Anderson R L 1982 Increased bactericidal activity of dilute preparations of povidone-iodine solutions. Journal of Clinical Microbiology 15: 635–639

Bicknell P G 1971 Sensorineural deafness following myringoplasty operations. Journal of Laryngology and Otology 85: 957–961

Blank I H 1969 Action of soaps and detergents on the skin. The Practitioner 202: 147–151

Brady L M, Thompson M, Palmer M A, Harkness J L 1990 Successful control of endemic MRSA in a cardiovascular unit. Medical Journal of Australia 152: 240–245

Brandberg Å, Andersson I 1981 Preoperative whole body disinfection by shower bath with chlorhexidine soap: effect on transmission of bacteria from skin flora. In: Maibach H I, Aly R (eds) Skin microbiology. Relevance to clinical infection. Springer-Verlag, New York, ch 12, p 92

Brandberg Å, Holm J, Hammarsten J, Schersten T 1981 Postoperative wound infections in vascular surgery: effect of preoperative whole body disinfection by shower-bath with chlorhexidine soap. In: Maibach H I, Aly R (eds) Skin microbiology. Relevance to clinical infection. Springer-Verlag, New York, ch 13, p 98

Broughall J M, Marshman C, Jackson B, Byrd P 1984 An automatic monitoring system for measuring handwashing frequency in hospital wards. Journal of Hospital Infection 5: 447–453

Butcher H R, Ballinger W F, Gravens D L, Dewar N E, Ledlie E F, Barthel W F 1973 Hexachlorophene concentrations in the blood of operating room personnel. Archives of Surgery 107: 70–74

Byatt M E, Henderson A 1973 Preoperative sterilization of the perineum: a comparison of six antiseptics. Journal of Clinical Pathology 26: 921–924

Bygdeman S, Hambraeus A, Hennigsson A, Nyström B, Skoglund C, Tunell R 1984 Influence of ethanol with and without chlorhexidine on the bacterial colonization of the umbilicus of newborn infants. Infection Control 5: 275–278

Byrne D J, Napier A, Cuschieri A 1990 Rationalizing whole body disinfection. Journal of Hospital Infection 15: 183–187

Calman R M, Murray J 1956 Antiseptics in midwifery. British Medical Journal 2: 200–204

Casewell M W, Desai N 1983 Survival of multiply-resistant Klebsiella aerogenes and other Gram-negative bacilli on finger-tips. Journal of Hospital Infection 4: 350–360

Casewell M W, Law M M, Desai N 1988 A laboratory model for testing agents for hygienic hand disinfection: handwashing and chlorhexidine for the removal of Klebsiella. Journal of Hospital Infection 12: 163–175

Champagne S, Fussell S, Scheifele D 1984 Evaluation of skin antisepsis prior to blood culture in neonates. Infection Control 5: 489–491

Chawla J C, Clayton C L, Stickler D J 1988 Antiseptics in the long-term urological management of patients by intermittent catheterisation. British Journal of Urology 62: 289–294

Cohen A 1985 A microbiological comparison of a povidone-iodine lubricating gel and a control as catheter lubricants. Journal of Hospital Infection 6 (Suppl): 155–161

Connolly R J, Shepherd J J 1972 The effect of preoperative surgical scrubbing with povidone-iodine on urinary iodine levels. Australian and New Zealand Journal of Surgery 42: 94–95

Curley A, Hawk R E, Kimbrough R D, Nathenson G, Finberg L 1971 Dermal absorption of hexachlorophene in infants. Lancet ii: 296–297

Daschner F D 1988 How cost-effective is the present use of antiseptics? Journal of Hospital Infection 11 (Suppl A): 227–235

Davies J, Babb J R, Ayliffe G A J, Wilkins M D 1978 Disinfection of the skin of the abdomen. British Journal of Surgery 65: 855–858

Davies J G, Babb J R, Bradley C R, Ayliffe G A J 1993 Preliminary study of test methods to assess the virucidal activity of skin disinfectants using poliovirus and bacteriophages. Journal of Hospital Infection 25: 125–131

Davies A J, Desai H N, Turton S, Dyas A 1987 Does instillation of chlorhexidine into the bladder of catheterized geriatric patients help reduce bacteriuria? Journal of Hospital Infection 9: 72–75

Davis G H G, Finlayson N, Kemp R 1985 Dilution of povidone-iodine. Medical Journal of Australia 143: 321

De Jong T E, Vierhout R J, van Vroonhoven T J 1982 Povidone-iodine irrigation of the subcutaneous tissue to prevent surgical wound infection. Surgery, Gynecology & Obstetrics 155: 221–224

Drewett S E, Payne D J H, Tuke W, Verdon P E 1972 Skin distribution of Clostridium welchii: use of iodophor as sporicidal agent. Lancet i: 1172–1173

Dubbert P M, Dolce J, Richter W, Miller M, Chapman S W 1990 Increasing ICU staff handwashing: effects of education and group feedback. Infection Control and Hospital Epidemiology 11: 191–193

Duignan N M, Lowe P A 1975 Pre-operative disinfection of the vagina. Journal of Antimicrobial Chemotherapy 1: 117

Eggers H J 1989 Handwashing and horizontal spread of viruses. Lancet i: 1452

Elliott T S J 1988 Intravascular-device infections. Journal of Medical Microbiology 27: 161–167

Evans C A, Mattern K L, Hallam S L 1978 Isolation and identification of Peptococcus saccharolyticus from human skin. Journal of Clinical Microbiology 7: 261–264

Faogali J, Fong J, George N, Mahoney P, O'Rourke V 1995 Comparison of the immediate, residual, and cumulative antibacterial effects of Novaderm R, Novascrub R, Betadine Surgical Scrub, Hibiclens, and liquid soap. American Journal of Infection Control 23: 337–343

Fares E, Selwyn S, Sethna T 1977 Chlorhexidine-detergent and other alternatives to hexachlorophane for use in maternity nurseries. Journal of Clinical Pathology 30: 785–786

Fawcett C, Chawla J C, Quoraishi A, Stickler D J 1986 A study of the skin flora of spinal cord injured patients. Journal of Hospital Infection 8: 149–158

Ferretti G A, Hansen I A, Whittenburg K, Brown A T, Lillich T T, Ash R C 1987 Therapeutic use of chlorhexidine in bone marrow transplant patients: case studies. Oral Surgery 63: 683–687

Fine P D 1985 A clinical trial to compare the effect of two antiseptic mouthwashes on gingival inflammation. Journal of Hospital Infection 6 (Suppl): 189–193

Flötra L, Gjermo P, Rölla G, Waerhaug J 1971 Side effects of chlorhexidine mouth washes. Scandinavian Journal of Dental Research 79: 119–125

Frost L, Pedersen M, Seiersen E 1989 Changes in hygienic procedures reduce infection following Caesarean section. Journal of Hospital Infection 13: 143–148

Galland R B, Saunders J H, Mosley J G, Darrell J H 1977 Prevention of wound infection in abdominal operations by peroperative antibiotics or povidone-iodine. A controlled trial. Lancet ii: 1043–1045

Gardner J F, Gray K G 1983 Chlorhexidine. In: Block S S (ed) Disinfection, sterilization, and preservation, 3rd edn. Lea & Febiger, Philadelphia, ch 12, p 251

Garibaldi R A 1988 Prevention of intraoperative wound contamination with chlorhexidine shower and scrub. Journal of Hospital Infection 11 (Suppl B): 5–9

Garibaldi R A, Skolnik D, Lerer T et al 1988 The impact of preoperative skin disinfection on preventing intraoperative wound contamination. Infection Control and Hospital Epidemiology 9: 109–113

Garner J S, Favero M S 1985 Guideline for handwashing and hospital environmental control, 1985. Centers for Disease Control, US Department of Health and Human Services, Atlanta, Georgia

Geiss H K, Heeg P 1992 Hand-washing agents and nosocomial infections. New England Journal of Medicine 327: 1390

Gillespie W A, Simpson R A, Jones J E, Nashef L, Teasdale C, Speller D C E 1983 Does the addition of disinfectant to urine drainage bags prevent infection in catheterised patients? Lancet i: 1037–1039

Gilmore O J A, Sanderson P J 1975 Prophylactic interparietal povidone-iodine in abdominal surgery. British Journal of Surgery 62: 792–799

Goldacre M J, Watt B, Loudon N, Milne L J R, Loudon J D O, Vessey M P 1979 Vaginal microbial flora in normal young women. British Medical Journal 1: 1450–1453

Gongwer L E, Hubben K, Lenkiewicz R S, Hart E R, Cockrell B Y 1980 The effects of daily bathing of neonatal rhesus monkeys with an antimicrobial skin cleanser containing chlorhexidine gluconate. Toxicology and Applied Pharmacology 52: 255–261

Greenstein G 1987 Chlorhexidine use. Journal of the American Dental Association 114: 292, 294

Guenthner S H, Hendley J O, Wenzel R P 1987 Gram-negative bacilli as nontransient flora on the hands of hospital personnel. Journal of Clinical Microbiology 25: 488–490

Hanson P J V, Gor D, Jeffries D J, Collins J V 1989 Chemical inactivation of HIV on surfaces. British Medical Journal 298: 862–864

Harper W E S 1981 An appraisal of 12 solutions used for bladder irrigation or instillation. British Journal of Urology 53: 433–438

Harrison L H 1980 Comparison of a microbicidal povidone-iodine gel and a placebo gel as catheter lubricants. Journal of Urology 124: 347–349

Hayek L J, Emerson J M, Gardner A M N 1987 A placebo-controlled trial of the effect of two preoperative baths or showers with chlorhexidine detergent on postoperative wound infection rates. Journal of Hospital Infection 10: 165–172

Hepsø H U, Bjørnland T, Skoglund L A 1988 Side-effects and patient acceptance of 0.2% versus 0.1% chlorhexidine used as post-operative prophylactic mouthwash. International Journal of Oral and Maxillofacial Surgery 17: 17–20

Hnatko S I 1977 Alternatives to hexachlorophene bathing of newborn infants. Canadian Medical Association Journal 117: 223–226

Holliman R, Seal D V, Archer H, Doman S 1987 Controlled trial of chemical disinfection of urinary drainage bags. Reduction in hospital-acquired catheter-associated infection. British Journal of Urology 60: 419–422

Hulka J F 1965 Peritoneal irritation due to an iodophor antiseptic solution. Archives of Surgery 90: 341–342

Junor B J R, Briggs J D, Forwell M A, Dobbie J W, Henderson I 1985 Sclerosing peritonitis — the contribution of chlorhexidine in alcohol. Peritoneal Dialysis Bulletin 5: 101–104

Kaiser A B, Kernodle D S, Barg N L, Petracek M R 1988 Influence of preoperative showers on staphylococcal skin colonization: a comparative trial of antiseptic skin cleansers. Annals of Thoracic Surgery 45: 35–38

Kimbrough R D 1973 Review of recent evidence of toxic effects of hexachlorophene. Pediatrics 51: 391–394

Kimbrough R D, Gaines T B 1971 Hexachlorophene effects on the rat brain. Archives of Environmental Health 23: 114–118

Kloos W E, Schleifer K H 1986 Genus IV. *Staphylococcus*. In: Sneath P H A, Mair N S, Sharpe M E, Holt J G (eds) Bergey's manual of systematic bacteriology. Williams & Wilkins, Baltimore, vol 2, p 1013

Knittle M A, Eitzman D V, Baer H 1975 Role of hand contamination of personnel in the epidemiology of gram-negative nosocomial infections. Journal of Pediatrics 86: 433–437

Kolari P J, Ojajärvi J, Lauharanta J, Mäkelä P 1989 Cleansing of hand with emulsion — a solution to skin problems of hospital staff? Journal of Hospital Infection 13: 377–386

Kopelman A E 1973 Cutaneous absorption of hexachlorophene in low-birth-weight infants. Journal of Pediatrics 82: 972–975

Kunin C M, Steele C 1985 Culture of the surfaces of urinary catheters to sample urethral flora and study the effect of antimicrobial therapy. Journal of Clinical Microbiology 21: 902–908

Larson D L 1968 Studies show hexachlorophene causes burn syndrome. Hospitals 42 (24): 63–64

Larson E 1990 clinical relevance of experimental models for testing efficacy of topical antimicrobial products. Infection Control and Hospital Epidemiology 11: 63–64

Larson E L 1995 APIC guideline for handwashing and hand antisepsis in health care settings. American Journal of Infection Control 23: 251–269

Larson E, Leyden J J, McGinley K J, Grove G L, Talbot G H 1986a Physiologic and microbiologic changes in skin related to frequent handwashing. Infection Control 7: 59–63

Larson E L, Eke P I, Laughon B E 1986b Efficacy of alcohol-based hand rinses under frequent-use conditions. Antimicrobial Agents and Chemotherapy 30: 542–544

Larson E L, Eke P I, Wilder M P, Laughon B E 1987 Quantity of soap as a variable in handwashing. Infection Control 8: 371–375

Larson E L, Butz A M, Gullette D L, Laughon B A 1990 Alcohol for surgical scrubbing? Infection Control and Hospital Epidemiology 11: 139–143

Laufman H 1989 Current use of skin and wound cleansers and antiseptics. American Journal of Surgery 157: 359–365

Leclair J M, Winston K R, Sullivan B F, O'Connell J M, Harrington S M, Goldmann D A 1988 Effect of preoperative shampoos with chlorhexidine or iodophor on emergence of resident scalp flora in neurosurgery. Infection Control and Hospital Epidemiology 9: 8–12

Leigh D A, Stronge J L, Marriner J, Sedgwick J 1983 Total body bathing with 'Hibiscrub' (chlorhexidine) in surgical patients: a controlled trial. Journal of Hospital Infection 4: 229–235

Lilly H A, Lowbury E J L 1978 Transient skin flora: their removal by cleansing or disinfection in relation to their mode of deposition. Journal of Clinical Pathology 31: 919–922

Lilly H A, Lowbury E J L, Wilkins M D 1979 Limits to progressive reduction of resident skin bacteria by disinfection. Journal of Clinical Pathology 32: 382–385

Lowbury E J L, Lilly H A 1973 Use of 4% chlorhexidine detergent solution (Hibiscrub) and other methods of skin disinfection. British Medical Journal 1: 510–515

Lowbury E J L, Lilly H A 1974 The effect of blood on disinfection of surgeons' hands. British Journal of Surgery 61: 19–21

Lowbury E J L, Lilly H A, Bull J P 1963 Disinfection of hands: removal of resident bacteria. British Medical Journal 1: 1251–1256

Lowbury E J L, Lilly H A, Bull J P 1964 Methods for disinfection of hands and operation sites. British Medical Journal 2: 531–536

Lowbury E J L, Lilly H A, Ayliffe G A J 1974 Preoperative disinfection of surgeons' hands: use of alcoholic solutions and effects of gloves on skin flora. British Medical Journal 4: 369–372

Lundström F, Krasse B 1987 *Streptococcus mutans* and lactobacilli frequency in orthodontic patients; the effect of chlorhexidine treatments. European Journal of Orthodontics 9: 109–116

Lustig F W 1963 A fatal case of hexachlorophene ('pHisoHex') poisoning. Medical Journal of Australia 1: 737

Mackenzie I 1988 Preoperative skin preparation and surgical outcome. Journal of Hospital Infection 11 (Suppl B): 27–32

Mackintosh C A, Hoffman P N 1984 An extended model for transfer of micro-organisms via the hands: differences between organisms and the effect of alcohol disinfection. Journal of Hygiene 92: 345–355

Maki D G 1989 The use of antiseptics for handwashing by medical personnel. Journal of Chemotherapy 1 (Suppl 1): 3–11

Maki D G, Ringer M, Alvarado C J 1991 Prospective randomised trial of povidone-iodine, alcohol, and chlorhexidine for prevention of infection associated with central venous and arterial catheters. Lancet 338: 339–343

Maloney M H 1975 Chlorhexidine, a hexachlorophane substitute in the nursery. Nursing Times (ICNA Suppl), 71(37): 21

Marcon M J, Powell D A 1992 Human infections due to *Malassezia* spp. Clinical Microbiology Reviews 5: 101–119

Martin-Bouyer G, Lebreton R, Toga M, Stolley P D, Lockhart J 1982 Outbreak of accidental hexachlorophene poisoning in France. Lancet i: 91–95

Matthews J A, Newsom S W B 1987 Hot air electric hand driers compared with paper towels for potential spread of airborne bacteria. Journal of Hospital Infection 9: 85–88

Meers P D, Leong K Y 1989 Hot-air hand driers. Journal of Hospital Infection 14: 169–171

Mitchell J P, Gillespie W A 1964 Bacteriological complications from the use of urethral instruments: principles of prevention. Journal of Clinical Pathology 17: 492–497

Montefiori D C, Robinson W E Jr, Modliszewski A, Mitchell W M 1990 Effective inactivation of human immunodeficiency virus with chlorhexidine antiseptics containing detergents and alcohol. Journal of Hospital Infection 15: 279–282

Montes L F, Wilborn W H 1970 Anatomical location of normal skin flora. Archives of Dermatology 101: 145–159

Morgan W J 1979 The effect of povidone-iodine (Betadine) aerosol spray on superficial wounds. British Journal of

Clinical Practice 33: 109–110

Mullick F G 1973 Hexachlorophene toxicity — human experience at the Armed Forces Institute of Pathology. Pediatrics 51: 395–399

Newsom S W B, Rowland C 1988 Studies on perioperative skin flora. Journal of Hospital Infection 11 (Suppl B): 21–26

Nyström B, Bygdeman S, Henningsson A, Tunell R, Berg U 1985 Influence of chlorhexidine in ethanol and in isopropanol on the bacterial colonization of the umbilicus of newborns. Infection Control 6: 186–188

O'Brien C A, Blumer J L, Speck W T, Carr H 1984 Effect of bathing with a 4 per cent chlorhexidine gluconate solution on neonatal bacterial colonization. Journal of Hospital Infection 5 (Suppl A): 141

O'Connor D O, Rubino J R 1991 Phenolic compounds. In: Block S S (ed) Disinfection, sterilization, and preservation, 4th edn. Lea & Febiger, Philadelphia, ch 12, p 218

Odds F C 1988 Candida and candidosis: a review and bibliography, 2nd edn. Baillière Tindall, London, p 74–75

Ojajärvi J, Mäkelä P, Rantasalo I 1977 Failure of hand disinfection with frequent hand washing: a need for prolonged field studies. Journal of Hygiene 79: 107–119

Okano M, Nomura M, Hata S et al 1989 Anaphylactic symptoms due to chlorhexidine gluconate. Archives of Dermatology 125: 50–52

Oneill J, Hosmer M, Challop R, Driscoll J, Speck W, Sprunt K 1982 Percutaneous absorption potential of chlorhexidine in neonates. Current Therapeutic Research 31: 485–489

Paulssen J, Eidem T, Kristiansen R 1988 Perforations in surgeons' gloves. Journal of Hospital Infection 11: 82–85

Pearman J W 1971 Prevention of urinary tract infection following spinal cord injury. Paraplegia 9: 95–104

Pearman J W, Bailey M, Harper W E S 1988 Comparison of the efficacy of 'Trisdine' and kanamycin-colistin bladder instillations in reducing bacteriuria during intermittent catheterization of patients with acute spinal cord trauma. British Journal of Urology 62: 140–144

Pecora D V, Landis R E, Martin E 1968 Location of cutaneous microorganisms. Surgery 64: 1114–1118

Peterson A F 1973 The microbiology of the hands: evaluating the effects of surgical scrubs. Developments in Industrial Microbiology 14: 125–130

Peterson A F, Rosenberg A, Alatary S D 1978 Comparative evaluation of surgical scrub preparations. Surgery, Gynecology & Obstetrics 146: 63–65

Pitcher D G, Noble W C 1978 Aerobic diphtheroids of human skin. In: Bousfield I J, Callely A G (eds) Coryneform bacteria. Academic Press, London, p 280–281

Platt J, Bucknall R A 1985 The disinfection of respiratory syncytial virus by isopropanol and a chlorhexidine-detergent handwash. Journal of Hospital Infection 6: 89–94

Plueckhahn V D 1973 Infant antiseptic skin care and hexachlorophene. Medical Journal of Australia 1: 93–100

Pollock A V, Evans M 1975 Povidone-iodine for the control of surgical wound infection: a controlled clinical trial against topical cephaloridine. British Journal of Surgery 62: 292–294

Powell H, Swarner O, Gluck L, Lampert P 1973 Hexachlorophene myelinopathy in premature infants. Journal of Pediatrics 82: 976–981

Price P B 1938 The bacteriology of normal skin: a new quantitative test applied to a study of the bacterial flora and the disinfectant action of mechanical cleansing.

Journal of Infectious Diseases 63: 301–318

Rahman M 1988 Hand scrubbing system in theatres and bacterial contamination. Journal of Hospital Infection 12: 327–328

Randall P E, Ganguli L A, Keaney M G·L, Marcuson R W 1985 Prevention of wound infection following vasectomy. British Journal of Urology 57: 227–229

Rodeheaver G, Bellamy W, Kody M et al 1982 Bactericidal activity and toxicity of iodine-containing solutions in wounds. Archives of Surgery 117: 181–185

Rosenberg A, Alatary S D, Peterson A F 1976 Safety and efficacy of the antiseptic chlorhexidine gluconate. Surgery, Gynecology & Obstetrics 143: 789–792

Rotter M 1988 Are models useful for testing hand antiseptics? Journal of Hospital Infection 11 (Suppl A): 236–243

Rotter M L 1990 Are experimental handwashing models a substitute for clinical trials to assess the efficacy of hand disinfectants? Infection Control and Hospital Epidemiology 11: 64–66

Rotter M L, Koller W, Wewalka G, Werner H P, Ayliffe G A J, Babb J R 1986 Evaluation of procedures for hygienic hand-disinfection: controlled parallel experiments on the Vienna test model. Journal of Hygiene 96: 27–37

Rotter M L, Larsen S O, Cooke E M et al 1988 A comparison of the effects of preoperative whole-body bathing with detergent alone and with detergent containing chlorhexidine gluconate on the frequency of wound infections after clean surgery. Journal of Hospital Infection 11: 310–320

Saatman R A, Carlton W W, Hubben K et al 1986 A wound healing study of chlorhexidine gluconate in guinea pigs. Fundamentals of Applied Toxicology 6: 1–6

Schaeffer A J, Jones J M, Amundsen S K 1980 Bactericidal effect of hydrogen peroxide on urinary tract pathogens. Applied and Environmental Microbiology 40: 337–340

Seal D V, Holliman R 1988 The role of antiseptics in the management of patients with long-term indwelling catheters. Journal of Hospital Infection 12: 334–336

Smerdely P, Lim A, Boyages S C et al 1989 Topical iodine-containing antiseptics and neonatal hypothyroidism in very-low-birthweight infants. Lancet ii: 661–664

Soriano F, Rodriguez-Tudela J L, Fernández-Roblas R, Aguado J M, Santamaría M 1988 Skin colonization by Corynebacterium groups D2 and JK in hospitalized patients. Journal of Clinical Microbiology 26: 1878–1880

Spradlin C T 1980 Bacterial abundance on hands and its implications for clinical trials of surgical scrubs. Journal of Clinical Microbiology 11: 389–393

Stickler D J 1990 The role of antiseptics in the management of patients undergoing short-term indwelling bladder catheterization. Journal of Hospital Infection 16: 89–108

Stickler D J, Thomas B 1980 Antiseptic and antibiotic resistance in Gram-negative bacteria causing urinary tract infection. Journal of Clinical Pathology 33: 288–296

Stickler D J, Chawla J C 1987 The role of antiseptics in the management of patients with long-term indwelling bladder catheters. Journal of Hospital Infection 10: 219–228

Stickler D J, Clayton C L, Chawla J C 1987a The resistance of urinary tract pathogens to chlorhexidine bladder washouts. Journal of Hospital Infection 10: 28–39

Stickler D J, Clayton C L, Chawla J C 1987b Assessment of antiseptic bladder washout procedures using a physical model of the catheterised bladder. British Journal of Urology 60: 413–418

Sweet D E, Goodpasture H C, Holl K, Smart S, Alexander

H, Hedari A 1985 Evaluation of H₂O₂ prophylaxis of bacteriuria in patients with long-term indwelling Foley catheters: a randomized controlled study. Infection Control 6: 263–266

Tuke W 1975 Hibiscrub in the control of staphylococcal infection in neonates. Nursing Times (ICNA Suppl), 71(37): 20

Ulrich J A 1981 Antimicrobial efficacy in the presence of organic matter. In: Maibach H I, Aly R (eds) Skin microbiology. Relevance to clinical infection. Springer-Verlag, New York, ch 18, p 149

Vorherr H, Vorherr U F, Mehta P, Ulrich J A, Messer R H 1980 Vaginal absorption of povidone-iodine. Journal of the American Medical Association 244: 2628–2629

Vorherr H, Vorherr U F, Mehta P, Ulrich J A, Messer R H 1984 Antimicrobial effect of chlorhexidine and povidone-iodine on vaginal bacteria. Journal of Infection 8: 195–199

Vorherr H, Vorherr U F, Moss J C 1988 Comparative effectiveness of chlorhexidine, povidone-iodine, and hexachlorophene on the bacteria of the perineum and groin of pregnant women. American Journal of Infection Control 16: 178–181

Walsh B, Blakemore P H, Drabu Y J 1987 The effect of handcream on the antibacterial activity of chlorhexidine gluconate. Journal of Hospital Infection 9: 30–33

Walter C W, Kundsin R B 1969 The bacteriologic study of surgical gloves from 250 operations. Surgery, Gynecology & Obstetrics 129: 949–952

Wear J B Jr, Shanahan R, Ratliff R K 1962 Toxicity of ingested hexachlorophene. Journal of the American Medical Association 181: 587–589

Webster J 1992 Handwashing in a neonatal intensive care nursery: product acceptability and effectiveness of chlorhexidine gluconate 4% and triclosan 1%. Journal of Hospital Infection 21: 137–141

Webster J, Faogali J L, Cartwright D 1994 Elimination of methicillin-resistant Staphylococcus aureus from a neonatal intensive care unit after hand washing with triclosan. Journal of Paediatrics and Child Health 30: 59–64

Winterbottom D R, Seal D V 1987 Comparison of flow rates into vented and non-vented urinary drainage bags: possible relevance to infection. Journal of Hospital Infection 10: 273–281

Wlodkowski T J, Speck W T, Rosenkranz H S 1975 Genetic effects of povidone-iodine. Journal of Pharmaceutical Sciences 64: 1235–1237

Yum S, Amkraut A, Dunn T, Chin I, Killian D, Willis E 1988 A disinfectant delivery system for control of micro-organisms in urine collection bags. Journal of Hospital Infection 11: 176–182

13. Microbial control of environments

In health care facilities, laboratories and certain processing, pharmaceutical and industrial settings, the immediate environment is a potential reservoir of microorganisms and source of infection or contamination. Of particular importance in this context are air and water and the mechanical systems associated with their handling, distribution and use. These systems may facilitate the transmission of infectious agents or the distribution of microbial contaminants. Minimizing the risk of infection or contamination from the environment requires the application of methods and the adoption of procedures for environmental microbial control.

INFECTION RISK

Infections in health care facilities

Health care facilities include hospitals, nursing homes, extended care facilities, medical and dental clinics, podiatry and acupuncture practices. Patients, occupants and users of these facilities may be susceptible to infection from their environment because of some degree of immunosuppression. The risk of nosocomial, or hospital-acquired, infection is highest where patients are severely immunosuppressed as a result of diseases, such as AIDS, congenital immunodeficiencies or immunosuppressive therapy. However, normal immunological responses are compromised also, to a lesser extent, by the natural process of ageing and activities such as smoking; both are identified as risk factors for Legionnaires' disease. In addition, the insertion of intravascular catheters and airway tubes tends to interfere with the body's defences, and even more so in the usual recipients of these devices, who are generally seriously ill. Consequently, nosocomial bacteraemias and pneumonias are well-recognized complications of the use of intravenous catheters for the administration of nutrients, fluids or therapeutic drugs (Elliott, 1988) and of mechanical ventilation in the treatment of patients in intensive therapy units (Cadwallader et al, 1990). Nosocomial infections are also associated with other indwelling medical devices and prostheses such as orthopaedic prostheses, prosthetic heart valves, ocular implants, central nervous system shunts, urinary and peritoneal dialysis catheters (Spencer, 1988; Bisno & Waldvogel, 1989). Urinary tract infections are the most common of the hospital-acquired infections and may also be a source of bacteraemias through extension to the blood stream (Jepsen et al, 1982).

Infections in health care workers

The increased risk of infection in health care workers is the result of their increased exposure. Of major concern is occupational exposure to blood-borne viruses and especially to HIV, as it becomes more prevalent in the health care environment. Needlestick injury with HIV-positive blood is the principal means of transmission of HIV in the health care setting. However, the rate of infection after accidental needlestick injury is low. Follow-up studies of more than 2000 such injuries have shown an infection rate of only 0.3 per cent (Henderson et al, 1990). Of concern also is the transmission of *Mycobacterium tuberculosis* (Centers for Disease Control and Prevention, 1994).

Laboratory-associated infections

Pike (1979) summarized publications and survey results from worldwide sources for his historical review of laboratory-associated infections in 1979. He reported a total of 4079 laboratory-associated infections, for more than 80 per cent of which no obvious laboratory accident could be recognized. A conservative estimate of the number of fatalities was 173. Regular surveys of infections in clinical laboratories covering two-year periods have been conducted in Britain (Grist, 1983; Grist & Emslie, 1985; 1987; 1989). From such reviews and surveys and the information amassed and analyzed by

Collins (1993) and Sewell (1995), certain infections have emerged as being of particular concern to laboratory workers. These include hepatitis B and C and infections due to species of *Mycobacterium* and *Brucella* and the enteric group. Among the latter, infections due to *Shigella* spp. are numerically predominant but salmonellosis, typhoid and paratyphoid fevers remain important laboratory-associated diseases. Cases of laboratory-acquired shigellosis, salmonellosis and typhoid fever in laboratory workers, or their close contacts, have resulted from the handling of test strains in laboratory proficiency testing programs (Blaser & Lofgren, 1981; Collins, 1993; Sewell, 1995). Laboratory technicians in morbid anatomy and mortuary attendants are at particular risk of acquiring tuberculosis (Grist & Emslie, 1985; 1987; 1989; Collins, 1993; Sewell, 1995).

Morbidity and mortality due to fungal infections in laboratory workers are also on record (Pike, 1979; Sewell, 1995). The main causal agents are the systemic mycotic pathogens for which the usual portal of entry is the respiratory tract. However, percutaneous inoculation through laboratory accidents also features as an important means of transmitting mycoses in laboratories. Cases of laboratory-acquired parasitic infections, including two fatal cases, have been reported (Herwaldt & Juranek, 1995; Sewell, 1995).

Disturbing reports of the occurrence of Creutzfeldt-Jakob disease in three histopathology technicians have been published (Miller, 1988; Sitwell et al, 1988). Routine formalin fixation does not inactivate prions (Taylor & McConnell, 1988) but Brown et al (1990) showed that prions in brain tissue could be reduced to a very low level of infectivity by combining exposure to concentrated formic acid with formalin fixation. However, combining formic acid with paraformaldehyde-lysine-periodate as fixative was not effective against mouse-passaged bovine spongiform encephalopathy agent (Taylor, 1995).

MICROBIAL CONTROL OF AIR

A variety of microorganisms and other particles are transmitted in air as, or in association with, droplets, droplet nuclei, dust particles, fibres, skin scales, bacteria-carrying particles, sporing bacteria, fungi and their spores, pollens and other allergens. Penetration of the respiratory tract depends on size; droplet nuclei and particles of 5 μm in diameter or less are most efficient at reaching the lungs. Their transmission may be prevented or reduced by aseptic filtration or ultraviolet disinfection of air.

Aseptic air filtration

The types of filters used for the aseptic filtration of air and the principles and parameters governing their operation and determining their efficiency have been described in Chapter 9. The general applications of air filtration have also been described in that chapter.

Air filtration on a large scale involves high efficiency HEPA filters and unidirectional, laminar air flow. In this system, the filtered air moves in one direction with uniform velocity along parallel flow lines. As shown in Figure 13.1, the air flow may be horizontal (crossflow) or vertical (downflow). These 'clean work stations' with laminar air flow provide a work space for the manipulation or assembly of non-hazardous materials in a high-quality, contamination-free environment. However, this type of work station

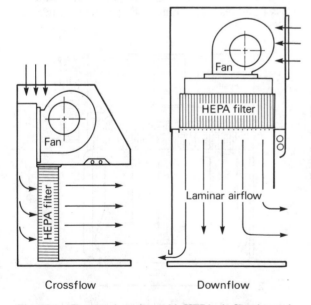

Fan

HEPA filter

Fan

HEPA filter

Laminar airflow

Crossflow   Downflow

Fig. 13.1 Clean work stations with HEPA air filtration and laminar air flow in a horizontal (crossflow) or vertical (downflow) direction.

must *not* be used for infectious, toxic or sensitizing materials because the operator is directly exposed to the immediate downstream exhaust.

Air filtration in health care facilities

The provision of protective environments by means of HEPA filtration is applicable to the removal of infectious aerosols in health care facilities. Enclosures consist of space contained by fixed or movable walls and a ceiling, all impervious to the air flow. The HEPA-filtered air originates at one wall or the ceiling. These laminar air flow enclosures are used in operating rooms for orthopaedic surgery or as isolation facilities for burns and immunosuppressed patients. The use of a five-bedded laminar flow enclosure successfully terminated an outbreak of invasive pulmonary aspergillosis among children in a bone marrow transplant unit (Barnes & Rogers, 1989).

HEPA filtration is recommended as a supplement to improved ventilation among the engineering controls designed to reduce or eliminate the transmission of *M. tuberculosis* in health care facilities (Centers for Disease Control and Prevention, 1994; Segal-Maurer & Kalkut, 1994). HEPA filters are installed in exhaust ducts to remove infectious aerosols before discharge of air from isolation units to other areas of the facility or to the general ventilation system. They are also used in ducts of enclosures such as sputum-induction booths which discharge into the surrounding room. For air recirculation within a room, the filters may be located in ducts or in ceiling- or wall-mounted units. HEPA filters are also available as portable units.

Laboratory applications of air filtration

Biological safety cabinets are widely used for the containment of infectious material and for protection against airborne, laboratory-acquired infections in microbiological laboratories. The control of microorganisms and particles in the air within the cabinet is effected through the use of vertical laminar flow and HEPA filtration of the air.

The three classes of biological safety cabinets have different performance characteristics and are intended for different purposes. Class I cabinets provide personnel protection while class II provides protection for both personnel and for the product and/or experiment. These cabinets are designed for the safe manipulation of microorganisms in the categories of 'ordinary' or 'special' hazard. Ordinary or potential hazard is defined as the risk level associated with agents which produce disease in humans, animals, or plants and which can be contained by normal microbiological techniques; special hazard is the risk level associated with agents which are highly infectious or toxic for humans, animals or plants with the production of dangerous disease. Also included are agents with genetic alterations and those which may have a synergistic effect with other materials (AS 2252.2 Part 1, 1994). The class III cabinet is a totally enclosed cabinet designed for the safe containment and handling of microbial agents of extreme hazard, the risk level associated with agents which are extremely dangerous for humans, animals, or plants, or cause serious epidemic disease (AS 2252.2 Part 1, 1994; BS 5726, 1992).

Class I biological safety cabinets provide personnel protection by the inward flow of air through the open front and away from the operator. The exhaust air is filtered through a HEPA filter before being discharged from the cabinet (Fig. 13.2). Class I cabinets may be fitted with a front panel with access ports which may, or may not, be equipped with gloves. Class II biological safety cabinets provide a HEPA-filtered recirculated vertical air flow within the work space. The exhaust air from the cabinet is filtered by a separate HEPA filter (Fig. 13.2). In the usual type of class II cabinet (type A), approximately 70 per cent of the total volume of cabinet air is recirculated through the supply HEPA filter and 30 per cent is exhausted (Stuart et al, 1982). Class III cabinets are totally enclosed and of gas-tight construction. The supply air is drawn into the cabinet through a HEPA filter and the exhaust air passes through two HEPA filters in series before discharge. All operations are conducted through attached rubber gloves and under conditions of negative pressure in the cabinet.

Biological safety cabinets must comply with the construction and performance specifications of relevant Standards, e.g. Australian Standards AS 2252.2 Part 1 (1994) and Part 2 (1994) for class I cabinets and class II cabinets respectively and British Standard BS 5726 (1992) for all three classes of cabinet. Biological safety cabinets should undergo testing with certification of performance on installation and annually thereafter. The proper use of biological cabinets is important, e.g. recommended practices include the avoidance of any unnecessary activities that might disrupt the inward flow of air through the front openings of class I and class II cabinets. Personnel who use the

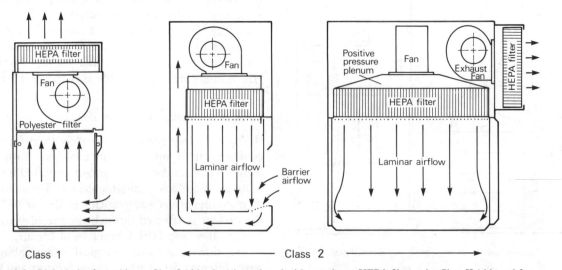

Fig. 13.2 Biological safety cabinets. Class I (side view) is equipped with an exhaust HEPA filter only; Class II (side and front views) has an additional HEPA filter for the provision of HEPA-filtered, recirculated air flow within the cabinet. Arrows indicate direction of air flow.

class III cabinet require a high level of competence in microbiology and special training in the handling of dangerous agents (BS 5726, 1992).

Pharmaceutical and industrial applications

Where contamination-free environments are required in pharmaceutical and allied industries, the increasing use of isolators incorporating HEPA filters and laminar air flow is gaining acceptance. The isolators are basically biological safety cabinets with modifications. Construction materials vary from stainless steel to clear, flexible film and front closures with sleeve ports and gloves are standard for sterile work. Other modifications to the basic design of a biological safety cabinet are the addition of pass-through boxes or transfer hatches on one or both sides of the main cabinet. The boxes and hatches are usually equipped with small, top-mounted HEPA filters and perforated bases through which the exhaust air passes to join the general exhaust system of the main cabinet. For sterility testing, ultraviolet lamps are supplied in the hatches for surface disinfection.

Apart from sterility testing, isolators are being used increasingly in the pharmaceutical industry for the aseptic preparation of:

1. Eyedrops
2. Injectables
3. Individually-formulated fluid diets for parenteral nutrition
4. Biologically active compounds
5. Cytotoxic drugs.

In most situations where a contamination-free environment is required, a piece of equipment or a filling station can be conveniently enclosed in an isolator. A suite of isolators may be custom-made for large-scale operations. Vertical laminar flow clean air modules are also used to provide particle-free environments for the micro-electronic, aircraft and spacecraft industries.

Ultraviolet (UV) disinfection of air

Ultraviolet (UV) radiation for disinfection is produced from a mercury vapour discharge tube at a peak wavelength of 254 nm. Only wavelengths in the 254 to 260 nm range have significant and powerful germicidal activity. In contrast, the wavelengths of the UV spectrum in sunlight are in the 290 to 400 nm band. Whereas UV radiation at 254 nm wavelength may cause skin and eye irritation, it does not cause the skin cancers and cataracts that are associated with prolonged exposure to solar radiation (NIOSH, 1972). Ozone production is negligible with currently available UV lamps.

UV irradiation damages the DNA of microorganisms. The most biologically significant lesions in microbial DNA are pyrimidine dimers, especially thymine dimers (Rubin, 1988). However, some bacteria possess enzymes which can excise the dimers and repair the damage. Although dark repair enzymes occur, enzymes that are activated on exposure to bright light are responsible for reversing most of the DNA damage. This process of light-activated DNA repair is termed photoreactivation.

Another important limitation on the efficacy of UV radiation is its poor penetrating ability. This means that any shielding, shadowing or clumping of microorganisms tends to provide protection against the biocidal action of UV radiation. In spite of these limitations, ultraviolet radiation at 254 nm wavelength can be used to kill or inactivate airborne microorganisms in droplet nuclei. The extent of inactivation of airborne microorganisms by UV irradiation depends on the intensity of the UV radiation, the nature of the microorganisms and the relative humidity of the environment. Above 70 per cent relative humidity, the biocidal activity of the UV radiation is significantly reduced (Riley & Kaufman, 1972). However, such high levels of humidity are not commonly encountered in indoor environments, except in tropical climates.

The UV tubes need to be replaced at the end of their rated useful life, which is usually one year for tubes used continuously. Alternatively, their output should be checked by a UV meter as germicidal power may be lost while the visible rays remain unchanged. Baffles are included in the fittings to protect against eye exposure and all UV installations should bear signs warning against eye and skin exposure.

Adjunct role of UV radiation in disease control

UV radiation can be used as an adjunct to other

engineering controls for preventing the transmission of M. tuberculosis. UV irradiation has a role to play in the decontamination of air from large, general areas, e.g. emergency and waiting rooms, where adequate ventilation is difficult to achieve and where undiagnosed tuberculosis may result in contamination (Centers for Disease Control and Prevention, 1994; Segal-Maurer & Kalkut, 1994). UV fixtures are placed in ducts or on the upper wall or ceiling of rooms. Placement in ducts minimizes human exposure. It is used for air recirculation of a room and its efficiency depends on all (or almost all) the room air passing through the duct. With upper room irradiation, the fixtures must be shielded. Efficiency depends on effective mixing of the upper and lower air. Mixing may be enhanced by introducing cool air at ceiling level and warm air at floor level (Segal-Maurer & Kalkut, 1994).

Adjunct role of UV radiation in clean rooms

UV irradiation contributes to the disinfection of air in clean rooms in microbiological laboratories, pharmaceutical processing facilities and certain industrial settings. It may also be used for the disinfection of clean surfaces, bench tops and the interior of biological safety cabinets as well as for surface disinfection prior to sterility testing.

MICROBIAL CONTROL OF WATER

Ecology and control of microorganisms in water

Prominent among the bacterial flora of water are Gram-negative rods belonging to the genera Legionella, Pseudomonas, Flavobacterium, Vibrio and the family Enterobacteriaceae. Water is the natural habitat and prime reservoir for some of these genera, including those with important pathogenic, or potentially pathogenic, species such as Legionella pneumophila and Pseudomonas aeruginosa. Other pathogens, e.g. species of Shigella and Salmonella, may be transmitted by water which has been polluted by faeces containing these enteric pathogens. Water may also contain non-tuberculous species of Mycobacterium and bacteria usually associated with soil, such as the sporing

Gram-positive rods of the genus Bacillus, as well as yeasts and fungi. Viruses, e.g. hepatitis A virus and rotavirus, may be present as a result of faecal contamination. Faecal pollution by man or animals is also responsible for contaminating water supplies with pathogenic parasites, e.g. Giardia, Cryptosporidium and Entamoeba histolytica.

Pseudomonas spp., which occur naturally in water, have simple nutritional requirements, along with considerable metabolic capabilities, and are easily cultured on ordinary laboratory media. They are resistant to a wide range of antibiotics, which probably reflects an evolutionary adaptation to antibiotic-producing environmental microorganisms but poses problems in the management and treatment of human diseases caused by pathogenic species, such as P. aeruginosa. P. aeruginosa is capable of multiplying in distilled water containing only traces of dissolved organic nutrients (Favero et al, 1971). As an important cause of nosocomial, water-associated infections, it must be controlled in the hospital environment by bacteria-retentive filters, heat or chemical disinfection. A limitation with the latter is that P. aeruginosa is much more resistant to chemical disinfection in a natural environment such as the distilled water reservoir of a hospital mist therapy unit than it is after culture, even once, on a laboratory medium (Carson et al, 1972). Moreover, P. aeruginosa is not unique in this respect as strains of L. pneumophila have been reported as showing enhanced resistance to chlorine disinfectant when adapted to tap water rather than agar-passaged (Kuchta et al, 1985).

Non-tuberculous mycobacteria, i.e. species of Mycobacterium other than Mycobacterium tuberculosis, occur commonly in natural and piped waters (Collins et al, 1984). Among these, M. fortuitum and M. chelonae are important opportunistic pathogens, the latter especially in haemodialysis patients (Silcox et al, 1981; Bolan et al, 1985). The source of infection for dialysis patients is the water used for rinsing dialyzers during reprocessing and for diluting chemical disinfectants. Carson et al (1978) showed that strains of M. chelonae isolated from the peritoneal fluids of patients and from dialysis machines were capable of multiplying to populations of 10^5–10^6 cells per millilitre in commercial distilled water. Furthermore, such strains were more resistant than were standard strains from the American Type Culture Collection to formaldehyde and glutaraldehyde disinfectants. Subsequently, Carson et al (1988) reported that the treated waters from 115 dialysis centres in the United States harboured non-tuberculous mycobacteria and showed that these bacteria were more numerous in the waters that had been treated in dialysis centres by softening, deionization and reverse osmosis than they were in the corresponding incoming municipal waters to those centres. The authors proposed that non-tuberculous mycobacteria be considered common bacterial contaminating flora of water used in dialysis centres. A formaldehyde concentration of at least 4 per cent w/v, or a chemical disinfectant of equivalent efficacy, should be used for the disinfection of dialyzers that are to be reused. Other non-tuberculous mycobacteria found in water include *M. avium* and *M. kansasii* which may cause pulmonary disease in immunocompromised hosts. The route of transmission of infection for these species is probably by inhalation of aerosols from showers, analogous to that for *Legionella* (Collins et al, 1984).

Standard methods of water treatment include filtration and chlorination and are intended to render the water safe for drinking. However, the standard water treatment will not remove parasitic cysts such as the cysts of *Giardia* and the oocysts of *Cryptosporidium* (Isaac-Renton et al, 1987), although the latter can be inactivated by use of an alternative water disinfectant such as ozone (Peeters et al, 1989).

In contrast to *Pseudomonas* and many other bacteria found in water, *Legionella* is difficult to grow in the laboratory and requires specific growth factors, such as cysteine and ferric pyrophosphate, and special growth conditions for successful cultivation. In its natural environment, *Legionella* obtains all its growth requirements through interactions with other microflora and by the utilization of organic and inorganic elements and constituents of its aquatic habitat. *L. pneumophila* multiplies in the temperature range of 20°C to 45°C but shows a preference for the upper limits of this range (Wadowsky & Yee, 1985; Peel et al, 1985). Artificial water systems, such as cooling towers and the

tanks and distribution systems for warm waters, promote the proliferation of legionellae and also provide the means by which these bacteria can be aerosolized for efficient dissemination and transmission of the infectious agents to the lungs. Of major concern with respect to the microbial control of water is the control of legionellae in water and water systems for the prevention of legionellosis, especially in health care establishments where vulnerable persons are congregated.

Legionellae and cooling towers

Structure and operation of cooling towers

In larger air-conditioning systems, heat is removed from the refrigeration system by means of a cooling tower. As shown in Figure 13.3, the heated water is circulated to the top of the tower and sprayed over fill material through which cooling air rises. The fill creates an extensive wetted surface through which the water and air pass in opposite directions (counter flow). In the process, the droplets in the water spray lose heat to the rising air through evaporation and convective and conductive heat exchange. The cooled water spray is collected in a water basin at the bottom of the tower and passed back to the refrigeration system. The air is drawn in from outside the tower through openings situated above the water basin by a fan located at the top of the tower, from where the air is finally discharged (induced draught type). Alternative arrangements for air flow are forced draught, with a fan located at the opening above the water basin forcing the air vertically through the tower; and crossflow, where air is induced or forced to flow across the falling water spray. The air stream entrains small water droplets which are then carried out of the tower to the environs. This drift contains chemicals and bacteria, including *Legionella* if present, and constitutes a loss of water to the system. Drift eliminators are designed to minimize the drift loss to less than 0.02 per cent of the total circulating water volume of the cooling tower. Water losses are replenished by the addition of make-up water to the system. *Legionella* may also occur in other similar heat-rejection systems, such as evaporative condensers.

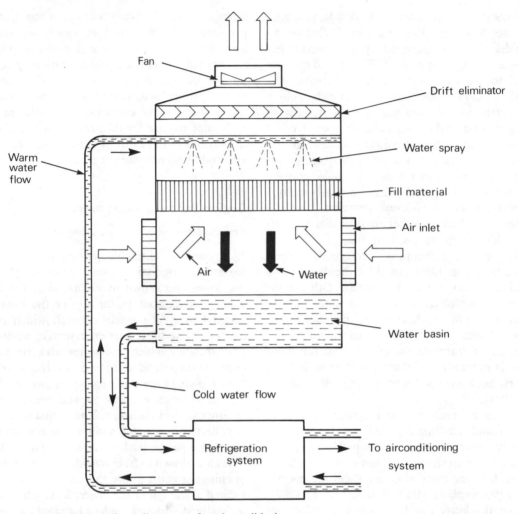

Fig. 13.3 Schematic diagram of a cooling tower of an air-conditioning system.

Ecology of legionellae in cooling towers

The incoming air provides a source of microorganisms and organic nutrients. Microorganisms may also gain access to the cooling tower waters through the make-up water. The microflora of the water may consist of algae, protozoa and bacteria, including legionellae.

L. pneumophila is able to grow in symbiosis with blue-green algae, utilizing their metabolic products of photosynthesis. The close association between *Legionella* and the blue-green algae was first described by Tison et al (1980), who proposed that it provided an explanation for the widespread distribution of legionellae in the waters of cooling towers and natural aquatic habitats.

Furthermore, protozoa can act as natural hosts and reservoirs of legionellae. *L. pneumophila* is able to multiply within single-celled amoebae and ciliates. Barbaree et al (1986) isolated protozoa from the waters of cooling towers actually implicated in an outbreak of Legionnaires' disease and showed that the protozoa could support the intracellular multiplication of an isolate of *L. pneumophila* from the same waters in co-culture in the laboratory. Protozoa, and especially their cysts, can apparently act as protective reservoirs of legionellae, allowing them to withstand the action of biocides and other environmental assaults and to multiply under conditions that might otherwise not support their growth.

The products of corrosion and inorganic elements in the water can also promote the growth of *L. pneumophila* (States et al, 1985). Legionellae occur particularly in association with biofilms, scale and sediments on the wetted structural surfaces of cooling towers.

Control of legionellae in cooling tower waters

The test conditions under which biocides are evaluated in the laboratory do not adequately reflect the complexities of the interactions between legionellae and the aquatic environments of cooling towers. Consequently, laboratory findings on the efficacy of chemical biocides in killing legionellae cannot be simply extrapolated and applied to the control of these bacteria in the waters of cooling towers (England et al, 1982).

An appreciation of the complexities of the interactions between legionellae and other microflora and the organic and inorganic constituents of cooling tower waters forms the basis for the recommendation that a multifaceted program of control be implemented. Regular cleaning for the removal of scale, slime, sediments and biofilms is of prime importance. Cleaning should be combined with an anti-algal, anti-bacterial and anti-corrosive treatment program. High-level chlorination is used, with cleaning, for the decontamination of cooling towers where indicated. Recent improvements in the design and construction of cooling towers promote access, facilitate draining, cleaning and flushing and reduce corrosion. Cooling towers should be sited downwind of air inlets on the same or adjacent buildings and the wetted surfaces should be protected from direct sunlight to discourage algal growths. Written policies and records for the cleaning and water treatment programs should be maintained.

Water distribution systems and legionellae

Because of their preference for warm temperatures, legionellae may proliferate to give high concentrations in hot water tanks that are maintained at 40–45°C rather than at 60–70°C (Stout et al, 1982; Plouffe et al, 1983; Peel et al, 1985) or allowed to stagnate out of use for some time (Fisher-Hoch et al, 1982). Bollin et al (1985) showed that shower heads and hot-water taps can generate aerosols containing viable *L. pneumophila* of a size that is small enough to penetrate to the lower respiratory tract of humans. Nonetheless, aspiration of contaminated potable waters has been proposed as the major mode of transmission for nosocomial legionellosis (Yu, 1993). Like aspiration pneumonia, the attack rate is low and risk factors similar, e.g. smoking, high alcohol intake and immunosuppression (Muder et al, 1986). Epidemiological data support the proposal (Johnson et al, 1985; Blatt et al, 1993; Mermel et al, 1995).

Ecology of legionellae in water distribution systems

Amoebae and ciliated protozoa, which can support the intracellular multiplication of *L. pneumophila*, have been isolated from hospital hot water tanks and plumbing systems (Fields et al, 1989; Nahapetian et al, 1991). Earlier, Skinner et al (1983) had proposed that chlorine-resistant cysts of protozoa may introduce *Legionella* into piped water systems. In addition, certain bacterial isolates from the waters of plumbing systems can provide nutrients which support the growth of *L. pneumophila*; such bacteria are more frequently isolated from the waters of hot water tanks than from cold water tanks (Stout et al, 1985a; Wadowsky & Yee, 1985).

Leached inorganic elements from water pipes and tanks and the products of corrosion in the waters of distribution systems also contribute to the growth of legionellae. Iron, zinc and potassium can each promote the multiplication of *L. pneumophila*, provided that their concentrations are not so high as to be toxic (States et al, 1985).

Colbourne et al (1984) reported that *L. pneumophila* is able to grow on the rubber components of washers in shower fittings. The use of, or replacement by, approved fittings of appropriate composition, e.g. those containing thiuram (Niedeveld et al, 1986), overcomes this problem.

The temperatures of warm water distribution systems promote the proliferation of *L. pneumophila*. However, Stout et al (1985b) have shown that significant contamination of cold water outlets in hospital can also occur.

Control of legionellae in water distribution systems

Thermal eradication. The 'heat-and-flush' method is effective in eradicating *L. pneumophila* from water distribution systems (Best et al, 1983; Muraca et al, 1990). In this method, the temperature of the hot water tanks is maintained at, or raised to, at least 70°C and all water outlets are flushed for a set period of time in order to kill legionellae colonizing distal sites. The temperature of the water issuing from the outlets should be checked to ensure that it is at least 60°C. It may be necessary to override or bypass thermostatic mixing valves and anti-scald devices to implement the heat-and-flush procedure. Water systems that remain contaminated after the heat-and-flush procedure should be checked for the presence of dead ends in the pipeline network. These sections of piping are not reached by the heated water and can act as a source for recolonizing the system (Groothius et al, 1985).

Instantaneous steam heating systems which disinfect incoming water by flash heating to 88°C are also available (Muraca et al, 1990). These systems obviate the need for hot water storage tanks which are often a reservoir of legionellae. However, the incoming cold water which is blended with the heated water is not treated and may contain legionellae.

Chemical disinfection. Hyperchlorination is suitable for the decontamination of cold waters which, unlike hot waters, do not readily drive off free chlorine (Fisher-Hoch et al, 1981; Muraca et al, 1987). Hyperchlorination involves the addition of hypochlorite to waters with an existing chlorine residual. For the inactivation of legionellae, a chlorine residual of more than 3 p.p.m. is required, whereas the chlorine residual in domestic water supplies is usually less than 1 p.p.m. (Skaliy et al, 1980). A problem with continuous use of high levels of chlorine is increased corrosion of water pipes, although this effect may be reduced by maintaining less acid pH levels or prevented, by coating the pipes with silicate (Helms et al, 1988).

The dynamics of inactivation of legionellae by ozone at a concentration of 1–2 p.p.m. are similar to those for chlorine (Muraca et al, 1987). As ozone is unstable, it must be generated on site, used immediately and has no residual. When combined with chlorine, it allows lower chlorine concentrations to be used (Muraca et al, 1990).

Copper and silver ions may also be used to promote the inactivation of *L. pneumophila* by low chlorine concentrations (Landeen et al, 1989). The installation of copper/silver ionization units into the contaminated hot water system of a hospital resulted in eradication of *L. pneumophila* once the levels of copper and silver reached 0.4 and 0.04 p.p.m. (Liu et al, 1994).

Ultraviolet radiation. *L. pneumophila* is inactivated by low doses of UV radiation (Antopol & Ellner, 1979). However, *L. pneumophila* and several other species of *Legionella* can repair much of the damage to their DNA by photoreactivation on subsequent exposure to indirect sunlight for 60 minutes (Knudson, 1985). This reversal of the UV damage indicates the need for caution in the application of UV irradiation to control *Legionella*. Another water bacterium, *Burkholderia cepacia*, has also been shown to be very efficient at photoreactivation on exposure to visible light after UV inactivation (Carson & Petersen, 1975). Legionellae and other environmental, water-associated bacteria might well be expected to have evolved efficient enzyme systems for coping with UV damage (Rubin, 1988).

UV light has the advantage of exerting no effect on the pH, odour or chemical composition of water. The UV disinfection unit consists of UV lamps housed in a quartz jacket through which the water flows past the lamps. Sensors are incorporated to monitor UV emission and to signal reduction of the emission, when the lamps need cleaning or replacement. Installation of the disinfection units is straightforward and annual replacement of the UV lamps is the only regular maintenance required.

A disadvantage of the use of ultraviolet radiation for water disinfection is its lack of residual action. However, this can be offset, to some extent, by using UV radiation in combination with some other form of disinfection such as chlorination. It is the usual practice to combine UV irradiation with filtration (e.g. by sand or clarifying filters) to minimize problems of the colour, turbidity and chemical constituents of the water interfering with UV transmission and protecting microorganisms (Muraca et al, 1990). Despite the disadvantages, the successful application of UV irradiation to the control of legionellae in water supplying a renal transplant unit has been reported (Farr et al, 1988). In this application, UV disinfection units were installed in both the hot and cold water pipes leading to the transplant area together with filters of 5 μm pore size and in combination with chemical disinfection of all the water pipes and outlets.

Other hospital sources of legionellae and their control

Respiratory devices have been implicated as a source of nosocomial pneumonias in hospitals. In 1980, legionellae were first detected in the water-filled reservoirs of nebulizers used in respiratory therapy (Gorman et al, 1980). Subsequently, nosocomial Legionnaires' disease was shown to be caused by aerosolized tap water from jet nebulizers and a room humidifier (Arnow et al, 1982) and aerosolized medications (Mastro et al, 1991). Sterile water only should be used for washing and filling such equipment (Mastro et al, 1991).

PROCEDURES FOR MINIMIZING THE RISK OF INFECTION

With the extraordinary advent and unparalleled impact of AIDS, attention and concern have focused on the need for effective care of immunosuppressed patients in health care establishments and minimization of the risk of infection to staff and other patients.

Minimizing the risk of blood-borne infections

Universal Precautions (USA)

In 1987, the Centers for Disease Control (CDC) in the United States recommended that blood and body fluid precautions to prevent parenteral, mucous membrane and non-intact skin exposure of health care workers be applied to the blood and body fluids of *all* patients (Centers for Disease Control, 1987). The application of precautions to all patients is referred to as 'Universal Blood and Body Fluid Precautions' or 'Universal Precautions'.

Subsequent publications clarified, updated and extended the original recommendations on Universal Precautions (Centers for Disease Control, 1988; 1989). In these publications, CDC reiterated that blood is the single, most important source of HIV, hepatitis B virus and other blood-borne pathogens in the occupational setting and emphasized that infection control efforts should focus primarily on the prevention of exposure to blood and the delivery of hepatitis B immunization.

The body fluids or substances to which the Universal Precautions apply are:

1. Blood and body fluids containing visible blood (most significant hazard)
2. Semen and vaginal secretions
3. Amniotic, cerebrospinal, pericardial and pleural fluids
4. Tissues.

The body fluids or substances to which the Universal Precautions do not apply include faeces, nasal secretions, sputum, sweat, tears, urine and vomitus. Breast milk and saliva are also in this category but blood and body fluid precautions apply to these body fluids in special settings. For example, the wearing of gloves is recommended for those handling breast milk for 'milk banks' and for those exposed to saliva in the course of digital examination of mucous membranes, endotracheal sectioning and during dental procedures.

Recommendations of the Hospital Infection Society (UK)

The recommendations of the Working Party of the Hospital Infection Society for the control of infections transmitted by inoculation of blood were published in 1990 (Speller et al, 1990). These recommendations differ from the single-tier approach of Universal Precautions in that, while certain control measures are applicable to all patients, special measures are recommended for patients at increased risk of being infected with HIV or hepatitis B virus, i.e. those patients identified as belonging to 'Inoculation Risk' categories.

The most important control measures for the prevention of blood-borne infection during the care of *all* patients are:

1. Prevention of inoculation injury
2. General care with blood or tissue fluid of whatever source.

In addition, supplementary precautions are applicable to those in the Inoculation Risk categories and to those for whom initial, automatic allocation to a category of inoculation risk is appropriate, e.g. patients presenting at accident and emergency departments or attending sexually transmitted diseases clinics.

Universal blood precautions. Protective clothing is recommended when there is a risk of contamination by blood, tissue or tissue fluids. The wearing of gowns, gloves and plastic aprons protects against direct contact. Masks and eye protection are added where there is a risk of splashing or spraying. Any skin contamination should be washed off immediately and the hands should be washed after removal of gloves (see Ch. 12). Cuts, abrasions and skin lesions should be covered by impermeable dressings. All staff should be immunized against hepatitis B and checked for seroconversion.

Sharps such as disposable needles, lancets, small pieces of broken glass and hard plastic should be discarded into a puncture-resistant sharps disposal container, situated as close as possible to the site of discard. A safe method for the transport and disposal of sharps is essential; incineration is recommended for disposal. Standards (e.g. AS 4031, 1992) apply to the requirements for safe design and construction of sharps disposal containers in health care areas. After use, needles should be discarded immediately into the sharps container without recapping, unless the recapping procedure can be carried out by a safe method with suitable equipment. Blood spillages should be covered with a chlorine disinfectant of 10 000 p.p.m. available chlorine, preferably in an absorbent granular or powdered form. The chlorine is allowed to act for 2–10 minutes, and is wiped up with paper towels in gloved hands.

National regulations and guidelines

In 1991, the American Occupational Safety and Health Administration (OSHA) issued a rule, for implementation by mid-1992, that required employers to take steps to protect health care workers who have occupational exposure to blood-borne pathogens. The rule mandates engineering controls, workplace practices and personal protective equipment, along with (free) employee training

and the offer of hepatitis B vaccination, for all employees who are exposed to blood and blood-borne pathogens. In addition, immediate post-exposure evaluation, prophylaxis (when indicated) and follow-up investigations must be available (Domin & Smith, 1992).

National Australian guidelines make similar recommendations, specifically that a 24-hour service be provided for the investigation and management of incidents which have the potential for blood-borne infection either to or from health care workers. The guidelines also advise against the performance of exposure prone procedures by health care workers and students infected with blood-borne viruses, if there is a reasonable risk of transmission of the infection (NHMRC/ANCA, 1996).

Minimizing the risk of nosocomial infections

Nosocomial, or hospital-acquired, infections can occur in health care facilities through the transmission of infectious agents from patient to health care worker, patient to patient and health care worker to patient. The carriage of microorganisms on the hands has long been recognized as the primary means by which infection is transmitted from patient to patient (Bruun & Solberg, 1973; Casewell & Phillips, 1977; Sakata et al, 1989). Frequent and efficient handwashing is considered to be the 'single most important measure' for reducing the risk of transmitting infectious agents from one person to another or from one place to another on the same person (Garner et al, 1996). Glove use should not be regarded as a substitute for handwashing (Garner et al, 1996; NHMRC/ANCA, 1996). Because of inapparent defects or the tearing of gloves, hands can become contaminated when gloves are being worn. Contamination is even more likely during removal of the gloves (Garner et al, 1996).

Body Substance Isolation (USA)

An alternative infection control system, also proposed in 1987, is Body Substance Isolation (Lynch et al, 1987). This system has broader aims than simply the protection of health care workers. It proposes the isolation of all moist and potentially infectious body substances through barrier precautions, mainly the wearing of gloves. Included among the moist body substances are faeces, saliva and oral secretions, sputum, urine and wound drainage. Health care workers don gloves before anticipated contact with such body substances or with mucous membranes or non-intact skin. In addition, they are required to respond to the presence of the alert signs, which are posted on the rooms of patients with diseases transmitted primarily by the airborne route, by checking the need to wear masks or the personal immunity requirements.

The intention of the Body Substance Isolation system was not only to reduce the risks of infection (including blood-borne infections) to health care workers but also to reduce the cross-transmission of infectious agents between patients (McPherson et al, 1988). Nonetheless, the system was deficient in that it did not promote handwashing after the removal of gloves; in this respect, it differed from Universal Precautions (Garner et al, 1996). Another disadvantage was the high cost of gloves (McPherson et al, 1988). However, the major problem was that the Body Substance Isolation system failed to make adequate provision for the prevention of certain infections, including emerging nosocomial infections of current concern (Garner et al, 1996). For example, the system does not provide adequate measures for the prevention of:

1. Droplet transmission of serious infections in paediatric patients, such as meningococcal meningitis and pertussis
2. Direct or indirect contact transmission of microorganisms from intact skin or the environment, such as vancomycin-resistant enterococci
3. Long- or short-range airborne transmission of infection in droplet nuclei, such as tuberculosis.

Standard Precautions (USA)

Clearly, a new infection control system, which provides guidelines for preventing nosocomial infections with diverse modes of transmission, was needed. That new system has now been developed and promulgated (Garner et al, 1996). It consists of two tiers of precautions. The first synthesizes the major features of Universal Precautions and Body Substance Isolation into a single set of precautions for use with all patients, irrespective of their diagnosis or presumed infection status. The precautions, termed Standard Precautions, are designed to reduce the risk of transmission of blood-borne and other pathogens in hospitals.

Standard Precautions apply to:

1. Blood
2. All body fluids, secretions and excretions (except sweat), regardless of whether or not they contain visible blood
3. Non-intact skin
4. Mucous membranes.

The Standard Precautions include handwashing and the use of personal protective equipment, which may include gloves, gowns, masks, eye protection and face shields; appropriate handling and disposal of sharps and other contaminated and infectious waste; appropriate cleaning and reprocessing of patient-care equipment and hygienic environmental control (Garner et al, 1996).

The second tier are precautions for use with patients who are known, or suspected, to be colonized or infected by epidemiologically significant pathogens that can be transmitted by the airborne, droplet or contact mode of transmission. These precautions are termed Transmission-Based Precautions, although Australian health and medical authorities prefer the term 'Additional Precautions' (NHMRC/ANCA, 1996). Transmission-Based Precautions comprise Airborne Precautions, Contact Precautions and Droplet Precautions. Examples of the application of Airborne Precautions and Contact Precautions to the control and prevention of nosocomial tuberculosis and vancomycin-resistant enterococci follow.

Minimizing the risk of nosocomial tuberculosis

Airborne Precautions apply to the control and prevention of tuberculosis which is transmitted in droplet nuclei by the airborne route. Both the reservoir and transmission of tuberculosis have increased significantly in hospitals and other health care facilities recently. A major contributing factor to this increase is the linkage between tuberculosis and HIV infection. A complication is the coincident rise of multidrug-resistant strains of *M. tuberculosis*. The increasing occurrence of the latter reduces the likelihood that initial anti-tuberculous therapy will be effective, thus the patient may remain infectious for a prolonged period (McGowan, 1995).

In dealing with these formidable problems, the Centers for Disease Control and Prevention advocate a hierarchy of control measures for preventing the transmission of *M. tuberculosis* in the health care setting (CDC, 1994). Heading the hierarchy are the administrative controls. These include the implementation of policies that ensure the rapid identification, isolation, diagnostic evaluation and treatment of persons with active tuberculosis; along with work practices (e.g. the closing of doors to the isolation rooms); and educational, counselling and screening programs for health care workers.

The second level of the hierarchy is use of engineering controls. These are designed to prevent the spread and to reduce the concentration of *M. tuberculosis* in droplet nuclei. They include the use of local exhaust ventilation in the immediate environment of the patient; airflow controls (e.g. negative pressure in isolation rooms); and general ventilation controls (e.g. 6 to 12 air changes per hour) for effective dilution of contaminated air. HEPA filtration and ultraviolet radiation are also used for microbial control of the air. Their contribution has been discussed in an earlier section of this Chapter.

The third level of control measures concerns the wearing of personal respiratory protection by health care workers who may be exposed to patients with infectious tuberculosis. Appropriate particulate respirators (masks) for this purpose should be capable of filtering particles of 1 μm in size with 95 per cent efficiency, when tested in the unloaded state, and of providing a tight facial seal, with no more than 10 per cent face-seal leakage (CDC, 1994).

When tested with a mycobacterial aerosol (*Mycobacterium chelonae*) and latex spheres of 0.804 μm diameter, five protective respiratory devices evaluated by Chen et al (1994) met the requirement for a filter efficiency of 95 per cent or better. The devices tested were: a submicron surgical mask, two dust/mist respirators, a dust/mist/fume respirator and a HEPA respirator. Filter efficiencies ranged from 97 per cent for the submicron surgical mask to 99.97 per cent for the HEPA respirator.

Minimizing the spread of vancomycin-resistant enterococci

Contact Precautions apply to the prevention of transmission of vancomycin-resistant enterococci (VRE), along with other strategies aimed specifically at interrupting the spread of vancomycin resistance (HICPAC, 1995; Garner et al, 1996).

The incidence of infection and colonization of hospitalized patients by VRE has increased dramatically over recent years. Two major problems arise. The immediate, practical problem is the treatment of patients infected by vancomycin-resistant strains of enterococci which already have high-level resistance to penicillins (and ampicillin) and the aminoglycosides. The future, potential consequence of concern is the possible genetic transmission of vancomycin resistance from VRE to *Staphylococcus aureus* and *S. epidermidis*.

As enterococci occur normally in the gastrointestinal tract, the source of VRE infection may be endogenous. The site of VRE colonization is generally the gastrointestinal tract. However, patient-to-patient transmission can occur through direct or indirect contact as the result of transient carriage of VRE on the hands of personnel or via contaminated patient-care equipment or environmental surfaces.

In response to the problems posed by the emergence of VRE, the American Hospital Infection Control Practices Advisory Committee recommends the following (CDC, 1995; HICPAC, 1995):

1. Responsible vancomycin use by clinicians
2. Education of health care workers regarding the problem of vancomycin resistance
3. Efficient, early detection and prompt reporting of vancomycin resistance
4. Implementation of Contact Precautions.

To prevent patient-to-patient transmission of VRE, Contact Precautions should be implemented immediately for patients with presumed or proven infection or colonization. These precautions are as follows:

1. Place the VRE-infected or colonized patient in a private room or in the same room as other patients with VRE (cohorting)
2. Wear gloves (e.g. clean, nonsterile gloves) when entering the room and change the gloves after contact with body substances that might contain high concentrations of VRE (e.g. faeces)

3. Wear a gown (e.g. a clean, nonsterile gown) when entering the room if significant contact with the patient, body substances or environmental surfaces is likely
4. Remove the gloves and gown before leaving the room and wash hands immediately with a skin disinfectant
5. After glove and gown removal, ensure that no incidental contact occurs with potentially contaminated, environmental surfaces
6. Dedicate the use of noncritical, patient-care equipment (e.g. stethoscope, rectal thermometer) to a single patient or cohort of patients who are infected or colonized by VRE; if such devices are to be used on other patients, clean and disinfect them first.

Additional measures are recommended for hospitals with endemic VRE or continued VRE transmission (CDC, 1995; HICPAC, 1995). These include the decontamination of environmental surfaces which play a role in the transmission of enterococci. Adequate procedures for the cleaning and disinfection of equipment, material supplies and environmental surfaces need to be in place and their performance verified. Appropriate procedures may need to take into account the relative thermotolerance of enterococci and susceptibility to chlorine disinfectants.

Kearns and others (1995) investigated the heat tolerance of six strains each of *Enterococcus faecium* and *E. faecalis*. Although *E. faecium* was found to be generally more thermotolerant than is *E. faecalis*, all strains of both species survived 65°C for 10 minutes and 71°C for 3 minutes. Of the six test strains of *E. faecium* investigated, all survived 65°C for 20 minutes and 75°C for 3 minutes; four of the six survived 80°C for 3 minutes and one strain survived 71°C for 10 minutes. However, all strains of both species were killed by exposure to 75 or 80°C for 10 minutes. These investigators also showed that available chlorine at a concentration of 500 p.p.m., but not 150 p.p.m., was effective in eliminating enterococci, provided that organic material does not interfere with the action of the disinfectant. It is important that bedpan and other washer/disinfectors operate at appropriate temperatures and holding times for effective elimination of enterococci.

CONTROLLED ENVIRONMENTS IN HEALTH-RELATED INDUSTRIES

Sterile products

The preparation and packaging of products that are to be sterilized involve strict control of environmental contamination levels and methods of processing. Sterile products may be divided into three groups:

1. Heat-stable pharmaceuticals that are terminally sterilized by heat in the final sealed containers
2. Heat-sensitive pharmaceuticals that are sterilized by filtration and then aseptically filled into the final containers
3. Therapeutic devices that are packaged then sterilized by ionizing radiation, ethylene oxide or steam under pressure.

Manufacturing process

The raw materials should have no significant microbial or particulate contamination. The time that elapses between the washing and the sterilization of processing equipment and containers, and also between the sterilization and the use of components in an aseptic process, should be minimized to prevent multiplication of bacteria and accumulation of their pyrogenic components. Large-volume parenterals (intravenous infusions) that are heat-sensitive should be sterilized by filtration immediately before aseptic filling into the final containers. The amount of solution that is prepared should not exceed the volume that can be filtered in one day or filled into the final containers and sterilized in one day. Water treatment plants should be free from U-bends, dead ends and poorly designed valves; the water should be maintained above 65°C and should be monitored for chemicals, microorganisms and pyrogenic components. Unsterilized distilled water should not be allowed to stand for more than a short time unless it is kept at a temperature above 65°C. Sterile equipment that is required in an aseptic processing area should be passed in through a double-ended autoclave. Written procedures for dealing with spillage or disposal of waste should be available.

Biological safety cabinets with vertical airflow should be used for manipulations involving pathogenic, toxic or radioactive materials. Killed vaccines and bacterial extracts may be processed in sterile product areas but production of live or attenuated vaccines should be separated in space or time. Animal tissue should also be processed separately. Sinks and drains should not be installed in aseptic processing areas and those in clean zones should be made from stainless steel, without overflow, and supplied with water of potable quality.

Quality of air

General or local control of airborne microorganisms and other particles is essential for the production of sterile pharmaceuticals and medical devices. The air pressure in special clean or aseptic zones should be positive in relation to surrounding areas, with a pressure indicator and warning signal installed. Special precautions apply to air locks at entrances and exits of changing rooms, hatches for passage of materials into the processing area and communication systems.

International Standard ISO 14644 Part 1 assigns ISO classification levels to the specification of air cleanliness in cleanrooms and associated controlled environments. A cleanroom is described as a room in which the concentration of airborne particles is controlled, and which is constructed and used in such a manner as to minimize the introduction, generation and retention of particles inside the room, and in which other relevant parameters, e.g. temperature, humidity and pressure, are controlled. The cleanliness levels are expressed in terms of ISO Class N, which represents the maximum allowable concentrations of airborne particles equal to or greater than a specified particle size per cubic metre of air (see Table 13.1). Particles are solid or liquid objects within the size range of 0.1 to 5 μm. Ultrafine particles are less than 0.1 μm in diameter, while macroparticles are more than 5 μm in diameter.

The designation of airborne particulate cleanliness for cleanrooms and clean zones must also include reference to occupancy state, as follows:

As-built. The condition where the installation is complete with all services connected and functioning but with no production equipment, materials or personnel present. This applies only to newly completed or newly modified cleanrooms or zones.

At-rest. The condition where the installation is complete with equipment installed and operating in a manner agreed between the customer and supplier but with no personnel present.

Operational. The condition where the installation is functioning in the specified manner, with the specified number of personnel present and working in the manner agreed upon.

Table 13.1 ISO classification for airborne particulate cleanliness of cleanrooms and clean zones

ISO classification number (N)	Maximum concentration limits per m³ for particles equal to or greater than the sizes specified below (ISO 14644.1)					
	0.1 μm	0.2 μm	0.3 μm	0.5 μm	1 μm	5 μm
ISO Class 1	10	2				
ISO Class 2	100	24	10	4		
ISO Class 3	1 000	237	102	35	8	
ISO Class 4	10 000	2 370	1 020	352	83	
ISO Class 5	100 000	23 700	10 200	3 520	832	29
ISO Class 6	1 000 000	237 000	102 000	35 200	8 320	293
ISO Class 7				352 000	83 200	2 930
ISO Class 8				3 520 000	832 000	29 300
ISO Class 9				35 200 000	8 320 000	293 000

Therapeutic devices

Sterile medical devices are subject to the same conditions as those which apply to pharmaceuticals. Plastic devices that are moulded at a high temperature carry few or no microorganisms unless they become contaminated from the environment or personnel during assembly and packaging. This should be minimized by maintenance of an appropriate clean air standard until the products are sealed into the final packages for sterilization by ionizing radiation, ethylene oxide or steam under pressure.

REFERENCES

Antopol S C, Ellner P D 1979 Susceptibility of *Legionella pneumophila* to ultraviolet radiation. Applied and Environmental Microbiology 38: 347–348

Arnow P M, Chou T, Weil D, Shapiro E N, Kretzschmar C 1982 Nosocomial Legionnaires' disease caused by aerosolized tap water from respiratory devices. Journal of Infectious Diseases 146: 460–467

AS 2252.1 Part 1 1994 Biological safety cabinets (Class I) for personnel and environment protection. Standards Association of Australia, Homebush, NSW

AS 2252.2 Part 2 1994 Laminar flow biological safety cabinets (Class II) for personnel, environment and product protection. Standards Association of Australia, Homebush, NSW

AS 4031 1992 Non-reusable containers for the collection of sharp medical items used in health care areas. Standards Australia, Sydney

Barbaree J M, Fields B S, Feeley J C, Gorman G W, Martin W T 1986 Isolation of protozoa from water associated with a legionellosis outbreak and demonstration of intracellular multiplication of *Legionella pneumophila*. Applied and Environmental Microbiology 51: 422–424

Barnes R A, Rogers T R 1989 Control of an outbreak of nosocomial aspergillosis by laminar air-flow isolation. Journal of Hospital Infection 14: 89–94

Best M, Yu V L, Stout J, Goetz A, Muder R R, Taylor F 1983 *Legionellaceae* in the hospital-water supply. Lancet ii: 307–310

Bisno A L, Waldvogel F A (eds) 1989 Infections associated with indwelling medical devices. American Society for Microbiology, Washington DC

Blaser M J, Lofgren J P 1981 Fatal salmonellosis originating in a clinical microbiology laboratory. Journal of Clinical Microbiology 13: 855–858

Blatt S P, Parkinson M D, Pace E et al 1993 Nosocomial Legionnaires' disease: aspiration as a primary mode of disease acquisition. American Journal of Medicine 95: 16–22

Bolan G, Reingold A L, Carson L A et al 1985 Infections with *Mycobacterium chelonei* in patients receiving dialysis and using processed hemodialyzers. Journal of Infectious Diseases 152: 1013–1019

Bollin G E, Plouffe J F, Para M F, Hackman B 1985 Aerosols containing *Legionella pneumophila* generated by shower heads and hot-water faucets. Applied and Environmental Microbiology 50: 1128–1131

Brown P, Wolff A, Gajdusek D C 1990 A simple and effective method for inactivating virus infectivity in formalin-fixed tissue samples from patients with Creutzfeldt-Jakob disease. Neurology 40: 887–890

Bruun J N, Solberg C O 1973 Hand carriage of Gram-negative bacilli and *Staphylococcus aureus*. British Medical Journal 2: 580–582

BS 5726 Parts 1, 2, 3, 4 1992 Microbiological safety cabinets. British Standards Institution, London

Cadwallader H L, Bradley C R, Ayliffe G A J 1990 Bacterial contamination and frequency of changing ventilator circuitry. Journal of Hospital Infection 15: 65–72

Carson L A, Bland L A, Cusick L B et al 1988 Prevalence of nontuberculous mycobacteria in water supplies of hemodialysis centers. Applied and Environmental Microbiology 54: 3122–3125

Carson L A, Favero M S, Bond W W, Petersen N J 1972 Factors affecting comparative resistance of naturally occurring and subcultured *Pseudomonas aeruginosa* to disinfectants. Applied Microbiology 23: 863–869

Carson L A, Petersen N J 1975 Photoreactivation of *Pseudomonas cepacia* after ultraviolet exposure: a potential source of contamination in ultraviolet-treated waters. Journal of Clinical Microbiology 1: 462–464

Carson L A, Petersen N J, Favero M S, Aguero S M 1978 Growth characteristics of atypical mycobacteria in water and their comparative resistance to disinfectants. Applied and Environmental Microbiology 36: 839–846

Casewell M, Phillips I 1977 Hands as route of transmission for *Klebsiella* species. British Medical Journal 2: 1315–1317

Centers for Disease Control 1987 Recommendations for prevention of HIV transmission in health-care settings. Morbidity and Mortality Weekly Report 36 (Suppl 2S): 3S–18S

Centers for Disease Control 1988 Update: Universal precautions for prevention of transmission of human immunodeficiency virus, hepatitis B virus, and other bloodborne pathogens in health-care settings. Morbidity and Mortality Weekly Report 37: 377–382, 387–388

Centers for Disease Control 1989 Guidelines for prevention of transmission of human immunodeficiency virus and hepatitis B virus to health-care and public-safety workers. Morbidity and Mortality Weekly Report 38 (Suppl S6): S1–S37

CDC 1994 Centers for Disease Control and Prevention Guidelines for preventing the transmission of *Mycobacterium tuberculosis* in health-care facilities. Morbidity and Mortality Weekly Report 43: RR–13

CDC 1995 Centers for Disease Control and Prevention Recommendations for preventing the spread of vancomycin resistance: recommendations of the Hospital Infection Control Practices Advisory Committee (HICPAC). Morbidity and Mortality Weekly Report 44: RR–12

Chen S–K, Vesley D, Brosseau L M, Vincent J H 1994 Evaluation of single-use masks and respirators for protection of health care workers against mycobacterial aerosols. American Journal of Infection Control 22: 65–74

Colbourne J S, Pratt D J, Smith M G, Fisher-Hoch S P, Harper D 1984 Water fittings as sources of *Legionella pneumophila* in a hospital plumbing system. Lancet i: 210–213

Collins C H 1993 Laboratory acquired infections, 3rd edn. Butterworths-Heinemann, Oxford

Collins C H, Grange J M, Yates M D 1984 A review. Mycobacteria in water. Journal of Applied Bacteriology 57: 193–211

Domin M A, Smith C E 1992 A report on recent regulatory action. OSHA's final rule on occupational exposure to bloodborne pathogens. Journal of Healthcare Materiel Management 10(2): 36–43

Elliott T S J 1988 Intravascular-device infections. Journal of Medical Microbiology 27: 161–167

England A C, Fraser D W, Mallison G F, Mackel D C, Skaliy P, Gorman G W 1982 Failure of *Legionella pneumophila* sensitivities to predict culture results from disinfectant-treated air-conditioning cooling towers. Applied and Environmental Microbiology 43: 240–244

Farr B M, Gratz J C, Tartaglino J C, Getchell-White S I, Gröschell D H M 1988 Evaluation of ultraviolet light for disinfection of hospital water contaminated with legionella. Lancet ii: 669–672

Favero M S, Carson L A, Bond W W, Petersen N J 1971 *Pseudomonas aeruginosa*: growth in distilled water from hospitals. Science 173: 836–838

Fields B S, Sanden G N, Barbaree J M et al 1989 Intracellular multiplication of *Legionella pneumophila* in amoebae isolated from hospital hot water tanks. Current Microbiology 18: 131–137

Fisher-Hoch S P, Bartlett C L R, Tobin J O'H et al 1981 Investigation and control of an outbreak of Legionnaires' disease in a district general hospital. Lancet i: 932–936

Fisher-Hoch S P, Smith M G, Colbourne J S 1982 *Legionella pneumophila* in hospital hot water cylinders. Lancet i: 1073

Garner J S Hospital Infection Control Practices Advisory Committee 1996 Guideline for isolation precautions in hospitals. Infection Control and Hospital Epidemiology 17: 53–80

Gorman G W, Yu V L, Brown A et al 1980 Isolation of Pittsburgh Pneumonia Agent from nebulizers used in respiratory therapy. Annals of Internal Medicine 93: 572–573

Grist N R 1983 Infections in British clinical laboratories 1980–81. Journal of Clinical Pathology 36: 121–126

Grist N R, Emslie J 1985 Infections in British clinical laboratories, 1982–3. Journal of Clinical Pathology 38: 721–725

Grist N R, Emslie J 1987 Infections in British clinical laboratories, 1984–5. Journal of Clinical Pathology 40: 826–829

Grist N R, Emslie J 1989 Infections in British clinical laboratories, 1986–87. Journal of Clinical Pathology 42: 677–681

Groothuis D G, Veenendaal H R, Dijkstra H L 1985 Influence of temperature on the number of *Legionella pneumophila* in hot water systems. Journal of Applied Bacteriology 59: 529–536

Helms C M, Massanari M, Wenzel R P et al 1988 Legionnaires' disease associated with a hospital water system (a five year progress report of continuous hyperchlorination). Journal of the American Medical Association 259: 2423–2427

Henderson D K, Fahey B J, Willy M et al 1990 Risk for occupational transmission of human immunodeficiency virus type 1 (HIV-1) associated with clinical exposures. Annals of Internal Medicine 113: 740–746

Herwaldt B L, Juranek D D 1995 Protozoa and helminths. In: Fleming D O, Richardson J H, Tulis J J, Vesley D (eds) Laboratory safety principles and practices, 2nd edn. ASM Press, Washington DC, ch 6, p 77

HICPAC 1995 Hospital Infection Control Advisory Committee Recommendations for preventing the spread of vancomycin resistance. Infection Control and Hospital Epidemiology 16: 105–113

Isaac-Renton J L, Fogel D, Stibbs H H, Ongerth J E 1987 *Giardia* and *Cryptosporidium* in drinking water. Lancet i: 973–974

ISO 14644–1 (draft) Cleanrooms and associated controlled environments — Part 1: Classification of airborne particulates. International Organization for Standardization, Geneva

Jepsen O B, Larsen S O, Dankert J et al 1982 Urinary-tract infection and bacteraemia in hospitalized medical patients — a European multicentre prevalence survey on nosocomial infection. Journal of Hospital Infection 3: 241–252

Johnson J T, Yu V L, Best M G et al 1985 Nosocomial legionellosis in surgical patients with head-and-neck cancer: implications for epidemiological reservoir and mode of transmission. Lancet ii: 298–300

Kearns A M, Freeman R, Lightfoot N F 1995 Nosocomial enterococci: resistance to heat and sodium hypochlorite. Journal of Hospital Infection 30: 193–199

Knudson G B 1985 Photoreactivation of UV-irradiated *Legionella pneumophila* and other *Legionella* species. Applied and Environmental Microbiology 49: 975–980

Kuchta J M, States S J, McGlaughlin J E et al 1985 Enhanced chlorine resistance of tap water-adapted *Legionella pneumophila* as compared with agar medium-passaged strains. Applied and Environmental Microbiology 50: 21–26

Landeen L K, Yahya M T, Gerba C P 1989 Efficacy of copper and silver ions and reduced levels of free chlorine in inactivation of *Legionella pneumophila*. Applied and Environmental Microbiology 55: 3045–3050

Liu Z, Stout J E, Tedesco L et al 1994 Controlled evaluation of copper-silver ionization in eradicating *Legionella pneumophila* from a hospital water distribution system. Journal of Infectious Diseases 169: 919–922

Lynch P, Jackson M M, Cummings M J, Stamm W E 1987 Rethinking the role of isolation practices in the prevention of nosocomial infections. Annals of Internal Medicine 107: 243–246

Mastro T D, Fields B S, Breiman R F, Campbell J, Plikaytis B D, Spika J S 1991 Nosocomial Legionnaires' disease and use of medication nebulizers. Journal of Infectious Diseases 163: 667–671

McGowan J E Jr 1995 Nosocomial tuberculosis: new progress in control and prevention. Clinical Infectious Diseases 21: 489–505

McPherson D C, Jackson M M, Rogers J C 1988 Evaluating the cost of the Body Substance Isolation system. Journal of Healthcare Materiel Management 6(6): 20–28

Mermel L A, Josephson S L, Giorgio C H, Dempsey J, Parenteau S 1995 Association of legionnaires' disease with construction: contamination of potable water? Infection Control and Hospital Epidemiology 16: 76–81

Miller D C 1988 Creutzfeldt-Jakob disease in histopathology technicians. New England Journal of Medicine 318: 853–854

Muder R R, Yu V L, Woo A H 1986 Mode of transmission of *Legionella pneumophila*. A critical review. Archives of Internal Medicine 146: 1607–1612

Muraca P, Stout J E, Yu V L 1987 Comparative assessment of chlorine, heat, ozone, and UV light for killing *Legionella pneumophila* within a model plumbing system. Applied and Environmental Microbiology 53: 447–453

Muraca P W, Yu V L, Goetz A 1990 Disinfection of water distribution systems for *Legionella*: a review of application procedures and methodologies. Infection Control and Hospital Epidemiology 11: 79–88

Nahapetian K, Challemel O, Beurtin D, Dubrou S, Gounon P, Squinazi F 1991 The intracellular multiplication of *Legionella pneumophila* in protozoa from hospital plumbing systems. Research in Microbiology 142: 677–685

NHMRC/ANCA 1996 Infection control in the health care setting. Guidelines for the prevention of transmission of infectious diseases. National Health and Medical Research Council, Australian National Council on AIDS, Australian Government Publishing Service, Canberra

Niedeveld C J, Pet F M, Meenhorst P L 1986 Effect of rubbers and their constituents on proliferation of *Legionella pneumophila* in naturally contaminated hot water. Lancet ii: 180–184

NIOSH 1972 Occupational exposure to ultraviolet radiation. National Institute of Occupational Safety and Health, US Department of Health, Education, and Welfare, Public Health Service, Washington, DC, No. (HSM) 73–110009

Peel M M, Calwell J M, Christopher P J, Harkness J L, Rouch G J 1985 *Legionella pneumophila* and water temperatures in Australian hospitals. Australian and New Zealand Journal of Medicine 15: 38–41

Peeters J E, Ares Mazás E, Masschelein W J, Villacorta Martinez de Maturana I, Debacker E 1989 Effect of disinfection of drinking water with ozone or chlorine dioxide on survival of *Cryptosporidium parvum* oocysts. Applied and Environmental Microbiology 55: 1519–1522

Pike R M 1979 Laboratory-associated infections: incidence, fatalities, causes, and prevention. Annual Review of Microbiology 33: 41–66

Plouffe J F, Webster L R, Hackman B 1983 Relationship between colonization of hospital buildings with *Legionella pneumophila* and hot water temperatures. Applied and Environmental Microbiology 46: 769–770

Riley R L, Kaufman J E 1972 Effect of relative humidity on the inactivation of airborne *Serratia marcescens* by ultraviolet radiation. Applied Microbiology 23: 1113–1120

Rubin J S 1988 Review. The molecular genetics of the incision step in the DNA excision repair process. International Journal of Radiation Biology 54: 309–365

Sakata H, Fujita K, Maruyama S, Kakehashi H, Mori Y, Yoshioka H 1989 *Acinetobacter calcoaceticus* biovar *anitratus* septicaemia in a neonatal intensive care unit: epidemiology and control. Journal of Hospital Infection 14: 15–22

Segal-Maurer S, Kalkut G E 1994 Environmental control of tuberculosis: continuing controversy. Clinical Infectious Diseases 19: 299–308

Sewell D L 1995 Laboratory-associated infections and biosafety. Clinical Microbiology Reviews 8: 389–405

Silcox V A, Good R C, Floyd M M 1981 Identification of clinically significant *Mycobacterium fortuitum* complex isolates. Journal of Clinical Microbiology 14: 686–691

Sitwell L, Lach B, Atack E, Atack D, Izukawa D 1988 Creutzfeldt-Jakob disease in histopathology technicians. New England Journal of Medicine 318: 854

Skaliy P, Thompson T A, Gorman G W, Morris G K, McEachern H V, Mackel D C 1980 Laboratory studies of disinfectants against *Legionella pneumophila*: Applied and Environmental Microbiology 40: 697–700

Skinner A R, Anand C M, Malic A, Kurtz J B 1983 Acanthamoebae and environmental spread of *Legionella pneumophila*. Lancet ii: 289–290

Speller D C E, Shanson D C, Ayliffe G A J, Cooke E M 1990 Acquired immune deficiency syndrome: recommendations of a Working Party of the Hospital Infection Society. Journal of Hospital Infection 15: 7–34

Spencer R C 1988 Infections in continuous ambulatory peritoneal dialysis. Journal of Medical Microbiology 27: 1–9

States S J, Conley L F, Ceraso M et al 1985 Effects of metals on *Legionella pneumophila* growth in drinking water plumbing systems. Applied and Environmental Microbiology 50: 1149–1154

Stout J, Yu V L, Vickers R M et at 1982 Ubiquitousness of *Legionella pneumophila* in the water supply of a hospital with endemic Legionnaires' disease. New England Journal of Medicine 306: 466–468

Stout J E, Yu V L, Best M G 1985a Ecology of *Legionella pneumophila* within water distribution systems. Applied and Environmental Microbiology 49: 221–228

Stout J E, Yu V L, Muraca P 1985b Isolation of *Legionella pneumophila* from the cold water of hospital ice machines: implications for origin and transmission of the organism. Infection Control 6: 141–146

Stuart D G, Greenier T J, Rumery R A, Eagleson J M 1982 Survey, use, and performance of biological safety cabinets. American Industrial Hygiene Association Journal 43: 265–270

Taylor D M 1995 Survival of mouse-passaged bovine spongiform encephalopathy agent after exposure to paraformaldehyde-lysine-periodate and formic acid. Veterinary Microbiology 44: 111–112

Taylor D M, McConnell I 1988 Autoclaving does not decontaminate formol-fixed scrapie tissues. Lancet i: 1463–1464

Tison D L, Pope D H, Cherry W B, Fliermans C B 1980 Growth of *Legionella pneumophila* in association with blue-green algae (cyanobacteria). Applied and Environmental Microbiology 39: 456–459

US Federal Standard 209 D 1988 Clean room and work station requirements, controlled environment. United States Federal Agencies, FSC 3694

Wadowsky R M, Yee R B 1985 Effect of non-*Legionellaceae* bacteria on the multiplication of *Legionella pneumophila* in potable water. Applied and Environmental Microbiology 49: 1206–1210

Yu V L 1993 Could aspiration be the major mode of transmission for *Legionella?* American Journal of Medicine 95: 13–15

14. Central sterilization and disinfection services

The underlying principles and the methods of application of the different sterilizing agents and chemical disinfectants have been covered in the foregoing chapters. The planning, administration and everyday working of central sterilizing departments in hospitals or regional service centres is the subject of this concluding chapter. The aim of central sterile supply is to provide reliably sterilized articles, including those obtained from commercial sources, for all departments requiring the service in hospitals or other health care institutions, as economically as possible under conditions that can be validated and controlled.

CENTRAL SERVICE

The advantages of centralization are as follows:

1. Coordinated installation of costly cleaning and sterilizing equipment where it can be fully utilized, correctly operated and regularly maintained
2. Employment of specially trained staff for departmental management, supervision of the work force and operation of the sterilizing equipment
3. Standardization of preparation and packaging of reusable medical and surgical equipment
4. Distribution of sterile supplies and supervision of storage conditions at the site of use.

Scope

The hospital sterilizing department is mainly concerned with the reprocessing and distribution of reusable equipment, such as sterile instrument trays and linen packs for operating theatres, ward procedure packs and disinfected medical equipment used for diagnosis or treatment.

A wide variety of sterile medical devices is now mass produced industrially, where the presterilization bioburden and the efficiency of the sterilization processes can be controlled with greater precision than is usually attainable in hospitals. These products, commonly termed 'disposable', are intended to be used once only and then discarded, unless the manufacturer provides instructions concerning their suitability for repacking, resterilization and reuse. Strategy on the part of the hospital administration is required to balance the convenience of these articles against the economic and safety factors involved in their use.

Functions

Definition of the scope and functions of a sterilizing department is a prerequisite for the architectural design of the department and the layout of each work area within it (Scott, 1988). The main functions are:

1. Reception, cleaning and disinfection of used equipment for reprocessing or reuse
2. Preparation and packaging for sterilization
3. Sterilization by the most suitable process for the particular articles
4. Monitoring the efficiency of sterilization
5. Maintenance and repair of sterilizers and cleaning equipment
6. Storage and distribution of sterile supplies to the user departments.

In addition, safety standards should be established and constantly supervised and all processes carried out in the department should be fully documented. The quality systems in use should be of the same standard as are those that apply to commercially sterilized products.

Terminology

The title of a hospital sterilizing department depends on the scope and functions; it is an administrative decision. The term SSD for sterile services department (HBN 13, 1992) will be used here. Other terms include: CSSD, CSD (central sterile supply, or sterilizing, department); SPS, SPC (sterile processing services or centre): and CPS (central processing services). TSSU (theatre sterile supply unit) refers to a separate unit, the scope of which is limited to surgical instruments and linen packs. An SDU (sterilizing and disinfecting unit) specializes in the cleaning and disinfection of special patient care equipment, particularly bulky items, to make them safe for reuse.

Staff establishment and education

Three general levels of staff are appointed:

1. Managers or superintendents (depending on terminology)
2. Area supervisors and/or specially trained technicians
3. General assistants (subject to inservice training).

Responsibilities and qualifications

The head of the department bears overall responsibility for its administration, the appointment of staff and supervision of all areas and processes. The necessary qualifications include education and experience in departmental management and a comprehensive understanding of sterilization technology. The successful applicant should continue to update knowledge by attendance or active participation in conferences or seminars and is responsible for education and inservice training programs for other staff members to whom the rationale of rules and regulations for their safety must be explained (DuMont, 1987). The manager or superintendent is usually supported by a deputy who has already acquired, or is in the process of acquiring, similar qualifications with a view to future promotion. A microbiologist who has special knowledge of the principles and practice of sterilization should be available for consultation when the efficiency of a process is in question.

Qualified technicians with appropriate knowledge and demonstrated competence should be placed in charge of operating, or directing the routine operation of, sterilizers and ancillary equipment. They should also be involved in the training of the general staff on whom the entire performance of the department depends. The responsibility for preventive maintenance and repair of such equipment is the province of engineers or other authorised persons (sterilizers) who understand the mechanical design and intended function of sophisticated sterilizers.

SSD assistants have an obligation to attend in-service training programs which are designed to promote their understanding of the various tasks that are carried out in different sections of the sterilizing department (Fluke, 1988a; 1988b; 1989). They should also appreciate the importance of their own special role in its overall operation and, in a wider sense, the infection control program of the hospital.

Sources of education and training

A scientifically based course for senior staff, combining relevant aspects of microbiology and detailed treatment of the principles and practice of sterilization, should be provided by an educational institution that is sponsored by the state or national health authority or an association of hospitals. The course should also include a section devoted to the relevance of sterilization in the infection control program, conducted by hospital microbiologists or infection control officers. A separate, appropriately designed course in departmental management, including the use of statistics in the design and interpretation of experiments or surveys, should also be included. A certificate based on assessment by assignments or projects and an adequate pass mark in written examinations should be awarded for successful completion of this course. The same type of educational institution may also offer a more technically oriented course for other levels of SSD staff with appropriate basic education.

Inservice training at the work bench in the various tasks, accompanied by appropriate classroom instruction within the hospital or, if space permits, within the SSD, is required for SSD assistants. This should be conducted by the SSD administrator or experienced technicians. Training manuals and work books have been prepared for this purpose (American Society for Healthcare Central Service Personnel, 1986; Institute of Sterile Services Management, 1990). The manuals provide straightforward explanations of underlying principles and recognized work practices, while leaving scope for variations with respect to differences in local practice.

Compliance with safety rules

The safety of all who work in the sterilizing department should be the subject of a special training program which is made available to all staff on acceptance of employment (Caporino, 1989). This should include the elements of microbiology and the potential hazards associated with the cleaning and disinfection of used equipment, especially when it is soiled with blood or other body fluids. With respect to personal hygiene, staff are expected to report for the treatment of any signs of infection and to pay meticulous attention to washing their hands at appropriate times, using the facilities provided in the recommended manner. Personal clothing should be changed daily; shoes should have non-slip soles for work in the cleaning section and be strong enough to protect against injury if articles are dropped accidentally.

Protective clothing is subject to strict rules, which may be for the protection of the worker or to avoid contributing to the bioburden of the articles during their preparation for sterilization or subsequent storage or for safety. Hair and beards should be covered and the wearing of jewellery when on duty may be discouraged. Protective clothing for workers who are involved in cleaning used equipment includes waterproof outer wear (apron or jumpsuit), supplemented by heavy duty gloves and safety glasses or face masks for manual or ultrasonic cleaning. This attire must be removed when leaving the area and replaced by fresh items on returning. All staff in the cleaning and decontamination area should be made aware of the risks associated with injury by dirty needles or sharp instruments and trained to avoid them (Beischer, 1987). Burn injuries may result from sealing machines or sterilizers lacking adequate insulation. Strong detergents or disinfectants may have adverse effects on the skin. Injury may also be caused by handling heavy loads. The safety training received by individual employees should be documented so that the departmental manager knows what a technician can be expected to know and do. Education should continue as new instruments and devices or new chemicals are introduced into the department (Caporino, 1989).

DESIGN OF A STERILIZING DEPARTMENT

Space allocation and work flow

The diagram of a medium-sized SSD in Figure 14.1 has been selected to show the different work sections and service areas that must be accommodated within the total space that is available for the department. Factors that must be considered in the general design and allotment of space include whether instruments will be processed, stored and issued from a separate TSSU; whether surgical linen will be packed in the SSD; and whether commercially sterilized devices will be accommodated in the storage area. Furthermore, the size of the anticipated work load is obviously an important factor.

The order of work flow and allocation of space for the different sections of the department are the principal features in the design and placement of the different processing areas. The first stage in the progression of equipment through the sterilizing department is the 'dirty' area for the reception, sorting, cleaning, disinfection and drying of incoming materials. This section may include adjacent areas for the cleaning and storage of containers and trolleys that have been used for transportation of contaminated equipment or waste material. The removal of outer transportation containers from incoming supplies of nonsterile or sterile materials may also be carried out in a separate annexe. The total area of the cleaning and decontamination section must allow for installation of the selected manual, mechanical and ultrasonic cleaning equipment. This section is physically separated from the 'clean' areas of the department.

The second section of the SSD accommodates work stations for inspection, assembly and packaging of the goods to be sterilized. Space is also required for storage of bulk supplies of clean materials and equipment to be included in composite packs and also for wrapping materials. If surgical

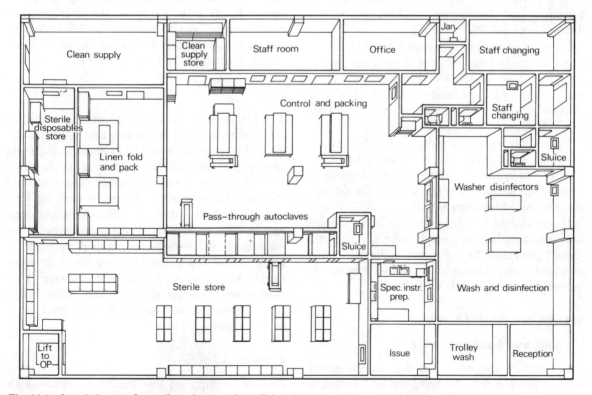

Fig. 14.1 Sample layout of a medium-size central sterilizing department (Courtesy of Getinge AB).

linen is folded and packed in the SSD, a separate room with lighted inspection tables and mending facilities is required. Steam and gas sterilizers, aeration cabinets and sterilizing ovens are installed in an area that communicates directly with the packing section. Adequate space is required for trolleys that convey the packaged goods to the sterilizers and on which they are left to cool before removal to the sterile store.

The store may be the largest single section of the SSD, with the possible exception of the packing area. The actual size depends on whether accommodation must be provided for commercially sterilized medical devices and/or bulky patient care equipment that is ready for return to the wards. Ample room for the movement and storage of the distribution trolleys must be allowed.

Provision of general services

In the planning stage for industrial type sterile services departments, consideration must be given to the provision of access roads, loading bays, collection and distribution facilities and service lifts or ramps (HBN 13, 1992).

Essential service requirements for a SSD include a steam supply from a boiler, a vacuum system, compressed air, distilled or demineralized water and controlled ventilation. Local dedicated exhaust ventilation is required in the vicinity of ethylene oxide sterilizers and aerators.

Favourable working conditions for the staff are 18–20°C and 35–70 per cent relative humidity. The level of lighting is important but the optimum depends on the nature of the task and the amount of reflectance from work benches.

Floors should be constructed so as to support the weight of heavy, loaded trolleys. The walls should preferably be solid (not hollow) in order to avoid being damaged by heavy trolleys or movable equipment (HBN 13, 1992).

SSD WORK PRACTICE

Cleaning and decontamination

The functions carried out in this section of the SSD commence with the reception and sorting of equipment and materials returned from wards and special departments around the hospital and conclude when reusable equipment that has been cleaned and disinfected is ready for transfer to the packaging area. Sorting, cleaning and disinfection present hazards to the staff but render the equipment safe for subsequent handling and in suitable condition for efficient sterilization or disinfection, whichever is appropriate for their intended use.

Reception

Transportation from the site of usage to the SSD involves the use of lidded containers, impermeable plastic bags and covered trolleys. The route should be planned to avoid contact with patients, visitors and hospital staff; designated lifts or dumbwaiters may be used. Liquids should be discarded into the sanitary system before the containers are dispatched from the department where they were used, and instruments soiled with blood may be decontaminated. Return of used articles in their original containers or packaging, with precautions against drying, is usually preferred because it eliminates the risk of infection being spread by nurses' hands in the wards and leaves decisions on processing to trained staff in the SSD. Articles that present an identifiable hazard should be identified according to the hospital policy.

Sorting

The first step in the sorting process is to discard waste material, used or unused, and single-use devices that have been stored or used in a patient care area; if they have been retained on the delivery trolley or in the departmental storage cupboard they may be returned to the sterile store for 'first out' redistribution if there is no evidence of damage or contamination. When sorting has been completed, the trolleys are washed in a special room that is connected to a hot water or steam supply and is provided with floor drainage. They should be tilted for draining and dried before reuse. Reusable transportation containers must also be cleaned.

Cleaning and disinfection

Reusable equipment that has been approved for reprocessing should be disassembled into its component parts whenever possible and allocated to the manual, mechanical or ultrasonic cleaning methods that have been described in Chapter 3. Ultrasonic cleaning is usually reserved for delicate articles that are difficult to clean manually, or as a supplement to the manual cleaning of some articles that have inaccessible crevices, such as hinges or box joints, which may harbour residual soil.

Gross soiling should be removed by rinsing or soaking the articles before any method of cleaning is undertaken. Soaking in an enzyme-containing detergent may be necessary if blood or tissue residues have dried, e.g. in hollow instruments or suction tubes. Disinfection may precede the cleaning of articles from wards that have been designated as isolation areas. Sterilization by steam is undesirable for decontamination because coagulation and hardening of organic material makes subsequent cleaning difficult. The use of an ethylene oxide sterilizer and aeration cabinet is not recommended because inclusion of the dirty articles in a cycle with clean, packaged equipment is unacceptable. Material that is suspected of containing viruses that cause hepatitis or AIDS should be immersed in a chlorine-based disinfectant containing 10 000 p.p.m. available chlorine or, if chlorine would be deleterious to the instruments, a solution of 2 per cent w/v activated glutaraldehyde. Activated glutaraldehyde has a labelled use life of 14–28 days but this time is reduced if the solution is diluted with added water or inactivated by organic soil that has been introduced with wet or inadequately cleaned equipment. The solution should be covered to prevent inhalation of the vapour and goggles and gloves should be worn. In the United Kingdom, glutaraldehyde is subject to occupational exposure limits of 0.2 p.p.m./8-h TWA and 2 p.p.m./10-min TWA. The use of a special machine that circulates the solution through instruments with hollow tubes is recommended.

The selection and use of detergents for manual, mechanical or ultrasonic cleaning are important and recommendations by the manufacturers of the equipment and the cleaning agents should be followed. The types of detergents and their applications have been discussed in Chapter 3 (Harrison et al, 1990). Neutral products (pH 7–9) are required for metal instruments, cleaned by any method. Alkaline products are suitable for mechanical cleaning of glassware but unsuitable for manual cleaning because of the risk of contact with the skin. Quaternary ammonium compounds, formulated by the manufacturer with compatible detergents, may be used. Cleaning should be done with a soft bristle brush; abrasive cleaners must not be used. Alcohols and phenolic disinfectants are unsuitable for the disinfection of plastics.

Surgical instruments that are assembled in sets for use in a particular operation may be kept together in a separate basket in a mechanical washer/disinfector. Ultrasonic cleaners do not disinfect the equipment but cleaning may be followed by disinfection in hot rinsing water. The baskets, with instruments in situ, may be immersed in a water-soluble instrument lubricant before they are dried. Cleaned equipment is usually dried by means of hot air and this may be included in the cycle of a washer/disinfector. Special cabinets are used in hot air drying of tubes, such as breathing circuits from anaesthetic or respiratory equipment, which are hung from nozzles of appropriate size. Electrical, mechanical and electronic equipment which cannot be immersed in cleaning solutions or disinfectants should be processed according to the manufacturers' instructions.

Assembly and packaging

Cleaned and disinfected equipment requiring preparation and packaging for sterilization is received from the cleaning and disinfection area. It is carefully inspected for cleanliness and proper function; defective or damaged instruments are sent to an on-site workshop or to the manufacturer. All mechanical and electrical equipment and electronic devices must be tested for safety and proper function by a qualified person; it is most important that all used equipment that is subjected to inspection and/or repair by experts has already been cleaned and disinfected.

Storage of bulk supplies

Wrapping materials and clean supplies for inclusion in procedure packs or trays should be stored in a section of the packing room after removal from the contaminated transportation containers elsewhere. The wrapping materials should be kept in an environment that will maintain their normal moisture content. If linen is folded and packed in the SSD, instead of the laundry, it should be delivered to a linen room where it is inspected and folded on lighted tables and folding and mending equipment are available.

Packaging materials and containers

The properties of packaging materials that meet the requirements for sterilization have been described in Chapter 3. Wrapping sheets of woven textiles (100 per cent cotton or a more closely woven blend of cotton and polyester) are used for large packs and instrument trays. These reusable wrappers are generally applied independently as two double-thickness layers to form a 'package within a package'. Nonwoven materials, which are used only once, may also be used; however, an outer layer of woven textile may be required to provide mechanical strength for large or heavy packs. Wrapping sheets may be folded by the square (parcel fold) or diagonal (envelope fold) method, depending on the size and composition of the pack, as illustrated in Chapter 3 (Fig. 3.1). Smaller articles may be packaged in preformed pouches, which are usually made from combined webs of chemically treated paper and transparent plastic. The pouch should be neither under- nor over-sized for the contents in order to avoid rupture of the seal. When plastic is bonded to paper, the pack should be removed from the heat sealer to cool; when two layers of plastic are bonded together it should be left to cool in the jaws to avoid stretching the seal while the material is melted. No type of pack, large or small, may be fastened by pins, staples, clips or any other device that pierces the wrapping material.

Method of packing

Large textile packs and instrument trays are subject to recommended limits of size and weight for sterilization by steam under pressure in prevacuum or downward displacement steam sterilizers (ANSI, ST46). Specially designed reusable containers made from metal or heat-stable plastic, are now widely used for large or small instrument sets for sterilization in prevacuum steam or ethylene oxide sterilizers (ANSI, ST33; Kneedler & Gattas, 1988). Perforated upper and lower panels are lined internally with microbial filter material which must be securely held in place. Alternatively, valves which are automatically opened and closed may be used to permit removal of air and entry of steam. The top and bottom parts must be securely fastened and locked in place. The containers should be disassembled, washed and rinsed after each use. The Edinburgh tray system (Bowie et al, 1963) has been described in Chapter 3. Sets of bowls should be nested in order of size and spaced by inserts of moisture-absorbing material, such as cotton towels or gauze sponges. Setting an instrument tray demands special knowledge of the instruments and the manner in which they must be presented on the tray.

Each set of instruments should be inspected before packing. Jointed instruments should be opened and unlocked; some may be disassembled, with the parts close together. Caution is required when packing textiles and metalware in the same pack, or as separate packs in the same sterilizer load, because the wrapping may be wetted by condensate that has coalesced and drained from the site at which it was formed, with liberation of latent heat, to another site where the latent heat is not available to vaporize it.

Linen should be prepared with the layers of cloth parallel and folds oriented alternately in either direction. Gowns should be folded inside out and drapes arranged in order of use. A towel may be placed on top of each gown for drying the hands. When the outer wrap has been removed, the inner one may be opened out on the table to serve as a sterile field.

Range of packs prepared in the SSD

It is recommended that the provision of trays and packs for operating rooms and special procedure packs for wards, departments and the community should be prepared in the SSD. Basic procedure packs may be prepared in the SSD or obtained commercially, depending on costs (HBN, 1992).

Labelling

Packs should be labelled before sterilization with a felt tip indelible ink marker on the tape securing the pack. Paper/plastic pouches should be labelled on the clear side as the ink may penetrate the paper. The label should identify the contents, sterilizer and cycle number, and the date of sterilization and should be initialled by the packer.

Sterilization

Prevacuum steam sterilizers are required for most of the work load. Ethylene oxide or a low-temperature steam and formaldehyde (LTSF) sterilizer should be installed only where operational expertise and prescribed safety measures are available (see Ch. 7). An ethylene oxide sterilizer and aeration cabinet should be provided with an exhaust hood; this is also a requirement for LTSF sterilizers since the need to eliminate the form-aldehyde vapours has been recognized (Alder, 1987; HTM, 1994). Adequate space should be allowed in the vicinity of the sterilizers for movement of load baskets and trolleys and also for cooling of the sterilized packs on trolleys or wire racks before they are moved to the sterile store. Packs should never be placed on a solid metal surface to cool. Clean (unused) plastic bags may be applied as dust covers to packs that are to be stored for an unpredictable time for use in emergency. Containerized articles should not be stacked in the sterilizer; they should be placed on well-spaced shelves. Unloaded packs should not be handled until they are cool and dry. It is the duty of the sterilizer operator, subject to supervision if necessary, to monitor the sterilization processes with test packs and thermocouples, biological and chemical indicators as recommended. Implantable devices should not be released until all monitoring tests have been completed.

A planned maintenance (PM) program which nominates the tests that are applicable to each type of steam or gas sterilizer and defines the responsibility for their performance at specified intervals is an essential component of sterilizing department policy (HTM, 1994). The physical, chemical and biological tests that are used to demonstrate the efficiency of a sterilization process have been described in detail in foregoing chapters. Some are classed as routine tests that are carried out by the sterilizer operator on a daily or weekly basis. A more comprehensive program of qualifying tests is required on commissioning a new sterilizer after installation in the hospital and this must be repeated on recommissioning after major repairs or modifications. The same tests are also performed annually.

Responsibility for carrying out the tests is shared by the sterilizer operator and the hospital maintenance engineer with advice, as required, from a specialist sterilizing engineer or the manufacturer of the sterilizer. Each of the persons involved in the maintenance program, including the manager of the sterilizing department and a consultant microbiologist, should have the knowledge and experience that is appropriate to their allotted tasks. Engineers should understand the design, construction and functions of the sterilizers and should also be familiar with the models that they service. The sterilizer operator should inspect the recorder chart or computer printout on conclusion of each sterilization cycle and, in conjunction with the manager of the department, should review these at least once a week. The advice of the consultant microbiologist may be required with respect to biological tests on gas sterilizers or when the results obtained from combined tests are not in accord.

Detailed records are an essential component of the planned maintenance program. The engineer is responsible for keeping a plant history record for each sterilizer. This should include the results of commissioning, recommissioning and regular yearly tests along with documents concerning the maintenance contract, the insurance surveyor's report and full details of maintenance, repairs and modifications of the sterilizer. A sterilizer process record is also required. This includes written procedures for all tests and the results obtained, the contents of each sterilizer load, the cycle number and date and a maintenance test certificate. Copies of these records, usually kept by the sterilizer engineer or the maintenance engineer, should be given to the manager of the sterilizing department, the sterilizer operator and the microbiologist or infection control officer. A process master record

(PMR) for each sterilizer and each type of load is prepared from the recording instrument or the computer memory bank of a cycle that has been proven satisfactory in a comprehensive testing schedule. A load may be described by the type or size of the batch or the types of equipment it contained. Alternatively, a PMR derived from a 'worst case' load may be used for several loading conditions. Each PMR should be selected from the result of two tests; the one that shows the shortest time at the sterilizing temperature is used.

Storage of sterilized supplies

The function of the 'sterile' store is to accommodate packs that have been produced in the SSD and, depending on hospital policy, supplies of sterile devices and procedure packs from commercial sources. Space may also be required for holding patient care equipment that has been disinfected and is ready for reuse in that condition. Provision is also required for the loading of trolleys for delivery of supplies to the operating room and other locations where they will be used.

Requirements for storage

The storage area should be clean, dry and well ventilated but free from draughts that could cause contamination of packs wrapped in paper or cotton fabric. Packs that may be stored for an unpredictable period should be protected by sealed plastic dust covers. Commercially produced devices, which are removed from the transportation container before they are admitted to the store, should not be removed from the shelf storage pack provided by the manufacturer until they are delivered to the user department. This secondary packaging fulfils the role of the outer layer of a double-wrapped pack. The store should be maintained at 18–22°C with the relative humidity between 35 and 75 per cent. The floor should be cleaned daily by damp mopping and shelves, delivery carts and containers should also be cleaned regularly. Handwashing by staff should be enforced.

Open shelf storage or closed cupboards may be used. The limited space provided by cupboards may be appropriate for supplies that are seldom used but fixed or movable (compactus) shelves are more commonly used. The lowest shelf should be solid and 20–25 cm above the floor, and the top of the stack 15 cm below the ceiling. Shelves should not be close to outside walls, sinks or sprinklers. Packs should be spaced to avoid friction when they are moved for rotation of stock. Rigid reusable containers may be stacked on the shelves. Entry to the store should be restricted and movement of persons within the area minimized. If packages are dropped in the store but are not damaged, those that are wrapped in plastic may be cleaned with disinfectant and returned to the shelf.

Shelf life

It is widely recognized that a time-related expiration date for the maintenance of sterility is meaningless (Mayworm, 1984). Standard et al (1973) found that packs which were wrapped in a double layer of woven material could become contaminated after 18–30 days in artificially created, worst-case storage conditions, but that the contamination-free period was extended to at least 9 months for products sealed in plastic dust covers and at least 1 year for paper/plastic pouches. However, maintenance of sterility depends primarily on the conditions of storage and frequency of handling. Microbial contamination of the storage environment, movements of air or personnel, temperature, moisture, location in the store and the barrier properties of the packaging material are contributing factors (Mayworm, 1984). The use of outmoded arbitrary expiration dating has given way to the concept that hospital products should be packaged so as to remain sterile until they are opened for use. If this is put into practice, it becomes feasible to use the label 'sterile unless opened or damaged', as is applied to industrially sterilized products. However, as dating is still common practice and may be required by hospital accreditation agencies, the emphasis has been changed and dates are now used to ensure stock rotation based on a 'first in, first out' system (Jevitt, 1984). It has been recommended that no date is required for double-wrapped articles that will be used within 24 hours (e.g. surgical instrument packs); 1 week is appropriate for articles with a high turnover rate; 6 months for those in rigid containers and 1 year for packs in sealed, plastic dust covers (Mayworm, 1984). Thus, expiration dating has been converted to an inventory control system. This system also provides a means of assessing the frequency of usage of packs and deciding whether the unused packs are no longer required.

Distribution of sterile supplies

The trolleys should be covered or closed, with a solid bottom shelf. Each article to be loaded must be inspected and handled with care; packs should not be crushed together in the boxes or bags. Several distribution systems are in use, depending on the size and operational policies of the hospital.

1. Requisition of supplies by the user department. This system has several disadvantages; it is unsuitable for large hospitals because it is labour intensive and the staff may lack the necessary time or training to implement the system without overstocking and hoarding.
2. Replenishment and replacement of packs as they are used. This system tends to be slow as it may involve repeated returns to the SSD for supplies unless requirements have been listed on a preliminary round.
3. Replacement of the whole day's supply by exchange carts. Special case carts (e.g. catheter carts or suture carts) may be devised by consultation between the user department and the SSD. This system may be wasteful but has some advantages and is applicable in both small and large hospitals. It requires duplication of stock and more space for handling the carts in the store.

Emergency carts for cardiac or respiratory arrest, which are required for a national disaster or large traffic accident, would be stored until needed. Transportation from the SSD store to the user departments may be by trolleys, dedicated lifts or pneumatic tubes. At the other extreme, the supplies are collected by the user. The success of any system depends on its reliability and timeliness; supplies should not run out before they are restocked.

Reuse of commercially sterilized devices

This is a controversial topic as most of the devices are intended for a single use only and failure to observe this instruction may result in illness of patients and possibly in legal action. Problems of allocating the cost of the article may also arise if some patients are treated with a new device and others with one that has been reprocessed.

Arguments for and against reuse are centered on two aspects:

1. Can the article be cleaned, repacked and resterilized successfully?
2. Will it still perform its function after reprocessing has been carried out?

Authorities in Britain and the United States have withdrawn total opposition to reuse of devices that are labelled 'single use only', leaving the decision and responsibility for reuse to the hospital. Such a decision should be based on investigation of the environment in which the pack was opened, the likely bioburden acquired and the manner in which it was handled (Reichert, 1988).

Situations that lead to consideration of reuse are:

1. The pack was not opened
2. The pack was opened but the device was not used
3. The article was used.

An unopened pack may be returned to the store if it is not soiled or damaged. Some devices undergo a second sterilization procedure when they are combined with other nonsterile components in a composite pack. Whatever reason is given for reuse, the effect of the sterilization procedure on the product or packaging material must be known and the cost of reprocessing versus replacement must also be considered.

Before a decision is made to rewrap and resterilize a device, the manufacturer should be asked if the effect of resterilization has been tested and if relevant information is available. It would be impractical for the hospital to carry out this type of study. A device that was originally double-wrapped and is still contained in the intact inner wrap is more suitable for resterilization than is a single-wrapped product. An article that has been used in the treatment of a patient must be cleaned, packaged and sterilized. It must also be pyrogen-free (Reichert, 1988). The new wrapping material, which may be different from that used by the manufacturer, must be compatible with the sterilization process that will be used in the hospital.

Requests for reprocessing should be reviewed by an appropriate hospital committee and refused if no information is available concerning the suitability of the proposed method of sterilization and its effect on the product and type of wrapping material. Deleterious effects on the product may be caused by contact with cleaning or sterilizing agents that could result in pinholes in ventilation circuits or the failure of balloons to inflate in cardiac catheters. If the manufacturer has evidence to show that the product will not be degraded, the economic aspects may be considered and, if these favour reuse, information may be sought on the method of reprocessing. The hospital's insurance company should also be consulted. If reuse is finally authorized, the level of quality control should be of the same standard as that which applies to the original commercial process. While the manufacturing process is subject to control, the manufacturer has no control over use of the device once it has been accepted by the hospital.

STERILIZATION AND DISINFECTION OF SPECIAL EQUIPMENT AND MATERIALS

Dental equipment and materials

Dental instruments and equipment should be either disposable ('single use') or capable of being sterilized by heat. Articles that are difficult to clean, e.g. saliva ejector tips, should also be disposable (Mulick, 1986). Before sterilization, all instruments and equipment should be thoroughly cleaned for the removal of saliva, blood and proteinaceous material which can act as a barrier to sterilization.

Dental burs

Burs should be disposable or sterilized after each use (Council on Dental Materials, Instruments, and Equipment, 1992). Dry heat is the usual agent used for sterilizing steel, carbon steel and tungsten-carbide burs. Sterilization is carried out

either in a hot air oven or in chairside glass bead units with extended exposure time (see Ch. 5). Patterson et al (1988) investigated the effects of up to 40 cycles of ultrasonic cleaning and autoclaving (at 134°C for 3.5 minutes) on two different types of tungsten-carbide burs. One type deteriorated rapidly whereas the other remained virtually unaltered.

Dental handpieces

Both air-turbine and conventional handpieces can now be sterilized by autoclaving, which is the method of choice for this type of equipment (Shovelton et al, 1984; Cottone & Molinari, 1987). Shovelton et al (1984) showed that lubrication before autoclaving at 134°C for 3.5 minutes did not interfere with sterilization when the instruments were additionally contaminated with a spore suspension of *Bacillus stearothermophilus*. However, they cautioned that lubrication might protect the spores if the suspension had been allowed to dry on the surfaces of the instrument. As stressed by the Council on Dental Materials, Instruments, and Equipment (1992) and Field et al (1988), the performance of autoclaves used in dental surgeries should be monitored, e.g. by process monitors for each load and biological indicators weekly.

Endodontic instruments

Dry heat sterilization is the preferred method for endodontic instruments, such as reamers and files, because this method of sterilization does not affect their sharpness or cutting ability. Forrester & Douglas (1988) rapidly sterilized endodontic reamers by holding them with forceps in a stream of air at a temperature of about 490°C produced by a chairside dental heating unit (see Ch. 5).

Dental impressions

Dental impressions should be washed free of saliva and blood immediately after removal from the mouth then decontaminated by immersion in a virucidal disinfectant that does not produce any dimensional change in the impression. Glutaraldehyde disinfectant at a 2 (or 2.2) per cent w/v concentration fulfils these requirements for both silicone-based and alginate impressions (Minagi et al, 1987; Tullner et al, 1988). Jones et al (1988) used a reflex plotter to show that no significant dimensional changes occurred with the latter. Alternative disinfectants, which may also be compatible with a wider range of impression materials, are sodium hypochlorite and iodophors (Miller & Palenik, 1991). A solution of 0.5 per cent w/v sodium hypochlorite (for 15 minutes) is often used.

Dental laboratory pumice

Pumice slurry is a recognized reservoir of oral and environmental bacteria in dental laboratories. Williams et al (1986) showed that such bacteria can survive, at high concentrations, for more than 3 months in untreated pumice slurry. To control this source of contamination, the pumice should be replaced after each use (Miller & Palenik, 1991).

General disinfection in dental surgeries

Water from the dental unit system is contaminated by the biofilm that forms along the luminal walls of tubing. The source of bacteria for the biofilm is the water supply, not aspirated oral fluids (Williams et al, 1995). *Legionella pneumophila*, which typically occurs in biofilms, may also be isolated (Challacombe & Fernandes, 1995). Weekly decontamination with 0.5 per cent w/v sodium hypochlorite is recommended. The system is flushed with the disinfectant, filled and allowed to stand for 10 minutes, then flushed with water (Williams et al, 1995). Operatory surfaces should be covered, e.g. with plastic film, or disinfected with iodophors, 0.05–0.5 per cent hypochlorite or phenolics (Council on Dental Materials, Instruments, and Equipment, 1992). Aerosol contamination of surfaces is reduced by a pre-rinse of the mouth with chlorhexidine (Logothetis & Martinez-Welles, 1995).

Endoscopes

Fibreoptic endoscopes have been implicated in the transmission of hepatitis B virus (Birnie et al, 1983) and *Mycobacterium* spp. (Wheeler et al, 1989) from infected patients to non-infected patients. In addition to cross-infection, endoscopes have also been responsible for transmitting opportunistic pathogens, e.g. *Pseudomonas aeruginosa* and non-tuberculous mycobacteria, from their aqueous environmental reservoir to patients (Classen et al, 1988: Spach et al, 1993). Serovars of *Salmonella* have also been prominent among agents transmitted by endoscopy from patient to patient (Spach et al, 1993). The clinical spectrum of infection ranges from colonization to serious, and sometimes fatal, disease. Moreover, pseudoinfections may entail unnecessary diagnostic and therapeutic interventions (Daschner, 1992; Spach et al, 1993).

Sterilization of operative endoscopes

Operative endoscopes that enter sterile body sites and cavities, e.g. arthroscopes and laparoscopes, should be sterile. Compact, benchtop autoclaves are available for point-of-use sterilization of endoscopes that can be autoclaved (Babb & Bradley, 1995a). They use a gentle method of steam injection based on the Joslyn process (see Ch. 6). The cycle time of about 16 minutes includes a sterilization time of 3 minutes at 134°C.

Sterilization is time-consuming and deemed to be unnecessary for bronchoscopes and gastroscopes which are not used in sterile body sites. These endoscopes are decontaminated by thorough cleaning and chemical disinfection. While cystoscopes are usually sterilized by the methods used for operative endoscopes, those used for flexible fibreoptic cystoscopy cannot withstand temperatures above 55–60°C. They are also decontaminated by cleaning and disinfection (Cooke et al, 1993).

Cleaning and disinfection of endoscopes

Glutaraldehyde is an effective disinfectant for endoscopes because it is active against a wide range of microorganisms, non-corrosive, and does not damage plastic, rubber or the cement mounting of lenses. The disadvantages of glutaraldehyde include its toxicity, which necessitates thorough rinsing of endoscopes after disinfection. Post-colonoscopy proctitis has been reported when the glutaraldehyde residues have not been properly removed (Spach et al, 1993). Glutaraldehyde is also an irritant to mucous membranes and may cause dermatitis and asthma-like reactions in handlers (Spach et al, 1993).

Endoscope cleaning and disinfection should be carried out in a dedicated room with exhaust ventilation to control glutaraldehyde vapours (Cowan et al, 1993). Where control measures are lacking or inadequate, personal protection is mandatory. This includes the wearing of long nitrile gloves, plastic aprons and eye protection (Cowan et al, 1993; Babb & Bradley, 1995a). Atmospheric levels of glutaraldehyde should be appropriately monitored to ensure that the occupational exposure levels remain below the recommended limits (Cowan et al, 1993).

The concentration of glutaraldehyde which is recommended for disinfection is 2 per cent. It is important that the concentration does not fall appreciably below 1.5 per cent; and that, for the alkali-activated glutaraldehyde, the use life does not exceed the post-activation life of 14 or 28 days (Babb et al, 1992). The repeated addition of washed endoscopes dilutes the glutaraldehyde solution which necessitates its replacement at time intervals that depend mainly on instrument throughput but which are usually shorter than the 14 or 28 day use life after activation.

The disinfection of endoscopes by glutaraldehyde should take place only in automated washer/disinfectors (Cowan et al, 1993). Suitable machines clean all channels as well as the insertion tube and the control head. Some incorporate an extraction/exhaust function. The cycle consists of washing in neutral or enzymatic detergent, disinfecting in glutaraldehyde and rinsing in water, with a final rinse in bacteria-free, filtered water. Some machines provide a drying facility that uses alcohol or hot air (Bradley & Babb, 1995). Manual pre-cleaning of endoscopes is required immediately after use and before automated processing (Bradley & Babb, 1995). In pre-cleaning, the valves are dismantled and brushed with a sterile or disinfected brush (Ayliffe et al, 1993) and all channels are flushed. Heat-stable accessories, e.g. biopsy forceps and cytology brushes, should be sterilized by autoclaving after each use, or they should be disposable (Cowan et al, 1993). Washer/disinfectors must have a self-disinfect function to prevent endoscope recontamination during processing (Babb & Bradley, 1995a).

The investigations of Hanson et al (1989) indicate that mechanical washing alone removes HIV from endoscopes. In 1992, Hanson et al reported that cleaning can achieve a 3.5 log reduction in the numbers of *Mycobacterium tuberculosis* experimentally applied to bronchoscopes.

All authorities agree that the thorough washing and cleaning of endoscopes before chemical disinfection is the single, most important procedure in decontamination. However, agreement is often lacking on the appropriate contact times for disinfection in 2 per cent glutaraldehyde. Reports of the isolation of glutaraldehyde-resistant strains of *Mycobacterium chelonae* by van Klingeren and Pullen (1993) have further complicated the issue.

Mycobacterium avium is more resistant to inactivation by glutaraldehyde than is *M. tuberculosis*. It is also an important pathogen for HIV-infected patients. To prevent environment-to-patient transmission of *M. avium*, the British Thoracic Society recommends that bronchoscopes be immersed in 2 per cent glutaraldehyde for a period of 60 minutes before use on immunocompromised patients. For other patients, immersion for a period of 20 minutes is recommended (Woodcock et al, 1989).

The British Association of Urological Surgeons recommends that the flexible, fibreoptic cystoscopes be decontaminated by exposure to 2 per cent glutaraldehyde for at least 10 minutes. Where urinary mycobacterial infection is diagnosed or suspected, an immersion period of 60 minutes is recommended (Cooke et al, 1993).

The British Society of Gastroenterology affirms that exposure of cleaned gastroscopes to 2 per cent glutaraldehyde for a period of 4 minutes should suffice to inactivate bacteria and viruses. However, a contact time of 20 minutes is advised if infection by *M. tuberculosis* is strongly suspected (Cowan et al, 1993). In Australia, Collignon & Graham have suggested the slightly longer contact time of 5 minutes, mainly for the more reliable inactivation of hepatitis B virus. However, the Australian authors concede that suggested contact times are largely arbitrary and conservatively based on the assumption that thorough cleaning, which will remove the bulk of the contaminants from endoscopes, precedes disinfection in glutaraldehyde (Collignon & Graham, 1989).

Chemical sterilization of endoscopes

Peracetic acid at a concentration of 0.2 per cent (Steris system) or 0.35 per cent (NuCidex) effectively destroys spores of *Bacillus subtilis*, as well as *M. tuberculosis*, *M. avium* and other species of *Mycobacterium*, when tested in the presence and absence of an organic load of 10 per cent serum (Babb & Bradley, 1995b). Although peracetic acid is potentially very corrosive, this property is virtually eliminated, for practical purposes, when the liquid sterilant is combined with a proprietary anti-corrosive chemical formulation in the commercially-developed system.

The Steris system is a self-contained, single-use, tabletop unit. Endoscopes must be cleaned before being placed in the sterilizer. The process operates at 50–55°C and terminates with rinsing in filter-sterilized water and drying by filter-sterilized air. Sterilization is accomplished in 12 minutes and the total cycle requires 20–30 minutes. Importantly, a temperature of 50–55°C is able to destroy oocysts of *Cryptosporidium* within 5 to 10 minutes whereas 2 per cent glutaraldehyde fails to inactivate them even after 30 minutes (Casemore et al, 1989). This anti-parasitic activity is advantageous since there is evidence that *Cryptosporidium* may have a significant intestinal carrier rate (Roberts et al, 1989) and cryptosporidiosis is a serious disease in AIDS patients.

NuCidex is another formulation of peracetic acid which contains proprietary corrosion inhibitors. It is used at a concentration of 0.35 per cent at ambient temperature and has a use life of 24 hours. NuCidex also differs from the Steris system in that it can be used in washer/disinfectors. However, peracetic acid is corrosive to copper and its alloys and, for this or other reasons, NuCidex is not compatible with all types of washer/disinfectors (Babb & Bradley, 1995b; Fraise, 1995).

Respiratory therapy equipment

Colonization of mechanical ventilators

The breathing circuits, humidifiers and other accessories of mechanical ventilators, which may be used on a continuous basis by seriously ill patients under intensive care, are readily colonized by microorganisms, especially in biofilms (Inglis, 1995). They are derived mainly from the patient's upper gastrointestinal (Inglis, 1995) or respiratory tracts. Gram-negative bacteria predominate in

the moist situation and can cause potentially fatal pneumonia in immunocompromised patients (Lichtenberg, 1988). This necessitates decontamination of the equipment after each use by different patients or at specified intervals if used by one patient.

Contamination levels in breathing circuits and humidifiers have been studied by Goularte et al (1987) and Cadwallader et al (1990). Each team of investigators arrived at the conclusion that the machine may be used continuously for 48 hours in adult patients as the contaminant population does not increase significantly during the second 24 hours. The type of humidifier influences the rate of colonization. Cold water humidifiers are rapidly colonized by Gram-negative bacteria but those equipped with a heated humidifier in the form of a bubbling cascade maintained at a temperature between 40°C and 60°C were considered to be an unlikely source of colonization or of dispersal of infective aerosols (Goularte et al 1987). However, Ayliffe et al (1993) recommend a temperature above 70°C in the humidifier. The need for a water humidifier may be overcome by the installation of a heat-moisture exchanger, which eliminates condensation in the breathing circuit. However, this may increase resistance in the circuit resulting in insufficient humidity for patients who are critically ill (Goularte et al, 1987).

Protection and decontamination

Small, multilayered, disposable filter units, with or without a heat-moisture exchange function, are available for installation in respiratory circuits. The filters in these units are hydrophobic membranes with a high electrostatic and mechanical filtering capability that allows them to act as bacteriological/viral filters. They are sterilized commercially by ethylene oxide and have a maximum service life of 24 hours. When used in anaesthesia or in intensive care (with the heat-moisture exchange function), these filters protect patients, equipment and health care personnel from environmental and cross contamination.

Anaesthetic and ventilatory equipment may be decontaminated by disinfection or sterilization, although the former only is indicated for these semicritical items. The method of choice is thermal disinfection in an automated washer/disinfector in which the disassembled equipment is cleaned, disinfected by hot water (e.g. 93°C for 10 minutes), rinsed and then dried (Geiss, 1995; AS 2711, 1993). The anaesthetic hoses are held in special cassettes or purpose-designed rotary supports and the breathing bags are placed on specialized jet nozzles. The programs are usually controlled by microprocessors. Total processing time is less than 1 hour.

Heat-stable components of respiratory therapy equipment are sterilized by steam at 134°C. Heat-labile equipment may be sterilized by gas plasma, low-temperature steam and formaldehyde or ethylene oxide. However, the aeration process does not always completely remove ethylene oxide from the interior of complex equipment such as small ventilators (Gschwandtner, 1990).

Equipment and infection risk

The term equipment has been frequently used in this book in two senses: equipment that is to be sterilized or disinfected for use and, in the other sense, the equipment required to process it for reuse. The complexity of modern surgical instruments and diagnostic devices has been matched by the sophistication of methods that are now employed to make them safe to handle by workers who are involved in preparing them for reuse and ultimately safe for use on the next patient. The development of prevacuum steam sterilizers for porous loads has now reached the peak of efficiency and reliability. The use of the gaseous sterilants, e.g. pure ethylene oxide and gas plasma, caters for heat-sensitive equipment. Ethylene oxide and ionizing radiation are used as industrial sterilants in the production of a wide range of sterile medical devices.

The validation of sterilization processes is seen as an essential component of modern sterilization practice. Validation refers to documented procedures for obtaining, recording and interpreting results needed to show that a process will consistently yield a product complying with pre-determined specifications. It encompasses the initial commissioning of processing equipment

and on-going performance qualification; which, for sterilization processes, comprises both physical and microbiological qualification.

Equipment for processing and reuse may be classified in three risk categories depending on their need for sterilization, disinfection or cleaning only. Items that enter the vascular system or sterile body cavities, such as surgical instruments and operative endoscopes, are in the high-risk category. For this category, cleaning followed by sterilization is mandatory. Items that contact intact mucous membranes, diseased or damaged skin or body fluids belong to the intermediate-risk group and require cleaning and disinfection (with sterilization as an option). Included in this category are bronchoscopes and gastro-intestinal endoscopes, vaginal speculae and clinical thermometers. In the low-risk group are items that make contact with intact skin. The group includes bedpans, urinals and eating utensils. Although cleaning is usually adequate for these items, disinfection may be indicated where an infection risk is identified or suspected. In practice, the processing of these items in efficient washer/disinfectors, as is usually recommended and performed, physically removes the bulk of the organic and microbial load by washing then disinfects by moist heat.

Developments in the field of chemical disinfection are less dramatic than those in sterilization processes. However, anti-corrosive formulations of peracetic acid have been developed commercially for application as high level disinfectants (or sterilants) for instrument reprocessing. A useful classification of disinfectants as high, medium or low level products is practised in the United States; high level disinfectants are those that can kill all types of microorganisms, including bacterial spores, under recommended conditions of concentration and time. Claims to this effect are based on the sterilization of all inoculated carriers in the AOAC sporicidal test. In Australia, a high level disinfectant claim can also be based on a demonstrated 6 $\log_{10}$ reduction in spore count in 3 to 5 hours (TGO, 1996). The principal high level disinfectants used for processing equipment such as flexible endoscopes for reuse are 2 per cent w/v activated or glycolated glutaraldehyde and peracetic acid in anti-corrosive formulations in the Steris system and as NuCidex.

REFERENCES

ANSI/AAMI ST33 — 1990 Good hospital practice: guidelines for the selection and use of reusable rigid sterilization container systems. American National Standards Institute, New York

ANSI/AAMI ST46 — 1993 Good hospital practice: steam sterilization and sterility assurance. American National Standards Institute, New York

AS 2711 1993 Washer/disinfectors for respiratory apparatus. Standards Australia, Homebush, NSW

Alder V G 1987 The formaldehyde/low temperature stream sterilizing procedure. Journal of Hospital Infection 9: 194–200

American Society for Healthcare Central Service Personnel 1986 Training manual for central service technicians. American Hospital Association, Chicago

Ayliffe G A J, Coates D, Hoffman P N 1993 Chemical disinfection in hospitals, 2nd edn. Public Health Laboratory Service, London

Babb J R, Bradley C R 1995a Endoscope decontamination: where do we go from here? Journal of Hospital Infection 30 Suppl: 543–551

Babb J, Bradley C R 1995b A review of glutaraldehyde alternatives. British Journal of Theatre Nursing 5(7): 20–24

Babb J R, Bradley C R, Barnes A R 1992 Question and answer. Journal of Hospital Infection 20: 51–54

Beischer N A 1987 How clean are your instruments? Australian and New Zealand Journal of Obstetrics and Gynaecology 27: 226–227

Birnie G G, Quigley E M, Clements G B, Follet E A C, Watkinson G 1983 Endoscopic transmission of hepatitis B virus. Gut 24: 171–174

Bowie J H, Campbell I D, Gillingham F J, Gordon A R 1963 Hospital sterile supplies: Edinburgh pre-set tray system. British Medical Journal 2: 1322–1327

Bradley C R, Babb J R 1995 Endoscope decontamination: automated vs. manual. Journal of Hospital Infection 30 Suppl: 537–542

Cadwallader H L, Bradley C R, Ayliffe G A J 1990 Bacterial contamination and frequency of changing ventilator circuitry. Journal of Hospital Infection 15: 65–72

Caporino P P 1989 Decontamination safety training for the CS technician. Journal of Healthcare Materiel Management 7(6): 40, 42, 44

Casemore D P, Blewett D A, Wright S E 1989 Cleaning and disinfection of equipment for gastrointestinal flexible endoscopy: interim recommendations of a Working Party of the British Society of Gastroenterology. Gut 30: 1156

Challacombe S J, Fernandes L L 1995 Detecting Legionella pneumophila in water systems: a comparison of various dental units. Journal of the American Dental Association 126: 603–608

Classen D C, Jacobson J A, Burke J P, Jacobson J T, Evans R S 1988 Serious Pseudomonas infections associated with endoscopic retrograde cholangiopancreatography. American Journal of Medicine 84: 590–596

Collignon P, Graham E 1989 How well are endoscopes cleaned and disinfected between patients? Medical Journal of Australia 151: 269–272

Cooke R P D, Feneley R C L, Ayliffe G, Lawrence W T, Emmerson A M, Greengrass S M 1993 Decontamination of urological equipment: interim report of a working group of the Standing Committee on Urological Instruments of the British Association of Urological Surgeons. British Journal of Urology 71: 5–9

Cottone J A, Molinari J A 1987 Selection for dental practice of chemical disinfectants and sterilants for hepatitis and AIDS. Australian Dental Journal 32: 368–374

Council on Dental Materials, Instruments, and Equipment 1992 Infection control recommendations for the dental office and the dental laboratory. Journal of the American Dental Association 123(8) Suppl: 1–8

Cowan R E, Manning A P, Ayliffe G A J et al 1993 Aldehyde disinfectants and health in endoscopy units. The report of the working party of the British Society of Gastroenterology Endoscopy Committee. Gut 34: 1641–1645

Daschner F D 1992 Nosocomial infection and pseudoinfection from contaminated endoscopes could have been avoided. Infection Control and Hospital Epidemiology 13: 254

DuMont P S 1987 Improving inservice effectiveness. Journal of Healthcare Materiel Management 5(5): 36–38, 40–41

Field E A, Field J K, Martin M V 1988 Time, steam, temperature (TST) control indicators to measure essential sterilisation criteria for autoclaves in general dental practice and the community dental service. British Dental Journal 164: 183–186

Fluke C 1988a Kits & trays: a perspective for employees. Journal of Healthcare Materiel Management 6(5): 102–104

Fluke C 1988b Exchange carts. What and why. Journal of Healthcare Materiel Management 6(3): 95–97

Fluke C 1989 CSR wrapping and packaging. Journal of Healthcare Materiel Management 7(6): 77–80

Forrester N, Douglas C W I 1988 Use of the 'Safe air' dental heater for sterilising endodontic reamers. British Dental Journal 165: 290–292

Fraise A P 1995 Disinfection in endoscopy. Lancet 346: 787–788

Geiss H K 1995 Reprocessing of anaesthetic and ventilatory equipment. Journal of Hospital Infection 30 Suppl: 414–420

Goularte T A, Manning M, Craven D E 1987 Bacterial colonization in humidifying cascade reservoirs after 24 and 48 hours of continuous mechanical ventilation. Infection Control 8: 200–203

Gschwandtner G 1990 Aeration of respiratory therapy items — are you really aerating? Journal of Healthcare Materiel Management 8(2): 48–49, 51

Hanson P J V, Chadwick M V, Gaya H, Collins J V 1992 A study of glutaraldehyde disinfection of fibreoptic bronchoscopes experimentally contaminated with Mycobacterium tuberculosis. Journal of Hospital Infection 22: 137–142

Hanson P J V, Jeffries D J, Batten J C, Collins J V 1988 Infection control revisited: dilemma facing today's bronchoscopists. British Medical Journal 297: 185–187

Hanson P J V, Gor D, Clarke J R et al 1989 Contamination of endoscopes used in AIDS patients. Lancet ii: 86–88

Harrison S K, Evans W J Jr, LeBlanc D A, Bush L W 1990 Cleaning and decontaminating medical instruments. Journal of Healthcare Materiel Management 8(1): 36–42

HBN 13 1992 Health Building Note 13 Sterile services department. NHS Estates, London

HTM 1994 Health Technical Memorandum 2010 Part 3: Validation and verification. Sterilization. NHS Estates, London

Inglis T J J 1995 New insights into the pathogenesis of ventilator-associated pneumonia. Journal of Hospital Infection 30 Suppl: 409–413

Institute of Sterile Services Management 1990 Teaching and training manual for sterile services personnel. ISSM, Manchester

Jevitt D 1984 Indefinite shelf life . . Amen! Journal of Healthcare Materiel Management 2(6): 36–37

Jones M L, Newcombe R G, Barry G, Bellis H, Bottomley J 1988 A reflex plotter investigation into the dimensional stability of alginate impressions following disinfection by varying regimes employing 2.2 per cent glutaraldehyde. British Journal of Orthodontics 15: 185–192

van Klingeren B, Pullen W 1993 Glutaraldehyde resistant mycobacteria from endoscope washers. Journal of Hospital Infection 25: 147–149

Kneedler J A, Gattas M 1988 A study of sterilization containers. Journal of Healthcare Materiel Management 6(4): 24–28, 30

Lichtenberg D 1988 Infection control in respiratory therapy. Journal of Healthcare Materiel Management 6(6): 42, 44, 46, 48, 50

Logothetis D D, Martinez-Welles J M 1995 Reducing bacterial aerosol contamination with a chlorhexidine gluconate pre-rinse. Journal of the American Dental Association 126: 1634–1639

Mayworm D 1984 Sterile shelf life and expiration dating. Journal of Hospital Supply, Processing and Distribution 2(6): 32–35

Miller C H, Palenik C J 1991 Sterilization, disinfection, and asepsis in dentistry. In: Block S S (ed) Disinfection, sterilization, and preservation, 4th edn. Lea & Febiger, Philadelphia, ch 39, p 676

Minagi S, Yano N, Yoshida K, Tsuru H 1987 Prevention of acquired immunodeficiency syndrome and hepatitis B. II: Disinfection method for hydrophilic impression materials. Journal of Prosthetic Dentistry 58: 462–465

Mulick J F 1986 Upgrading sterilization in the orthodontic practice. American Journal of Orthodontics 89: 346–351

Patterson C J W, McLundie A C, Mackay A M 1988 The effect of ultrasonic cleansing and autoclaving on tungsten carbide burs. British Dental Journal 164: 113–115

Reichert M 1988 Another look at reuse. Journal of Healthcare Materiel Management 6(1): 24–28, 30–32

Roberts W G, Green P H R, Ma J, Carr M, Ginsberg A M 1989 Prevalence of cryptosporidiosis in patients undergoing endoscopy: evidence for an asymptomatic carrier state. American Journal of Medicine 87: 537–539

Scott S B R 1988 Health building note No. 13. Sterilising and disinfecting unit. Journal of the Institute of Sterile Services Management 1(2): 10–15

Shovelton D S, Plant C G, Burdon D W, Brown R M 1984 The sterilisation of dental handpieces: an account of a trial. British Dental Journal 157: 325–327

Spach D H, Silverstein F E, Stamm W E 1993 Transmission of infection by gastrointestinal endoscopy and bronchoscopy. Annals of Internal Medicine 118: 117–128

Standard P G, Mallison G F, Mackel D C 1973 Microbial penetration through three types of double wrappers for sterile packs. Applied Microbiology 26: 59–62

TGO 1996 Therapeutic Goods Order No. 54 Standard for composition, packaging, labelling and performance of disinfectants and sterilants. Therapeutic Goods Administration, Canberra

Tullner J B, Commette J A, Moon P C 1988 Linear dimensional changes in dental impressions after immersion in disinfectant solutions. Journal of Prosthetic Dentistry 60: 725–728

Wheeler P W, Lancaster D, Kaiser A B 1989 Bronchopulmonary cross-colonization and infection related to mycobacterial contamination of suction valves of bronchoscopes. Journal of Infectious Diseases 159: 954–958

Williams H N, Baer M L, Kelley J I 1995 Contribution of biofilm bacteria to the contamination of the dental unit water supply. Journal of the American Dental Association 126: 1255–1260

Williams H N, Falkler W A, Hasler J F, Romberg E 1986 Persistence of contaminant bacteria in dental laboratory pumice. Quintessence of Dental Technology 10(6): 385–388

Woodcock A, Campbell I, Collins J V C et al 1989 Bronchoscopy and infection control. Lancet ii: 270–271

Index

TO THE OWNER OF THIS BOOK

We are interested in your reaction to *Sterilization, disinfection and infection control 3/e,* by Joan Gardner and Margaret Peel.

1. What was your reason for using this book?

    ____ university course ____ continuing education course
    ____ college course ____ personal interest
    ____ TAFE course ____ other (specify)

2. In which school are you enrolled? _____

3. Approximately how much of the book did you use?
    ____ 1/4 ____ 1/2 ____ 3/4 ____ all

4. What is the best aspect of the book?

5. Have you any suggestions for improvement?

6. Would more diagrams / illustrations help?

7. Is there any topic that should be added?

Fold here

(Tape Shut)

No postage stamp required
if posted in Australia

|||

REPLY PAID 5
Acquisitions Editor, College Division
Harcourt Brace & Company, Australia
Locked Bag 16
MARRICKVILLE, NSW 2204